D1340007

Antihypertensives

ACE inhibitors	fetal renal failure, teratogenic (3% risk)	Avoid	methyldopa	captopril safe
Methyldopa	nil known	nifedipine, Best 1st line	N/A	safe
β-Blockers	possible IUGR if early	Caution, 3rd line	methyldopa	safe
Ca antagonists	nil known	Best 2nd line (eg nifedipine)	N/A	safe
Thiazide diuretics	maternal hypovolaemia, Fetal thrombocytopenia	Avoid	methyldopa	safe

Fundamentals: Severe hypertension in pregnancy is common and life threatening and requires treatment. Avoid ACE inhibitors prenatally

Endocrine/ Hormone treatments

Thyroid hormone	(replacement therapy)	Use if indicated	N/A	safe
Propylthiouracil	fetal hypothyroidism (rare)	Use, minimum dose	N/A	monitor
Carbimazole	fetal hypothyroidism (rare), aplasia cutis	Use, minimum dose	Propylthiouracil	monitor
Insulin	(replacement therapy)	Use with usual precautions	N/A	safe
Metformin	maternal hypoglycaemia, probably safe, little data	Caution	Insulin	safe

Fundamentals: Treatment of underlying disease greatly reduces maternal and fetal risks.

Immunosuppresants

Ciclosporin	nil known	Continue, monitor levels	N/A	probably s...
Azothioprine	minimal	Continue if indicated	N/A	safe
Prednisolone	no fetal effects	Use minimum dose	N/A	safe
	maternal gestational diabetes, hypertension			

Fundamentals: Treatment of underlying disease (eg transplant) imperative and reduces maternal and therefore fetal risks.

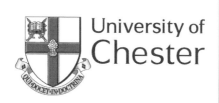

University of
Chester

LIS Library

Chester 01244 511234
Warrington 01925 534284
lis.helpdesk@chester.ac.uk

OXFORD MEDICAL PUBLICATIONS

Oxford Handbook of
Obstetrics and Gynaecology

Published and forthcoming Oxford Handbooks

Oxford Handbook of
Obstetrics and Gynaecology

SECOND EDITION

Sally Collins

Specialist Registrar in Obstetrics and Gynaecology,
The John Radcliffe Hospital,
Oxford, UK

Sabaratnam Arulkumaran

Professor of Obstetrics and Gynaecology,
St George's Hospital Medical School,
University of London, UK

Kevin Hayes

Senior Lecturer/Honorary Consultant in Obstetrics
and Gynaecology, and Medical Education,
St George's Hospital and Medical School,
University of London, UK

Simon Jackson

Consultant Gynaecologist,
The John Radcliffe Hospital,
Oxford, UK

Lawrence Impey

Consultant in Obstetrics and Fetal Medicine,
The John Radcliffe Hospital,
Oxford, UK

OXFORD
UNIVERSITY PRESS

OXFORD

UNIVERSITY PRESS

Great Clarendon Street, Oxford OX2 6DP

Oxford University Press is a department of the University of Oxford.
It furthers the University's objective of excellence in research, scholarship,
and education by publishing worldwide in

Oxford New York

Auckland Cape Town Dar es Salaam Hong Kong Karachi
Kuala Lumpur Madrid Melbourne Mexico City Nairobi
New Delhi Shanghai Taipei Toronto

With offices in

Argentina Austria Brazil Chile Czech Republic France Greece
Guatemala Hungary Italy Japan Poland Portugal Singapore
South Korea Switzerland Thailand Turkey Ukraine Vietnam

Oxford is a registered trade mark of Oxford University Press
in the UK and in certain other countries

Published in the United States
by Oxford University Press Inc., New York

© Oxford University Press, 2008

The moral rights of the author have been asserted
Database right Oxford University Press (maker)

First edition published 2005;
Second edition published 2008;
Reprinted 2009, with corrections
Reprinted 2010

British Library Cataloguing in Publication Data
Data available

Library of Congress Cataloguing in Publication Data
Data available

Typeset by Cepha Imaging Private Ltd., Bangalore, India
Printed in China
on acid-free paper through
Asia Pacific Offset

ISBN 978-0-19-922724-2

10 9 8 7 6 5 4 3

Contents

Preface

Welcome to the completely re-written, second edition of this Oxford Handbook. In Obstetrics and Gynaecology, as in all fields of medicine, the available evidence, technology and guidelines move forward at a rapid pace and can often prove difficult to keep up with. As the majority of junior doctors are well aware, the gaps in our knowledge often become apparent at the most inopportune moments; this book seeks to fill those gaps rapidly and effectively. It uses the well-known Oxford Handbook format to facilitate easy navigation around concise, clinically relevant, evidence-based information. It can be quickly dipped into for specific answers between seeing patients in clinic or on delivery suite, as well as providing a solid, general grounding for those just beginning in the specialty. It also has sufficient depth and detail to provide a good starting point in the preparation for postgraduate exams. To ensure the most up-to-date information is always available, emphasis has been placed on providing relevant web addresses, especially for guidelines and useful organisations. Text boxes have also been employed to help highlight some of the more important pieces of information.

Although this handbook is most likely to be used by trainees within the specialty, we envisage it will be useful for all those involved in women's health, including GPs, midwives and medical students. We hope you find it a helpful resource and that it proves to be a valuable companion and guide in your everyday practice of obstetrics and gynaecology.

Acknowledgements

It is always difficult to try to improve on a popular textbook and we owe a huge debt of gratitude to the editors and authors of the first edition. We would also like to thank all our second edition authors, especially the trainees at the John Radcliffe and St George's hospitals. Additionally, we are very grateful to the doctors of all grades who anonymously reviewed the text for us and provided valuable feedback, further fine-tuning the finished manuscript. To conform to the Oxford Handbook style and to avoid overlap and repetition, some contributions have been considerably edited and we thank all our authors for their understanding. We are most grateful to Mr Basky Thilaganathan for providing many of the ultrasound images. Thank you also to Sue Cunningham at St George's and Tracey Shepherd at the John Radcliffe, for the invaluable secretarial support which they have so generously provided. We cannot fail to mention the marvellous team at OUP including Kate Wilson and Susan Crowhurst, but especially Mark Knowles, whose endless patience, expert guidance and great sense of humour have kept this book on track. Last, but definitely not least, we would like to thank our partners and families who have remained so patient and supportive throughout this project, especially Berni O'Connor and David Reynard.

Sally Collins, Sabaratnam Arulkumaran, Kevin Hayes, Simon Jackson and Lawrence Impey
London and Oxford, January 2008

Abbreviations

ABG	arterial blood gases
AC	abdominal circumference
AFE	amniotic fluid embolism
AIS	androgen insensitivity syndrome
APH	antepartum haemorrhage
APTT	activated partial thromboplastin time
ARDS	adult respiratory distress syndrome
ARM	artificial rupture of membranes
ART	assisted reproductive technologies
AVM	arteriovenous malformations
bd	twice daily
BM	blood sugar monitoring
BMD	bone mineral density
BMI	body mass index
BP	blood pressure
BPD	biparietal diameter
BV	bacterial vaginosis
CAH	congenital adrenal hyperplasia
CBT	cognitive-behavioural therapy
CCT	controlled cord traction
CHD	congenital heart disease
CHD	coronary heart disease
CIN	cervical intraepithelial neoplasia
CMV	cytomegalovirus
CP	cerebral palsy
CPP	chronic pelvic pain
CRL	crown–rump length
CS	Caesarean section
CSE	combined spinal epidural
CTG	cardiotocography
CVA	cerebrovascular accident
CVD	cardiovascular disease
CVP	central venous pressure
CVS	chorionic villus sampling
CXR	chest radiograph
DIC	disseminated intravascular coagulation

DSD	disorders of sex development
DUB	dysfunctional uterine bleeding
DVT	deep vein thrombosis
ECG	electrocardiograph
ECV	external cephalic version
EDD	expected date of delivery
EPAU	early pregnancy assessment unit
ETT	endotracheal tube
ERPC	evacuation of retained products of conception
ESR	erythrocyte sedimentation rate
FBC	full blood count
FDPs	fibrin degradation products
FFN	fetal fibronectin
FFP	fresh frozen plasma
FHR	fetal heart rate
FISH	fluorescent in situ hybridization
FL	femur length
FSD	female sexual dysfunction
FSE	fetal scalp electrode
FSH	follicle stimulating hormone
FVS	fetal varicella syndrome
GA	general anaesthesia
GBS	group B streptococcus
GDM	gestational diabetes
GFR	glomerular filtration rate
GnRH	gonadotrophin releasing hormone
GTD	gestational trophoblastic disease
GUM	genitourinary medicine
HAART	highly active antiretroviral therapy
HBV	hepatitis B virus
HC	head circumference
hCG	human chorionic gonadotrophin
HCT	haematocrit
HDU	high dependency unit
HFEA	Human Fertilisation and Embryology Authority
HPV	human papillomavirus
HSG	hysterosalpingography
HSV	herpes simplex virus
HyCoSy	hysterosalpingo-contrast-sonography
IBD	inflammatory bowel disease

ICSI	intracytoplasmic sperm injection
ICU	intensive care unit
IMB	intermenstrual bleeding
IOL	induction of labour
ITP	idiopathic thrombocytopaenic purpura
IUCD	intrauterine contraceptive device
IUD	intrauterine death (of the fetus)
IUGR	intrauterine growth restriction
IV	intravenous
IVF	in vitro fertilization
JVP	Jugular venous pressure
LAVH	laparoscopic assisted vaginal hysterectomy
LDH	lactate dehydrogenase
LFTs	liver function tests
LH	luteinizing hormone
LLETZ	large loop excision of the transformation zone
LMP	last menstrual period
LMWH	low molecular weight heparin
LVS	low vaginal swab
MA	mentoanterior
MAS	meconium aspiration syndrome
MI	myocardial infarction
MMP	matrix metalloproteinase
MMR	maternal mortality ratio
MP	mentoposterior
MSAF	meconium-stained amniotic fluid
MSU	midstream urine (sample)
MTCT	mother-to-child transmission
NBM	nil by mouth
od	once daily
OHSS	ovarian hyperstimulation syndrome
PCA	patient-controlled analgesia
PCB	postcoital bleeding
PCOS	polycystic ovary syndrome
PDA	patent ductus arteriosus
PE	pulmonary embolism
PEP	postexposure prophylaxis
PEFR	peak expiratory flow rate
PGD	pre-implantation genetic diagnosis
PID	pelvic inflammatory disease

PIGF	placental growth factor
PMB	postmenopausal bleeding
PO	Per oral (by mouth)
POF	premature ovarian failure
PPH	postpartum haemorrhage
PPROM	preterm prelabour rupture of membranes
PROM	prelabour rupture of membranes
PV	per vaginam
Q	ventilation
qds	four times daily
RCT	randomized controlled trials
ROM	rupture of the membranes
SAH	subarachnoid haemorrhage
SCBU	special care baby unit
SFH	symphysis fundal height
SIDS	sudden infant death syndrome
SOL	space-occupying lesion
SPD	symphysis pubis dysfunction
SROM	spontaneous rupture of membranes
STI	sexually transmitted infection
$t_{1/2}$	half-life
T_3	triiodothryonine
T_4	thyroxine
TAH & BSO	total abdominal hysterectomy with bilateral salpingo-oopherectomy
TBG	thyroid-binding globulin
tds	three times daily
TIBC	total iron binding capacity
TFTs	thyroid function tests
TOP	termination of pregnancy
TTP	thrombotic thrombocytopaenic purpura
U+Es	urea and electrolytes
UC	ulcerative colitis
UFH	unfractionated heparin
UPSI	unprotected sexual intercourse
USS	ultrasound scan
UTI	urinary tract infections
V/Q scan	ventilation/perfusion
VBAC	vaginal birth after Caesarean
VE	vaginal examination

VEGF	vascular endothelial growth factor
VIN	vulval intraepithelial neoplasia
VSD	ventricular septal defects
VTE	venous thromboembolism
VZV	varicella zoster virus

Contributors

Editors

Miss Sally Collins
Specialist Registrar rotation,
Oxford Deanery

Professor Sabaratnam Arulkumaran
St George's Hospital Medical
School, London

Mr Kevin Hayes
St George's Hospital Medical
School, London

Mr Simon Jackson
John Radcliffe Hospital, Oxford

Mr Lawrence Impey
John Radcliffe Hospital, Oxford

Contributors

Dr Christian Becker
Nuffield Department of
Obstetrics and Gynaecology,
John Radcliffe Hospital, Oxford

Mrs Rebecca Black
John Radcliffe Hospital, Oxford

Dr Shabana Bora
Department of Early Pregnancy
and Gynaecological Ultrasound,
St George's Healthcare NHS Trust,
Tooting, London

Dr Brian Brady
John Radcliffe Hospital, Oxford

Mr Paul Bulmer
St George's Hospital, Tooting,
London

Mr Edwin Chandraharan
Delivery Suite, St George's
Healthcare NHS Trust, Tooting,
London

Dr Noan-Minh Chau
Specialist Registrar rotation
in Medical Oncology, London
Deanery

Dr Mellisa Damodaram
Queen Charlotte's and Chelsea
Hospital, London

Miss Claudine Domoney
Chelsea and Westminster
Hospital, London

Dr Stergios K. Doumouchtsis
Department of Obstetrics and
Gynaecology, St George's Hospital,
Tooting, London

Dr Cleave W. J. Gass
Department of Anaesthesia,
St George's Hospital, Tooting,
London

Dr Ingrid Granne
John Radcliffe Hospital, Oxford

Miss Catherine Greenwood
John Radcliffe Hospital, Oxford

Mr Manish Gupta
John Radcliffe Hospital, Oxford

Miss Pauline Hurley
John Radcliffe Hospital, Oxford

Dr Nia Jones
Queens Medical Centre, Nottingham

Miss Brenda Kelly
Nuffield Department of
Obstetrics and Gynaecology,
John Radcliffe Hospital, Oxford

Dr Nigel Kennea
St George's Hospital, Tooting,
London

Dr Andy Kent
St George's Hospital, Tooting,
London

Dr Su-Yen Khong
Women's Centre, John Radcliffe
Hospital, Oxford

Dr Emma Kirk
Acute Gynaecology Unit,
St George's Healthcare NHS Trust,
Tooting, London

Dr Samatha Low
Royal Berkshire Hospital, Reading

Dr Jo Morrison
Nuffield Department of
Obstetrics and Gynaecology,
University of Oxford

**Dr Neelanjana
Mukhopadhaya**
St George's Hospital, Tooting,
London

Dr Faizah Mukri
Specialist Registrar rotation,
London Deanery

Dr Santosh Pattnayak
Neonatal Unit, St George's
Hospital, Tooting, London

Dr Natalia Price
Women's Centre, John Radcliffe
Hospital, Oxford

Dr Aysha Qureshi
John Radcliffe Hospital, Oxford

Dr Devanna Rajeswari
St George's Hospital, Tooting,
London

Dr Gowri Ramanathan
St George's Hospital, Tooting,
London

Dr Margaret Rees
Women's Centre, John Radcliffe
Hospital, Oxford

Dr Lisa Story
John Radcliffe Hospital, Oxford

Ms Louise Strawbridge
University College London

Dr Alex Swanton
Specialist Registrar rotation,
Oxford Deanery

Dr Linda Tan
Acute Gynaecology Unit,
St George's Healthcare NHS Trust,
Tooting, London

Dr Katy Vincent
John Radcliffe Hospital, Oxford

Dr Niraj Yanamandra
Department of Obstetrics and
Gynaecology, St Peter's Hospital,
Chertsey

Normal pregnancy

Obstetric history: current pregnancy

Obstetric history taking has many features in common with most other sections of medicine, along with certain areas specific to the specialty. The basic framework can be easily learned; however, competence requires good clinical knowledge and a lot of practice. As obstetrics often requires intimate examination and discussion of sensitive information, it is important to ensure privacy and to demonstrate respect and confidentiality.

A carefully obtained history taken in a logical sequence avoids inadvertent omission of important details, and guides the examination to follow.

Current pregnancy

Much of this information will be contained in the patients 'hand-held' notes.
- Name.
- Age.
- Occupation.
- Relationship status.
- Gravidity (i.e. number of pregnancies including the current one).
- Parity (i.e. number of births beyond 24 weeks gestation).

The expected date of delivery (EDD) can be calculated from the last menstrual period (LMP) using Naegele's rule (add 1 year and 7 days to the LMP and subtract 3 months) most often done with an obstetric calendar ('wheel'). Enquire details that may affect the validity of the patient's EDD as calculated from her LMP including:
- Long cycles.
- Irregular periods.
- Recent use of the combined oral contraceptive pill (COCP).

▶ Dating scans between 8 and 13 weeks are more reliable than LMP and should be used to provide an EDD where possible.

Enquire about the current pregnancy, including:
- General health (tiredness, malaise, and other non-specific symptoms).
- If >20 weeks, enquire about fetal movements.
- General details of pregnancy to date (previous admissions and current problems).
- Results of all antenatal blood tests—routine and specific.
- Results of anomaly and other scans (details of results can be cross-checked with the notes).
- If she is postnatal:
  - labour and delivery
  - history of the postnatal period.

An obstetric history should include:

- Current pregnancy details.
- Past obstetric history.
- Past gynaecological history.
- Past medical and surgical history.
- Drug history and allergies.
- Family history—especially multiple pregnancy, diabetes, hypertension, chromosome or congenital malformations.
- Social history.

Gravidity and parity explained

The terminology used is gravida x, para $a+b$:
- x is the total number of pregnancies (including this one).
- a is the number of births beyond 24 weeks gestation.
- b is the number of miscarriages or termination of pregnancies before 24 weeks gestation.

Example

A woman who is pregnant for the 4th time with 1 normal delivery at term, 1 termination at 9 weeks and 1 miscarriage at 16 weeks would be gravida 4, para 1 + 2.

Obstetric history: other relevant features

> **Past obstetric history includes:**
> - Details of all previous pregnancies (including miscarriages and terminations).
> - Length of gestation.
> - Date and place of delivery.
> - Onset of labour (including details of induction of labour).
> - Mode of delivery.
> - Sex and birth weight.
> - Fetal and neonatal life.
> - Clear details of any complications or adverse outcomes (such as shoulder dystocia, postpartum haemorrhage, or stillbirth).

▶ History often repeats itself, so previous antenatal, intrapartum, or postpartum complications should influence the management of this pregnancy.

Past gynaecological/medical/surgical history
- Method of contraception before conception.
- Previous gynaecological procedures.
- Cervical smear history.
- Medical conditions such as hypertension, epilepsy, or diabetes.
- Details of any consultations with other physicians (neurologist or endocrinologist).
- Involvement of multidisciplinary teams.
- Details of any previous surgery.

Drug and allergy history
- Current medications
- Medications taken at any time during the pregnancy
- Any allergies and their severity (anaphylaxis or a rash?).

Family history
Any history of hereditary illnesses or congenital defects is important and is required to ensure adequate counselling and screening is offered.
- Familial disorders such as thrombophilias,
- Previously affected pregnancies with any chromosomal or genetic disorders,
- Consanguinity,

Social history
- Smoking.
- History of drug or alcohol abuse.
- Plans for breastfeeding.
- Social aspects such as plans for childcare arrangements.
- Domestic violence screening.

Obstetric physical examination

At the initial visit, a complete physical examination should be undertaken.

Abdominal examination—inspection

- Note the apparent size of the abdominal distension.
- Note any asymmetry.
- Fetal movements.
- Cutaneous signs of pregnancy:
  - linea nigra (dark pigmented line stretching from the xiphi sternum through the umbilicus to the suprapubic area)
  - striae gravidarum (recent stretch marks are purplish in colour)
  - striae albicans (old stretch marks are silvery-white)
  - flattening/eversion of umbilicus (due to ↑intra-abdominal pressure).
- Superficial veins (alternate paths of venous drainage due to pressure on the inferior vena cava by a gravid uterus).
- Surgical scars (a low Pfannenstiel incision may be obscured by pubic hair, and laparoscopy scars hidden within the umbilicus).

Abdominal examination—palpation

- Symphysis–fundal height (SFH):
  - palpated <20 weeks
  - measured in cm >20 weeks.
- Estimation of number of fetuses:
  - ?multiple fetal poles.
- Fetal lie (relationship of longitudinal axis of fetus to that of the uterus):
  - longitudinal—fetal head or breech palpable over pelvic inlet
  - oblique—the head or breech is palpable in the iliac fossa
  - transverse—fetal poles felt in flanks
- Presentation (part of the fetus overlying the pelvic brim):
  - cephalic
  - breech
  - other (shoulder, compound)
- Amniotic fluid volume:
  - ↑ tense abdomen with fetal parts not easily palpated
  - ↓ compact abdomen with fetal parts easily palpable.

Auscultation of the fetal heart

The fetal heart is best heard at the anterior shoulder of the fetus using:
- A Doppler ultrasound device (Sonicaid) from about 12 weeks gestation.
- A fetal stethoscope (Pinard) from about 24 weeks gestation
- In a breech presentation it is often heard at, or above, the level of the maternal umbilicus.
- The rate and the rhythm of the fetal heart should be determined over 1 minute.

Vaginal examination

A vaginal examination (speculum or digital examination) is not part of a routine obstetric examination but may be indicated to diagnose rupture of membranes or onset of labour.

General examination

- Body mass index (BMI) calculated [weight (kg)/height (m)^2].
- ⚠ Pregnancy complications are increased with a BMI <18.5 and >25.
- Blood pressure measured in the semi-recumbent position (45° tilt)
- ⚠ Use an appropriate size cuff: too small a cuff gives a falsely high BP.
- Auscultation of the heart and lungs:
  - flow murmurs are common in pregnancy and are not significant
  - cardiac murmurs may be detected for the first time in pregnancy.
- Thyroid gland (exclude a goitre).
- Breasts (exclude any lumps).
- Varicose veins and skeletal abnormalities (kyphosis or scoliosis):
  - normal pregnancy is associated with an increase in lumbar lordosis which can lead to lower backache.

Normal uterine size

- The uterus normally becomes palpable at 12 weeks gestation.
- It reaches the level of the umbilicus at 20 weeks gestation.
- It is at the xiphi sternum at 36 weeks gestation.

Symphysis–fundal height

▶The SFH detects approximately 40–60% of small-for-gestational age fetuses but its predictive value in detecting large-for-dates fetuses is considerably less.

The uterine size is objectively measured with a tape measure from the highest point of the fundus to the upper margin of the symphysis pubis (see Fig. 1.1).

Appropriate growth is usually estimated to be the number of weeks gestation in centimetres (at 30 weeks the SFH should be 30 cm ± 2 cm):

- ± 2 cm from 20 until 36 weeks gestation.
- ± 3 cm between 36 and 40 weeks.
- ± 4 cm at 40 weeks.

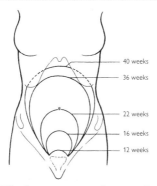

Fig. 1.1 Typical fundal heights at various stages of pregnancy. Reproduced from Wyatt JP, Illingworth RN, Graham CA *et al.* (eds) *Oxford handbook of emergency medicine*, OUP, 2006. By permission of Oxford University Press.

Engagement of the fetal head

Conventionally, engagement or the passage of the maximal diameter of the presenting part beyond the pelvic inlet, is estimated using the palm width of the five fingers of the hand (Fig. 1.2). If five fingers are needed to cover the head above the pelvic brim, it is five-fifths palpable, and if no head is palpable, it is zero-fifths palpable.

- Normally, the fetus engages in an attitude of flexion in the transverse diameter of the pelvic inlet, unless the pelvis is very roomy where it may engage in any diameter. See Fig. 1.3.
- In nulliparous women, engagement usually occurs by 37 weeks but in multiparous women it may not occur until the onset of labour.
- Rare causes of non-engagement should always be considered and investigated with an ultrasound scan (USS) (including placenta praevia and fetal abnormality)
- In women of Afro-Caribbean origin, engagement may only occur at the onset or during the course of labour, even in nulliparous women.

Paulik's grip

This is a one-handed technique that uses a cupped right hand to grasp and assess the lower pole of the uterus (usually the fetal head).

▶ This can be very uncomfortable and is not necessary if the head can be palpated using two hands.

Engagement
- A head that is only two-fifths palpable is usually considered to be engaged (and therefore fixed in the pelvis). See Fig. 1.2.
- Put simply: an easily palpable head is not engaged, whereas a head more difficult to palpate is more likely to be deeply engaged.

⚠ Care must be taken, as a breech presentation can sometimes be mistaken for a deeply engaged head.

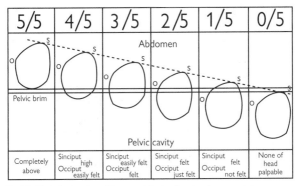

5/5	4/5	3/5	2/5	1/5	0/5
Completely above	Sinciput high Occiput easily felt	Sinciput easily felt Occiput felt	Sinciput felt Occiput just felt	Sinciput felt Occiput not felt	None of head palpable

Fig. 1.2 Clinical estimation of descent of the fetal head and engagement. Reproduced from Arulkumaran S, Symonds IM, Fowlie A. *Oxford handbook of obstetrics and gynaecology*, OUP, 2004. By permission of Oxford University Press.

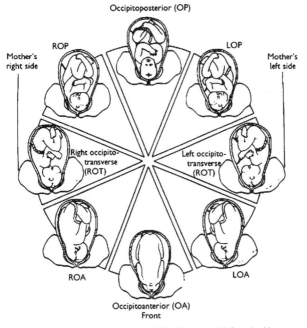

Fig. 1.3 Fetal position. Reproduced from Collier J, Longmore M, Brinsden M. *Oxford handbook of clinical specialties*, 7th edn, OUP, 2006. By permission of Oxford University Press.

The female pelvis

The bony ring of the pelvis is made up of two symmetrical innominate bones and the sacrum. Each innominate bone is made up of the ilium, ischium and the pubis, which are joined anteriorly at the symphysis pubis and posteriorly to the sacrum at the sacroiliac joints.

The female pelvis has evolved for giving birth, and differs from the male pelvis in the following ways:

- The female pelvis is broader, and the bones more slender than those of the male.
- The male pelvic brim is heart shaped and is widest towards the back, whereas the female pelvic brim is oval shaped transversely and is widest further forwards because the sacral promontory is less prominent.
- The female pelvic cavity is more roomy and has a wider outlet than the male pelvis.
- The subpubic angle is rounded in a female pelvis (like a Roman arch) and more acute in the male pelvis (like a Gothic arch).

Pelvic muscles and ligaments

The pelvis gains its strength and stability through numerous muscles and ligaments. The inner aspect of the pelvic bones is covered by muscles. Above the pelvic brim are the iliacus and psoas muscles; the obturator internus and its fascia occupies the side walls; the posterior wall is covered by the pyriformis; and the levator ani and coccygeus with their opposite counterparts constitute the pelvic floor.

Pelvic ring stability is provided by the following ligaments:

- **Sacrospinous ligament:** extending from the lateral margin of the sacrum and coccyx to the ischial spine.
- **Sacrotuberous ligament:** extending from the sacrum to the ischial tuberosity.
- **Iliolumbar ligament:** extending from the spine to the iliac crest at the back of the pelvis.
- **Dorsal sacroiliac ligament:** a heavy band passing from the ilium to the sacrum posterior to the sacroiliac joint.
- **Ventral sacroiliac ligament:** bridging the sacroiliac joint anteriorly, and is an important stabilizing structure of the joint.
- **Inferior and superior pubic ligament:** a band across the lower and upper part of the symphysis respectively, providing further strength to the joint.
- **Inguinal ligament:** running from the anterior superior iliac spine of the ilium to the pubic tubercle of the pubic bone.

The remaining ligaments that surround the pelvis are ligaments that do not provide stabilization of the pelvis.

Pelvic boundaries

The pelvis is divided by an oblique plane passing through the prominence of the sacrum, the arcuate and pectineal lines, and the upper margin of the symphysis pubis, into the greater and the lesser pelvis. The circumference of this plane is termed the pelvic brim. This pelvic brim separates the false pelvis above from the true pelvis below. The plane of the pelvis is at an angle of 55° to the horizontal.

Pelvic shapes

There are four basic shapes of the female pelvis, as illustrated in Fig. 1.4.
- **Gynaecoid:** the classical female pelvis with the inlet transversely oval and a roomier pelvic cavity.
- **Anthropoid:** a long, narrow and oval shaped pelvis due to the assimilation of the sacral body to the fifth lumbar vertebra.
- **Android:** the inlet is heart shaped and the cavity is funnel shaped with a contracted outlet.
- **Platypolloid:** a wide pelvis flattened at the brim with the sacral promontory pushed forward.

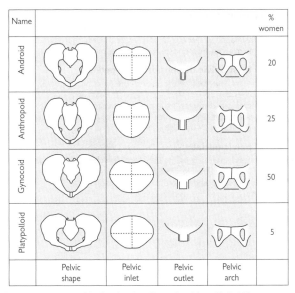

Name	Pelvic shape	Pelvic inlet	Pelvic outlet	Pelvic arch	% women
Android					20
Anthropoid					25
Gynocoid					50
Platypolloid					5

Fig. 1.4 Basic shapes of the female pelvis. (Reproduced from Abitbol M, Chervenak F, Ledger WJ, *Birth and human evolution: anatomical and obstetrical mechanics in primates*, Bergin & Garvey 1996).

Diameters of the female pelvis

The female bony pelvis is not distensible, and only very minor degrees of movement are possible at the symphysis pubis and the sacroiliac joints. Its dimensions are hence critical for normal childbirth.

▶ The diameters of the female pelvis vary at different parts of the pelvis.
- The true pelvis is bound anteriorly by the symphysis pubis (3.5 cm long) and posteriorly by the sacrum (12 cm long).
- The superior circumference of the true pelvis is the pelvic inlet and the inferior circumference is the outlet (Fig. 1.5).

The true pelvis has four planes:

Plane of pelvic inlet
- This is bound anteriorly by the upper border of the pubis, laterally by the iliopectineal line, and posteriorly by the sacral promontory.
- The average transverse diameter is ~13.5 cm and the average anteroposterior diameter is 11 cm (obstetric conjugate diameter).
- It is not possible to measure these diameters clinically, and the only diameter at the pelvic inlet amenable to clinical assessment is the distance from the inferior margin of the pubic symphysis to the mid-point of the sacral promontory (the diagonal conjugate) which is ~1.5 cm greater than the obstetric conjugate diameter.

Plane of greatest pelvic dimensions/cavity
- This is the roomiest part of the pelvis and has little clinical significance.
- It is almost round in shape with an average transverse diameter of 13.5 cm and an average anteroposterior diameter of 12.5 cm.

Plane of least pelvic dimensions/mid-pelvis
- This is bound anteriorly by the apex of the pubic arch, laterally by the ischial spines and posteriorly by the tip of the sacrum.
- The interspinous diameter is the narrowest space in the pelvis (10 cm) and represents the level at which impaction of the fetal head is most likely to occur.

Plane of pelvic outlet
- This is bound anteriorly by the pubic arch which should have a desired angle of >90°, posterolaterally by the sacrotuberous ligaments and ischial tuberosities leading to the coccyx posteriorly.
- The average intertuberous diameter is 11 cm.

Assessment of 'pelvic adequacy'

Examination of the pelvis before labour does not accurately discriminate between those who will achieve vaginal birth and those who will not. Even CT or MRI scanning, together with ultrasound of the fetal head, is not helpful, unless there is a gross abnormality which will be evident from the history or gait. This is because the head 'moulds' and the joints of the pelvis can move slightly.

The ideal female pelvis has the following features:
- Oval brim.
- Shallow cavity.
- Non-prominent ischial spines.
- Curved sacrum with large sciatic notches (>90°).
- Sacrospinous ligament >3.5 cm long.
- Rounded subpubic arch >90°.
- Intertuberous distance of at least 10 cm.
- Diagonal conjugate diameter of at least 12 cm.

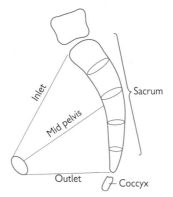

Fig. 1.5 Median sagittal section of the female pelvis showing the pelvic inlet and outlet. Reproduced from Collier J, Longmore M, Brinsden M. *Oxford handbook of clinical specialties*, 6th edn, OUP, 2003. By permission of Oxford University Press.

Fetal head

Anatomy of the fetal skull

The fetal cranium is made up of five main bones, two parietal bones, two frontal bones, and the occipital bone. These are held together by membranous areas called **sutures**, which permits movement during birth (Fig. 1.6).

- The **coronal suture** separates the frontal bones from the parietal bones.
- The **sagittal suture** separates the two parietal bones.
- The **lambdoid suture** separates the occipital bone from the parietal bones.
- The **frontal suture** separates the two frontal bones.

When two or more sutures meet, there is an irregular membranous area between them called a **fontanelle** (Fig 1.6).

- The **anterior fontanelle** or **bregma** is a diamond-shaped space at the junction of the coronal and sagittal sutures, this measures about 3 cm in anteroposterior and transverse diameters, and usually ossifies at ~18 months after birth.
- The **posterior fontanelle** or the **lambda** is a smaller triangular area that lies at the junction of the sagittal and lambdoid sutures.

⚠ The position of the sutures and fontanelles play a very important role in identifying the position of the fetal head in labour.

Regions of the fetal head

The fetal head has different regions assigned to help in the description of the presenting part felt during vaginal examination in labour.

- The **occiput** is the bony prominence that lies behind the posterior fontanelle.
- The **vertex** is the diamond-shaped area between the anterior and posterior fontanelles, and between the parietal eminences.
- The **bregma** is the area around the anterior fontanelle.
- The **sinciput** is the area in front of the anterior fontanelle, which is divided into the brow (between the bregma and the root of the nose) and the face (lying below the root of the nose and the supraorbital ridges).

Caput and moulding of the fetal head

During labour, the dilating cervix may press firmly on the fetal scalp preventing venous blood and lymphatic fluid from flowing normally. This may result in a tissue swelling beneath the skin called **caput succedaneum**. It is soft and boggy to touch and usually disappears within 24 hours of birth.

There is usually some alteration in the shape of the fetal head and a reduction in the head circumference in labour by a process of overlapping of the cranial bones (a reduction of up to 4 cm is possible). This moulding is physiological and disappears a few hours after birth. The frontal bones can slip under the parietal bones, and in addition one parietal bone can override the other and in turn slip under the occipital bone.

The degree of moulding can be assessed vaginally:
- No moulding: when the suture lines are separate.
- 1+ moulding: when the suture lines meet.
- 2+ moulding: when the bones overlap but can be reduced with gentle digital pressure.
- 3+ moulding: when the bones overlap and are irreducible with gentle digital pressure.

▶ The presence of caput and moulding can play an important part in diagnosing obstructed labour.

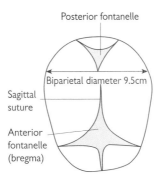

Fig. 1.6 Fontanelles, sagittal suture and biparietal diameter. Reproduced from Collier J, Longmore M, Brinsden M. *Oxford handbook of clinical specialties*, 6th edn, OUP, 2003. By permission of Oxford University Press.

Diameters and presenting parts of the fetal head

The region which presents in labour depends on the degree of flexion or deflexion of the fetal head on presentation to the maternal pelvis. The important diameters of the fetal head as well as the presenting parts are as described below (Fig. 1.7):

- **Suboccipitobregmatic diameter** (9.5 cm): the presentation of a well-flexed vertex. The diameter extends from the middle of the bregma to the undersurface of the occipital bone where it joins the neck. The fetal head circumference is smallest at this plane and measures 32 cm.
- **Suboccipitofrontal diameter** (10.5 cm): a partially flexed vertex, with the diameter extending from the prominent point of the mid frontal bone to the undersurface of the occipital bone where it joins the neck.
- **Occipitofrontal diameter** (11.5 cm): the presentation of a deflexed head. The diameter extends from the prominent point of the mid frontal bone to the most prominent point on the occipital bone. The fetal head circumference at this plane measures 34.5 cm.
- **Mentovertical diameter** (13 cm): a brow presentation, with the diameter extending from the chin to the most prominent point of the midvertex. This presents with the largest anteroposterior diameter.
- **Submentobregmatic diameter** (9.5 cm): a face presentation, with the diameter extending from just behind the chin to the middle of the bregma.

Other noteworthy diameters of the fetal head include:

- **Biparietal diameter** (9.5 cm): the greatest transverse diameter of the head, extending from one parietal eminence to the other.
- **Bitemporal diameter** (8 cm): the greatest distance between two temporal eminences.
- **Bimastoid diameter** (7.5 cm): the distance between the tips of the two mastoid processes.

See Chapter 6, Malpresentations in labour, 📖 p. 313.

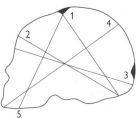

1 Suboccipitobregmatic 9.5cm
  flexed vertex presentation
2 Suboccipitofrontal 10.5cm
  partially deflexed vertex
3 Occipipitofrontal 11.5cm deflexed vertex
4 Mentovertical 13cm brow
5 Submentobregmatic 9.5cm face

Fig. 1.7 Different presenting diameters of the fetal head. Reproduced from Collier J, Longmore M, Brinsden M. *Oxford handbook of clinical specialties*, 6th edn, OUP, 2003. By permission of Oxford University Press.

Placenta: early development

The placenta is the organ responsible for providing endocrine secretions and selective transfer of substances to and from the fetus. It serves as an interface between the mother and the developing fetus. Understanding the development of the placenta is important, as it is the placental trophoblasts that are critical for a successful pregnancy.

Embryological development

- After fertilization, the zygote enters the uterus in 3–5 days and continues to divide to become the blastocyst.
- Implantation of the blastocyst starts on day 7 and is finished by day 11:
  - the inner cell mass of the blastocyst forms the embryo, yolk sac, and amniotic cavity
  - the trophoblast forms the future placenta, chorion and extraembryonic mesoderm.
- When the blastocyst embeds into the decidua, trophoblastic cells differentiate and the embryo becomes surrounded by two layers of trophoblasts:
  - the inner mononuclear cytotrophoblast
  - the outer multinucleated syncytiotrophoblast.
- The invading trophoblast penetrates endometrial blood vessels forming intertrophoblastic maternal blood-filled sinuses (lacunar spaces).
- Trophoblastic cells advance as early or primitive villi, each consisting of cytotrophoblast surrounded by the syncytium.
- These villi mature into secondary and tertiary villi and the mesodermal core develops to form fetal blood vessels (completed by day 21).
- On day 16–17, the surface of the blastocyst is covered by branching villi which are best developed at the embryonic pole:
  - the chorion here is known as chorionic frondosum; the future placenta develops from this area.
- Simultaneously, the lacunar spaces become confluent with one another and by weeks 3–4, form a multilocular receptacle lined by syncytium and filled with maternal blood:
  - this becomes the future intervillous space.
- With further growth of the embryo the decidua capsularis becomes thinner and both villi and the lacunar spaces in the decidua are obliterated, converting the chorion into chorionic levae.
- The villi in the chorionic frondosum show exuberant division and subdivision and with the accompanying proliferation of the decidua basalis, the future placenta is formed.
- This process starts at 6 weeks and the definitive numbers of stem villi are established by 12 weeks.

Placenta: later development

Placental growth continues to term.

- Until week 16 the placenta grows both in thickness and circumference due to the growth of the chorionic villi with accompanying expansion of the intervillous space.
- After 16 weeks growth occurs mainly circumferentially.

Placental villi

- These are the functional units of the placenta.
- There are approximately 60 stem villi in human placenta with each cotyledon containing 3–4 major stem villi.
- Despite their close proximity (0.025 mm), there is no mixing of maternal and fetal blood.
- This placental barrier is made of outer syncytiotrophoblast which is in direct contact with maternal blood, the cytotrophoblast layer, basement membrane, stroma containing mesenchymal cells, and the endothelium and basement membrane of fetal blood vessels.

The placenta at term

- Circular, diameter 15–20 cm, thickness ~2.5 cm at the centre
- Weight ~500 g (the ratio of fetal:placental weight at term is about 6:1)

It occupies about 30% of the uterine wall at term and has two surfaces:

Fetal surface

- Covered by a smooth, glistening amnion with the umbilical cord usually attached at or near its centre.
- The branches of the umbilical blood vessels are visible beneath the amnion as they radiate from the insertion of the cord.
- The amnion can be peeled off from the underlying chorion except at the insertion of the cord.

Maternal surface

- Has a rough and spongy appearance and is divided into several velvety bumps called the cotyledons (15–20) by septa arising from the maternal tissues.
- Each cotyledon may be supplied by its own spiral artery.
- Numerous small greyish spots may be visible on the maternal surface representing calcium deposition in degenerated areas.

Umbilical cord

- Vascular cable that connects the fetus to the placenta.
- Varies from 30 to 90 cm long, covered by amniotic epithelium.
- Contains two umbilical arteries and one umbilical vein embedded into the Wharton's jelly.
- The arteries carry deoxygenated blood from the fetus to the placenta and the oxygenated blood returns to the fetus via the umbilical vein.
- In a full-term fetus, the blood flow in the cord is approximately 350 mL/min.

Placenta: circulation

The placental circulation consists of two distinctly different systems: the uteroplacental circulation and the fetoplacental circulation.

Uteroplacental circulation

The uteroplacental circulation is the maternal blood circulating through the intervillous space (Table 1.1). The intervillous blood flow at term is estimated to be 500–600 mL/min, and the blood in the intervillous space is replaced 3–4 times per minute. The pressure and concentration gradients between fetal capillaries and the intervillous space favours placental transfer of oxygen and other nutrients.

Arterial system

- The spiral arteries respond to the ↑ demand of blood supply to the placental bed by becoming low-pressure, high-flow vessels.
- They become tortuous, dilated and less elastic by trophoblastic invasion which starts early in pregnancy and occurs in two stages:
  - in the first trimester the decidual segments of the spiral arterioles are structurally modified
  - in the second trimester the second wave of trophoblastic invasion occurs resulting in invasion of the myometrial segments of the spiral arteries.

▶ Failure of this physiological change, particularly the second wave of trophoblastic invasion, is implicated in development of pre-eclampsia.

Venous system

- Blood entering the intervillous space from the spiral artery becomes dispersed to reach the chorionic plate and gradually the basal plate, being facilitated by mild movements of the villi and uterine contractions.
- From the basal plate, the uterine veins drain the deoxygenated blood.
- Venous drainage only occurs during uterine relaxation.
- Spiral arteries are perpendicular and veins are parallel to the uterine wall, enabling large volumes of blood available for exchange at the intervillous space even though the rate of flow is decreased during contraction.

Fetoplacental circulation (see Table 1.2)

- Two umbilical arteries carry deoxygenated blood *from* the fetus and enter the chorionic plate underneath the amnion.
- The arteries divide into small branches and enter the stem of the chorionic villi, where further division to arterioles and capillaries takes place.
- The blood then flows to the corresponding venous channel and subsequently to the umbilical vein.
- Maternal and fetal bloodstreams flow side by side and in opposite directions, this counterflow facilitates exchange between mother and fetus.

Table 1.1 Haemodynamics of uteroplacental circulation

Volume of blood in the intervillous space	150 mL
Blood flow in the intervillous space	500–600 mL/min
Pressure changes in the intervillous space	
Height of uterine contraction	30–50 mmHg
Uterine relaxation	10–15 mmHg
Pressure in the spiral artery	70–80 mmHg
Pressure in the uterine veins	8–10 mmHg

Table 1.2 Haemodynamics in the fetoplacental circulation

Fetal blood flow through placenta	400 mL/min
Pressure	
In the umbilical artery	60–70 mmHg
In the umbilical vein	10 mmHg
Oxygen saturation and partial pressure of oxygen	
In the umbilical artery	60%; 20–25 mmHg
In the umbilical vein	70–80%; 30–40 mmHg

Placenta: endocrine functions

The placenta is directly responsible for mediating and/or modulating the maternal environment necessary for normal fetal development.

Principle functions of the placenta

- To anchor the fetus and establish the fetoplacental unit.
- To act as organ for gaseous exchange.
- Endocrine organ to bring the needed changes in pregnancy.
- Transfer of substances to and from the fetus.
- Barrier against infection.

The placenta as an endocrine organ

As an active endocrine organ, the placenta produces a number of hormones, growth factors and cytokines. The production of human chorionic gonadotrophin (hCG), oestrogens, and progesterone by the placenta is vital for the maintenance of pregnancy.

hCG

- Primarily produced by syncytiotrophoblasts.
- Detected from 6 days after fertilization and forms the basis of modern pregnancy testing.
- Concentrations reach a peak at 10–12 weeks gestation then plateau for the remainder of the pregnancy.

The placenta as a barrier

The placenta acts as a barrier for the fetus against pathogens and the maternal immune system.

Infection

The placenta forms an effective barrier against most maternal blood-borne bacterial infections. However some important organisms such as syphilis, parvovirus, hepatitis B and C, rubella, HIV, and cytomegalovirus (CMV) are able to cross it and infect the fetus during pregnancy.

Drugs

Many drugs administered to the mother will pass across the placenta into the fetus, exceptions include low-molecular weight heparin (LMWH).

Some drugs may have little effect on the fetus and be considered 'safe' (e.g. paracetamol), but others (e.g. warfarin) may significantly affect the development, structure and function of the fetus—a process known as **teratogenesis**.

Before prescribing any drug to a pregnant woman it is the prescriber's obligation to ensure that it is considered safe for that stage of pregnancy

See Chapter 5, Drugs in pregnancy, 📖 p. 258.

Placental transfer

Although the placenta acts as a barrier to most substances, it allows exchange of gases, transfer of fetal nutrition, and removal of waste products in a highly effective manner. The speed of exchange and concentration of substance exchanged depends upon:

- The concentration of the substance on each side of the placenta.
- Molecular size.
- Lipid solubility.
- Ionization.
- Placental surface area.
- Maternofetal blood flow.

A low-molecular-weight lipid-soluble substance with a high concentration gradient across the placenta, for example, will be transferred quickly to the fetus. The actual transfer occurs by simple diffusion, facilitated diffusion, active transport and/or endocytosis (Table 1.3).

Table 1.3 Transfer mechanisms across the placenta for common anabolites and catabolites

Substance	Transfer mechanism(s)	Direction of transfer
Oxygen	Simple diffusion	To fetus
Carbon dioxide	Simple diffusion	From fetus
Glucose	Simple and facilitated diffusion	To fetus
Amino acids	Facilitated diffusion	To fetus
Iron	Endocytosis	To fetus
Fatty acids	Facilitated diffusion	To fetus
Water	Simple diffusion	To and from fetus
Electrolytes	Counter-transport mechanism	To and from fetus
Urea and creatinine	Simple diffusion	From fetus

Physiology of pregnancy: endocrine

Physiological and anatomical changes occur during the course of pregnancy to provide a suitable environment for the growth and development of the fetus. Early changes are due, in part, to the metabolic demands brought on by the fetus, placenta and uterus and, in part, to the increasing levels of pregnancy hormones, particularly those of progesterone and oestrogen. Later changes are more anatomical in nature and are caused by mechanical pressure from the expanding uterus.

Endocrine changes

Progesterone ↑ throughout pregnancy

- Synthesized by the corpus luteum until day 35 days and by the placenta thereafter.
- Progesterone promotes smooth muscle relaxation (gut, ureters, uterus) and raises body temperature.

Oestrogens, mainly oestradiol (90%)

- ↑ breast and nipple growth and pigmentation of the areola.
- Promote uterine blood flow, myometrial growth, cervical softening.
- ↑ sensitivity and expression of myometrial oxytocin receptors.
- ↑ water retention and protein synthesis.

Human placental lactogen (hPL)

- Has a structure and function similar to growth hormone.
- modifies maternal metabolism to ↑ the energy supply to the fetus.
- ↑ insulin secretion but ↓ insulin's peripheral effect (liberating maternal fatty acids and sparing glucose enabling it to be diverted to the fetus).

The pituitary gland in pregnancy

- Enlarges mainly due to changes in the anterior lobe.
- Prolactin levels increase substantially probably due to oestrogen stimulation of the lactotrophes.
- Gonadotrophin secretion is inhibited whilst plasma adrenocortico-trophic hormone (ACTH) levels ↑
- Maternal plasma cortisone output ↑ but the unbound levels remain constant.

The posterior pituitary releases oxytocin principally during the first stage of labour and during suckling.

Effect of pregnancy on the thyroid

- The maternal thyroid gland enlarges due to ↑ demand in pregnancy.
- ↑ renal clearance of iodine results in a relative iodide deficiency.
- The thyroid responds by tripling its iodide uptake from the blood which results in follicular enlargement.
- Thyroid-binding globulin (TBG) is doubled by the end of the first trimester due to high oestrogen levels.
- As a result, total T_3 (triiodothryonine) and T_4 (thyroxine) levels rise early in pregnancy and then fall to remain within the normal non-pregnant range.
- Thyroid-stimulating hormone (TSH) may decrease slightly in early pregnancy but tends to remain within the normal range.
- T_3 and T_4 cross the placental barrier in very small amounts.

⚠ Iodine, antithyroid drugs, and long-acting thyroid stimulator (LATS) or antibodies associated with Graves' disease can cross the placenta.

Physiology of pregnancy: haemodynamics

Plasma volume
- ↑ by 10–15% at 6 to 12 weeks of gestation.
- Expands rapidly until 30–34 weeks.
- Total gain at term ~1100–1600 mL (total plasma volume of 4700–5200 mL, a 30–50% ↑ from the non-pregnant state).
- Acute excessive weight gain is commonly due to oedema.

Red cell volume (or red cell mass)
- Rises from 1400 mL to 1640 mL at term (↑ 18%).
- With iron and folate supplementation, an ↑ of 30% has been reported.

▶The discrepancy between the rate of ↑ of plasma volume and that of red cell mass results in a relative haemodilution or 'physiological anaemia' with the haemoglobin concentration, haematocrit and red cell counts all ↓ (particularly in the second trimester).

▶ Mean corpuscular haemoglobin concentration remains constant.

Total white cell count
- ↑ mainly due to the ↑ in neutrophil polymorphonuclear leucocytes which peaks at 32 weeks.
- A further massive neutrophilia occurs during labour.
- Eosinophils, basophils and monocytes remain relatively constant but there is a profound ↓ in eosinophils during labour, being virtually absent at delivery.
- Although the lymphocyte count and the number of B and T cells remain constant, lymphocyte function and cell-mediated immunity are profoundly depressed, giving rise to a lowered resistance to viral infections.

Platelets
- ↓ slightly during pregnancy.
- Platelet function is unchanged.

Clotting factors
- Pregnancy is a hypercoagulable state.
- Most clotting factors ↑, especially fibrinogen.

▶ Erythrocyte sedimentation rate (ESR) levels can also be elevated up to fourfold in pregnancy.

Physiology of pregnancy: cardio-respiratory

Cardiovascular changes

Major changes occur in the cardiovascular system in pregnancy, the most significant of these changes occurring within the first 12 weeks.

- Cardiac output ↑ from 5 to 6.5 L/min by ↑ stroke volume (10%) and pulse rate (~15 beats/min).
- During labour, contractions may ↑ cardiac output by 2 L/min probably due to injection of blood from the distended intervillous space.
- With progressive enlargement of the uterus, the heart and diaphragm are displaced upwards.
- The heart enlarges and ↑ in volume by 70–80 mL due to ↑ diastolic filling and muscle hypertrophy.

▶ Pregnancy may proceed normally even when the mother has an artificial cardiac pacemaker, compensation occurring mainly from increased stroke volume.

Blood pressure in pregnancy

- Peripheral resistance ↓ by nearly 50% (probably due to the ↑ production of vasodilator prostaglandins).
- Blood pressure (most noticeably diastolic), ↓ mid-pregnancy by 10–20 mmHg, ↑ to non-pregnant levels by term.
- Profound ↓ can occur late in pregnancy when lying supine, due to compression of the inferior vena cava leading to ↓ venous return and ↓ cardiac output (supine hypotension syndrome).
- Aortic compression may also occur causing a conspicuous difference between brachial and femoral pressures giving a pressure difference of 10–15% from the supine to the lateral position.
- The balance of vasoconstrictor and vasodilator factors regulating peripheral resistance may be the basis of blood pressure regulation in pregnancy and implicated in development of pregnancy induced hypertension.
- Vasodilatation and hypotension also stimulates renin–angiotensin release which plays a part in blood pressure regulation.

Respiratory system changes

- The level of the diaphragm rises in pregnancy and the intercostal angle ↑ from 68° in early pregnancy to 103° in late pregnancy:
  - breathing becomes more diaphragmatic than costal.
- Tidal volume ↑~40% (500–700 mL) due to the effect of progesterone
- Inspiratory capacity (tidal volume plus inspiratory reserve volume) ↑ progressively in late pregnancy (Fig. 1.13).
- Respiratory rate changes slightly, hence the resting pregnant woman ↑ ventilation by breathing more deeply and not more frequently.
- Breathlessness is common in pregnancy as maternal pCO$_2$ (partial pressure of carbon dioxide) is set lower to allow the fetus to offload CO$_2$.

Physiology of pregnancy: genital tract and breast

Uterus
- Undergoes a 10-fold ↑ in weight to 1000 g at term.
- Muscle hypertrophy occurs up to 20 weeks, after which stretching of the muscle fibres occurs.
- Uterine blood flow has been shown to ↑ from ~50 mL/min at 10 weeks to 500–700 mL/min at term.
- The uterine and ovarian arteries, and branches of the superior vesical arteries undergo massive hypertrophy.

The uterus is divided functionally and morphologically into three sections:
- Cervix
- Isthmus (which later develops into the lower segment)
- Body of the uterus (corpus uteri).

Cervix
- Reduction in cervical collagen towards term enables its dilatation.
- Hypertrophy of cervical glands leads to the production of profuse cervical mucus and the formation of a thick mucus plug or operculum that acts as a barrier to infection.
- Vaginal discharge ↑ due to cervical ectopy and cell desquamation.

Uterine body
- ↑ in size, shape, position, and consistency.
- Uterine cavity expands from 4 to 4000 mL.

Vagina
- A rich venous vascular network in the connective tissue surrounds the vaginal walls with blood and gives rise to a slightly bluish appearance.
- High oestrogen levels stimulate glycogen synthesis and deposition:
  - action of lactobacilli on glycogen in vaginal cells produces lactic acid
  - lactic acid lowers the vaginal pH to keep the vagina relatively free from any bacterial pathogens.

Breast
- The lactiferous ducts and alveoli develop and grow under the stimulus of oestrogen, progesterone, and prolactin.
- From 3–4 months, colostrum (thick, glossy, protein-rich fluid) can be expressed from the breast.
- Prolactin stimulates the cells of the alveoli to secrete milk:
  - this effect is blocked during pregnancy by the peripheral action of oestrogen and progesterone.
  - shortly after delivery the sudden ↓ in these hormones enables prolactin to act uninhibited on the breast, and lactation begins
- Suckling further stimulates prolactin and oxytocin release:
  - oxytocin stimulates contraction of the myoepithelial cells to cause ejection of milk.

Physiology of pregnancy: other changes

Urinary tract

Various anatomical and physiological changes in occur in pregnancy:
- Kidney size ↑ by about 1 cm in length.
- Marked dilatation of the calyces, renal pelvis, and ureter from the first trimester.
- Vesicoureteric reflux occurs sporadically:
  - a combination of reflux and ureteric dilatation leads to urinary stasis and ↑ infection
- Although bladder muscle relaxes in pregnancy, residual urine is not normally present after micturition.
- Uric acid clearance increases from 12 to 20 mmol/mL causing a reduction in plasma uric acid levels:
  - as pregnancy progresses the filtered load of uric acid ↑ while the excretion remains constant resulting in plasma levels returning to non-pregnant values.
- Renal blood flow ↑ by 30–50% in the first trimester in line with the ↑ in cardiac output that occurs, and remains elevated:
  - results in ↑ glomerular filtration rate (GFR) and effective renal plasma flow, causing a ↓ in plasma levels of urea and creatinine
  - plays an important role in the variable glycosuria and urinary frequency that occurs in pregnancy.

⚠ Creatinine within the normal range for non-pregnant women may indicate renal impairment in pregnancy.

Alimentary system

- ↓ tone of oesophageal sphincter and displacement through the diaphragm due to ↑ abdominal pressure causes reflux oesophagitis (heartburn).
- Gastric mobility is low and gastric secretion is reduced, resulting in delayed gastric emptying.
- Gut motility is generally ↓ and with possible ↑ sodium and water absorption in the large bowel, there is a tendency to constipation.

Skin

- Pigmentation in linear nigra, nipple, and areola or chloasma (brown patches of pigmentation seen especially on the face).
- Palmar erythema and spider naevi are also common.
- Incidence of striae varies in different populations:
  - represents the effect of disruption of collagen fibres in the subcuticular zone
  - probably related to the effect of ↑ production of adrenocortical hormones as well as to the actual stress in the skin associated with expansion of the abdomen.

Preparing for pregnancy

A woman's body undergoes significant changes in pregnancy, with the developing fetus making increasing demands. Preparation for pregnancy should begin before conception, as fetal development begins from the third week after the last menstrual period and damaging effects (e.g. exposure to drugs) may occur before the woman is even aware she is pregnant. Being as fit and healthy as possible before conception maximizes the chances of a healthy pregnancy, although not all poor obstetric outcomes can be avoided. Prepregnancy counselling by a specialist team is recommended where specific risks and diseases are identified.

Specific risks for older mothers

- Advanced maternal age is a risk factor for adverse outcome.
- A woman >35 years old has a reduced chance of conceiving and this rate of decline drops very quickly by 40 years of age.
- Age also carries an increased risk of chromosomal abnormalities in the baby (most common abnormality being Down's syndrome).
- Older mothers are more likely to develop complications in pregnancy, e.g. pre-eclampsia and diabetes mellitus.

Exercise and stress

- Moderate exercise should be encouraged, as it improves a woman's cardiovascular and muscular fitness.
- Women should be reassured that beginning or continuing a moderate course of exercise during pregnancy is not associated with adverse outcome.
- The best exercises are low impact aerobics, swimming, brisk walking and jogging.
- Contact sports, high-impact sports and vigorous racquet sports that may involve the risk of abdominal trauma should be avoided.
- Exercise is also associated with higher self-esteem and confidence.
- Relaxation and avoiding stress should be encouraged when planning for pregnancy.

⚠ Scuba diving may result in fetal birth defects and fetal decompression disease, therefore is not recommended.

Stopping contraception

- There is no delay in return to fertility after stopping the pill or having the coil removed.
- Women who use the contraceptive injection may experience a delay for up to several months.
- It is often recommended that women wait 3 months after stopping the pill before trying to conceive.

Supplements and lifestyle advice

Folic acid and other vitamins

Folic acid is the only vitamin supplement that is recommended to be taken before pregnancy and up to 12 weeks of gestation for women who are otherwise eating a healthy balanced diet.

Recommended doses of folic acid

- 400 micrograms/day of folic acid has been shown to reduce the occurrence of neural tube defects.
- For women at higher risk (e.g. previous affected child, women with epilepsy), a dose of 5 mg/day is recommended.

- **Iron:** routine supplementation is not necessary and should be prescribed when medically indicated. However, it may be considered as routine in areas where the incidence of iron-deficiency anaemia is high.
- **Calcium:** supplementation may be necessary if the intake of calcium is low; however, the ideal is increased calcium from dietary sources.
- **Iodine:** deficiency is endemic in some parts of the world, and can cause cretinism and neonatal hypothyroidism. Supplementation with iodinized salt or oil should be considered.
- **Zinc:** low serum levels have been associated with an increased risk of preterm labour and growth restriction, but increased intake from dietary sources such as milk and dairy products should be sufficient.

⚠ Vitamin A supplementation (intake >700 micrograms/day) might be teratogenic and should be avoided, as should consumption of products high in vitamin A such as liver and pate.

Alcohol, smoking, and recreational drugs

Excessive alcohol intake has been conclusively shown to cause fetal malformations. The exact threshold of alcohol that will cause malformation in the fetus has not been established.

⚠ Avoid alcohol whenever possible, or limit consumption to one standard unit per day.

Smoking during pregnancy has an adverse effect on the developing fetus (e.g. preterm labour, low birth weight). Women should be encouraged to stop and supported through smoking cessation. If they cannot stop, reduction should be promoted.

▶ Stopping smoking at any stage has a beneficial effect.

⚠ Recreational and illegal drugs cause significant problems including miscarriage, preterm birth, poor fetal development, and intrauterine death. Help and support for dealing with any addiction should be sought from the appropriate agencies.

Weight and diet

- Fertility may be reduced in women who are significantly overweight (BMI >30) or underweight (BMI <18.5).
- Obesity is the most common nutritional disorder in the industrialized world, with increased risks including gestational diabetes and hypertension; also, monitoring and assessment may be difficulty during pregnancy and labour (see Chapter 5: Obesity in pregnancy, 📖 p. 254).
- Obesity has been recognized by CEMACH as carrying a greater risk of maternal death (see Chapter 11: The confidential enquiry, 📖 p. 410).
- Malnutrition, on the other hand, is a major life hazard in the developing world and is a cause of other problems such as anaemia which has its own inherent risk for both mother and fetus.
- Poor nutrition in pregnant women is associated with the delivery of low birth weight (<2500 g) babies, and improving the nutritional status and maternal weight can have a positive effect on the birth outcome.
- Weight gain should be around 11–16 kg during pregnancy, and women should consume an additional 350 kilocalories (1500 kJ) a day.
- A nutritious, well-balanced diet includes foods rich in protein, dairy foods (which supply calcium), starchy foods, and plenty of fruit and vegetables that supply vitamins and fibre.
- It is best to avoid a lot of sugary, salty, or fatty foods.
- Food delicacies such as undercooked meats and eggs, pates, soft cheeses, shellfish and raw fish, and under-pasteurized milk should be avoided as they are potential sources of *Listeria* and *Salmonella*.

⚠ Listeriosis in pregnancy is a known, but rare cause of poor obstetric outcome and fetal death.

General health check

Planning a pregnancy provides a good opportunity for a general health check by the GP and may identify any potential obstetric risk factors well in advance.

A pre-pregnancy general health check may include:

- A general examination including blood pressure, heart, and lungs.
- Family history of inherited disorders or congenital abnormalities.
- Urine dipstick.
- Blood tests such as thalassaemia and sickle cell disease may be offered if at risk.
- Rubella (and hepatitis) status should be ascertained and vaccination given if not immune (women should be advised to avoid pregnancy for 3 months after immunization).
- HIV screening if at risk.
- Dental examination.

Pre-existing medical disorders (see Chapter 5)

Pregnancy can have an adverse effect on pre-existing medical disorders.
- The effect may be transient, returning to normal after delivery (e.g. diabetes mellitus), or it may be permanent and progressive, leading to maternal mortality (e.g. severe renal impairment or severe cardiac disease).
- For a woman with a pre-existing disorder contemplating pregnancy, the advice of a specialist should be sought early. If the risk is very high, pregnancy may be discouraged altogether.
- Optimal control of certain diseases before conception may be very important to avoid the risk of fetal malformation or adverse outcome (e.g. diabetes mellitus).
- Some medications may be changed before conception to reduce the risk of teratogenesis (e.g. antiepileptics).
- Pregnancy undertaken when the illness is in remission, stable or cured will ensure a better outcome.

Medication

In general, both prescription drugs and over-the-counter medication should be used as little as possible. Most drugs carry warnings about use in pregnancy. However, the benefit may outweigh the risks, even in pregnancy, so a doctor should be consulted before stopping or starting any medication in pregnancy or before conception.

Working during pregnancy

- Women should be reassured that it is safe to continue working before and during pregnancy.
- Some workplaces are more likely to present hazards (e.g. chemical factories, operating theatres, X-ray departments), hence precautions may be necessary—specific advice should be sought from the employer's occupational health department.
- Women should be reassured that the use of computers and video display units has not been proven to be linked with any adverse outcome.
- See Chapter 4: Vaccination and travel, 📖 p. 174.

Diagnosis of pregnancy

The most obvious symptom of pregnancy is cessation of periods, i.e. a period of amenorrhoea in a woman having regular menstruation.

Other common symptoms of early pregnancy

Nausea and vomiting (morning sickness)
- Common in the 1st trimester.
- May occur at any time of the day.
- May sometimes persist throughout pregnancy.

Frequency of micturition
- ↑ plasma volume and ↑ urine production.
- Pressure effect of the uterus on the bladder.

Excessive lassitude or fatigue
- Common in early pregnancy.
- Tends to disappear after 12 weeks gestation.

Breast tenderness or 'heaviness'
- Often seen early in pregnancy, particularly in the month after the first period is missed.

Fetal movements or quickening
- ~20 weeks gestation in the nullipara.
- 18 weeks in the multipara.
- Many women may experience fetal movements earlier than this and some may not perceive movements until term.

Occasionally a pregnant woman may experience an abnormal desire to eat something not normally regarded as nutritive (such as dirt). This is known as **pica.**

Clinical examination
- The vagina and cervix have a bluish tinge due to blood congestion.
- The size of the uterus may be estimated by bimanual examination (reasonably accurate in early pregnancy).
- After 12 weeks uterus is palpable abdominally and the fetal heart may be heard using a hand-held Doppler.

The pregnancy test
- The hormone hCG is secreted by trophoblastic tissue:
  - ↑ exponentially from ~ 8 days after ovulation
  - peaks at 8–12 weeks gestation
- hCG levels can be measured in blood or urine.
- Test kits are available commercially (home pregnancy tests)
  - can show a positive result with urinary hCG levels >50 IU/L.
  - some 'early' pregnancy test kits will detect levels of >25 IU/L.
- These tests can confirm pregnancy within 1 week of a missed period.

Dating of pregnancy

Menstrual history

- The first day of the LMP may be used to calculate the gestational age and the EDD (📖 p. 02), but this may be inaccurate as:
  - many women may not be certain of their LMP
  - ovulation does not always occur on day 14 and the proliferative phase may vary considerably in shorter or longer menstrual cycles
- The EDD can be calculated using Naegele's formula (📖 p. 02)
- About 40% of women will deliver within 5 days of the EDD and about 2/3 within 10 days.

⚠ 11–42% of gestational age estimates from LMP may be inaccurate.

▶ Pregnancies resulting from in-vitro fertilization (IVF) can be dated using the day of embryo transfer.

Dating ultrasound scan

Between 8 and 13 weeks USS provides the most accurate measure of gestational age and, where possible, should be used to calculate EDD.
- Before 8 weeks it is unreliable due to the small size of the gestation sac and fetal pole.
- After 13 weeks other factors may affect fetal growth, therefore, although an estimate can be made using BPD and FL, it may be unreliable.

Crown–rump length (CRL) (Fig. 1.8) is used to calculate gestation between 8 and 13 weeks. It is measured from one fetal pole to the other along its longitudinal axis in a straight line.

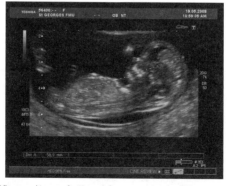

Fig. 1.8 Ultrasound image of a 12 week fetus measuring the CRL.

Ultrasound assessment of fetal growth

Any clinical suspicion that the fetus may be small or large for gestational age should be followed by a formal US assessment of fetal growth and amount of amniotic fluid (liquor volume).

The measurements used are (Fig. 1.9):

Biparietal diameter (BPD) and head circumference (HC)

- The anatomical landmarks used to ensure the accuracy and reproducibility of the measurement are a midline falx, the thalami symmetrically positioned on either side of the falx, the visualization of the cavum septum pellucidum at one third the frontooccipital distance and the lateral ventricles with their anterior and posterior horns identifiable.
- The calipers are placed between the leading edge of the proximal and distal skull bones (BPD) and circumferentially around the head (HC).

Abdominal circumference (AC)

- The abdominal circumference is the single most important measurement in assessing fetal size and growth.
- It is measured where the image of the stomach and the portal vein is visualized in a tangential section.

Femur length (FL)

- By convention, measurement of the FL is considered accurate only when the image shows two blunted ends.

⚠ FL can be underestimated if the correct plane is not obtained.

See Chapter 3: IUGR, 📖 p. 140.

The uterus may measure small for dates because of:

- Wrong dates.
- Oligohydramnios.
- Intrauterine growth restriction.
- Presenting part deep in the pelvis.
- Abnormal lie of the fetus.

The uterus may measure large for dates because of:

- Wrong dates.
- Macrosomia.
- Polyhydramnios.
- Multiple pregnancy.
- Presence of fibroids.

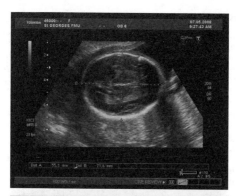

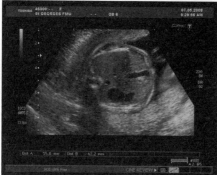

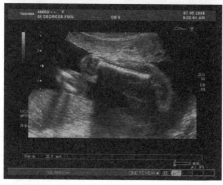

Fig. 1.9 Ultrasound measurement of biparietal diameter, abdominal circumference and femur length.

Booking visit

The needs of each pregnant woman should be assessed at the first appointment and a plan of care made for her pregnancy. This should be reassessed at each appointment throughout pregnancy as new problems can arise at any time. Many women in the UK have 'shared obstetric care' whereby the woman's GP and community midwife undertake most of the obstetric care with a limited number of visits to the hospital to see a consultant.

Routine involvement of an obstetrician in the care of women with an uncomplicated pregnancy does not appear to improve perinatal outcomes compared with involving obstetricians when complications arise.

There should be continuity of care throughout the antenatal period and this should be provided by a small group of carers with whom the woman feels comfortable. The environment in which antenatal appointments take place should enable women to discuss sensitive issues such as domestic violence, sexual abuse, psychiatric illness, and illicit drug use. Women should be given the information needed for in order to choose giving birth at home, in a midwifery-led unit, or in hospital.

Booking should ideally be early in pregnancy (prior to 12 weeks) in order to take full advantage of antenatal care. However, many women are seen for the first time in the second trimester.

⚠ Children born to very late bookers or unbooked women have a higher risk of perinatal mortality (4–5 fold) and morbidity, with an attendant increase in maternal morbidity and mortality.

Booking visit: history

A comprehensive history should be elicited (see Obstetric history, 📖 p. 2) and a full physical examination undertaken (see Obstetric examination, 📖 p. 6).

- Risk factors from past history should be highlighted.
- An effort should be made to obtain past obstetric notes if it is thought that this information may change the management.
- History of inheritable diseases in close relatives should be sought, as well as history of migration and travel: this may identify risk for diseases such as haemoglobinopathies, some forms of hepatitis, and HIV infection.
- History of alcohol abuse, smoking and addictive drug use are useful behavioural markers of other potential risks (e.g. fetal abnormalities, impaired fetal growth, and preterm labour).
- It is important to identify women at risk of postnatal depressive illness:
  - women should be asked about previous psychiatric disorders, social problems including domestic violence and previous self-harm
  - women at risk should have full psychiatric care and social support.
- Advice and support should be given on healthy lifestyles (including diet and exercise), pregnancy care services available, maternity benefits, and sufficient information to enable informed decision-making on screening tests.

Antenatal care: planning

The basic aims of antenatal care are:
- To provide evidence-based information and support to women and their partners, to enable them to make informed decisions regarding their care.
- To advise on minor problems and symptoms of pregnancy.
- To assess maternal and fetal risk factors at the onset of pregnancy.
- To facilitate provision of prenatal screening and subsequent management of any abnormalities detected.
- To monitor fetal and maternal well-being throughout pregnancy and screen for commonly occurring complications (most notably a BP and urine check at every visit to detect signs of developing pre-eclampsia)
- To determine timing and mode of delivery when complications arise or if pregnancy continues after the EDD.

A schedule of antenatal appointments with specific aims for each appointment should be discussed. A nulliparous woman with an uncomplicated pregnancy should need ten appointments, whereas in a parous woman, seven antenatal appointments should be adequate.

The needs of each pregnant woman should be assessed at each appointment as new problems can arise at any stage in pregnancy.

⚠ Urine should be dipstick tested and blood pressure measured at every antenatal visit.

Screening for chromosomal and structural abnormalities

Ideally, screening should be offered to all women at the time of booking. Detailed, unbiased, written information should be provided about the conditions being screened for, types of test available, and the implications of the results.

⚠ It is important for a woman to understand that a negative result in any screening test does not guarantee that her baby does not have that or another abnormality.

For full details on current UK screening see 📖 Chapter 3: Prenatal diagnosis: overview, p. 106.

Antenatal care: routine blood tests

Antenatal care starts once the pregnancy is confirmed, and a referral is made by the GP to the community midwife for booking.

Routine blood tests

Full blood count (FBC)

- Physiological anaemia means the lower limit for a 'normal' haemoglobin (Hb) is 10.5 g/dL in pregnancy as opposed to 11.5 g/dL in a non-pregnant woman.
- The commonest cause of anaemia is iron deficiency. Anaemia is investigated by assessment of haematinic indices such as ferritin and total iron binding capacity (TIBC) in microcytic hypochromic anaemia and serum and red cell folate and serum B_{12} levels in macrocytic anaemia.

Blood grouping and antibody screen

- Determining the blood group at booking makes it possible to identify rhesus-negative women who are at risk of rhesus isoimmunization (see 📖 Chapter 3: Rhesus isoimmunization, p. 133).

Rubella screen

- Around 2% of nulliparous and 1% of multiparous women are not immune to rubella, and it is recommended that these women receive postpartum rubella vaccination.

Syphilis screen

- Although the incidence of syphilis in the UK is low, outbreaks of the disease do occur.
- Early treatment can prevent congenital syphilis in the neonate.

Hepatitis B screen

- Screening for hepatitis B is performed on all women in pregnancy at booking so that effective postnatal intervention can be offered.
- In the adult the virus is cleared within 6 months in 90% of infected individuals.
- In infected neonates 90% become chronic carriers with the risk of postinfective hepatic cirrhosis and hepatocellular carcinoma—hence the need to screen and prevent.

HIV screen

- The recommendation for all maternity units in the UK is for universal screening for HIV at the booking visit ('opt out' policy).
  - Vertical transmission from mother to fetus can be significantly reduced (by two-thirds) by treatment of the mother with antiretrovirals in pregnancy and labour and of the infant for 6 weeks postnatally.
  - The risk of transmission is reduced by Caesarean section (CS) and avoidance of breast-feeding. (See 📖 Chapter 4:HIV, p. 166)

Antenatal care: specific blood tests

Haemoglobin electrophoresis
This should be routinely performed in women of minority ethnic or racial origins with high incidence of haemoglobinopathies.

Some ethnic origins at high risk of thalassaemia
- Cyprus
- Eastern Mediterranean.
- Middle Eastern.
- Indian subcontinent.
- South-east Asia.

▶ Women of African or Afro-Caribbean origin are at risk of sickle cell disease or trait.

▶ If a woman is affected, testing her partner's status would enable appropriate counselling and further prenatal testing.

⚠ Persistent anaemia, where a cause cannot be identified, may be an indication for haemoglobin electrophoresis in any woman regardless of racial origin.

Miscellaneous tests
A variety of other blood tests may be indicated on an individual basis. Examples include thyroid function tests (history of thyroid disease), HbA1c (to assess long term control of diabetes), or baseline urea and creatinine (in chronic hypertensives with renal complications).

Screening for gestational diabetes (GDM)
There is little consensus as to who, when, how, or even whether to screen for GDM. At present there is insufficient evidence to support routine screening for GDM. The timing of any screening is equally controversial as the later the test is performed, the higher the detection rate since glucose tolerance progressively deteriorates. On the other hand, the earlier in pregnancy GDM is diagnosed and hyperglycaemia treated, the greater the likelihood of positively influencing the outcome.

Most units currently use targeted screening based on known risk factors.

Risk factors for gestational diabetes (GDM)
- Previous GDM.
- Family history of diabetes (first-degree relative with diabetes).
- Previous macrosomic baby.
- Previous unexplained stillbirth.
- Obesity (BMI>30).
- Glycosuria on more than one occasion.
- Polyhydramnios.
- Large for gestational age fetus in current pregnancy.

Antenatal care: preparing for delivery

- In the early 3rd trimester, women are seen monthly and at each visit BP, urinalysis, and fundal height measurement, as well as enquiry about maternal well-being and fetal activity, are recorded.
- FBC and antibody screen is repeated at 28 and 34 weeks gestation, and rhesus-negative women are given anti-D prophylaxis at these times.
- From 36 weeks onwards, fetal presentation as well as growth is assessed, and an ultrasound assessment performed if indicated.
- Preparation for labour and delivery should be discussed.
- The final routine visit between 40 and 41 weeks includes discussions on induction of labour after 41 weeks gestation.
- In women who wish to avoid induction, the risks of prolonging pregnancy should be discussed and a plan for increased fetal surveillance with cardiotocography and ultrasound assessment of fetal growth and liquor volume can be made.

Pregnancy complications

Minor symptoms of pregnancy: gastrointestinal

These symptoms are mostly related to the hormonal, physiological, and increased weight-bearing aspects of pregnancy. Although they are usually mild and self-limiting, some women may experience severe symptoms which can effect their ability to cope with activities of daily living.

📖 www.rcog.org.uk/resources/Public/pdf/Antenatal_Care.pdf

Nausea and vomiting (morning sickness)
- Most common complaint in pregnancy, especially in the first trimester:
  - nausea 80–85%
  - vomiting 52%.
- Believed to be caused by hormones of pregnancy especially hCG.
- Increased in multiple and molar pregnancies.
- May be severe enough to warrant hospital admission—hyperemesis gravidarum (see Hyperemesis, 📖 p. 518).
- Not usually associated with poor pregnancy outcome.
- Tends to resolve spontaneously by 16–20 weeks.
- Management:
  - lifestyle modification (e.g. eating small meals, increasing fluid intake)
  - ginger
  - acupressure (P6)
  - antiemetics (prochlorperazine, promethazine, metoclopramide).

Gastro-oesophageal reflux (heartburn)
- Very common complaint at all stages of pregnancy:
  - 1st trimester 22%
  - 2nd trimester 39%
  - 3rd trimester 72%.
- Progesterone relaxes the oesophageal sphincter allowing gastric reflux, this gradually worsens with increasing intra-abdominal pressure from the growing fetus.
- Management:
  - lifestyle modification (e.g. sleeping propped up, avoiding spicy food)
  - alginate preparations and simple antacids
  - if severe, H_2 receptor antagonists (ranitidine).

Constipation
- Common complaint which appears to decrease with gestation:
  - 1st trimester 39%
  - 2nd trimester 30%
  - 3rd trimester 20%.
- Progesterone reduces smooth muscle tone, affecting bowel activity.
- Often made worse by iron supplementation.
- Management:
  - lifestyle modification (e.g. increasing fruit, fibre. and water intake)
  - fibre supplements
  - osmotic laxatives (lactulose).

Minor symptoms of pregnancy: musculoskeletal and vascular

Symphysis pubis dysfunction (SPD)
- Describes a collection of signs and symptoms producing pelvic pain.
- Usually mild but can present with severe and debilitating pain.
- Incidence up to 10%.
- Management:
  - physiotherapy advice and support
  - simple analgesia
  - limit abduction of legs at delivery
  - Caesarean section (CS) not indicated.

□ www.pelvicpartnership.org.uk

Backache and sciatica
- Common complaint, attributed to hormonal softening of ligaments exacerbated by altered posture due to the weight of the uterus.
- Prevalence estimated between 35% and 61%
- Pressure on the sciatic nerves may also produce neurological symptoms (sciatica).
- Management:
  - lifestyle modification (e.g. sleeping positions)
  - alternative therapies including relaxation and massage
  - physiotherapy input (e.g. back care classes)
  - simple analgesia.

Carpal tunnel syndrome
- Occurs due to oedema compressing the median nerve in the wrist.
- Usually resolves spontaneously after delivery.
- Management:
  - sleeping with hands over the side of the bed may help
  - wrist splints may be of benefit
  - if evidence of neurological deficit, surgical referral may be indicated.

Haemorrhoids
- Tend to occur in the 3rd trimester.
- 8–30% of pregnant women.
- Management:
  - avoid constipation from early pregnancy
  - ice packs and digital reduction of prolapsed haemorrhoids
  - suppositories and topical agents for symptomatic relief
  - if thrombosed, may require surgical referral.

Varicose veins
- Common complaint which increases with gestation
- Thought to be due to progesterone relaxing the vasculature and the fetal mass effect decreasing pelvic venous return.
- Management:
  - regular exercise
  - compression hosiery
  - consider thromboprophylaxis if other risk factors are present.

Minor symptoms of pregnancy: genitourinary and others

Urinary symptoms
- Frequency in the 1st trimester results from increased glomerular filtration rate and the uterus pressing against the bladder.
- Stress incontinence may occur in the 3rd trimester as a result of pressure on the pelvic floor.

△ Urinary tract infections (UTI) are common in pregnancy.
- Management:
  - screen for UTI (urine dipstick testing: nitrite analysis is best)
  - avoid caffeine and fluid late at night.

Vaginal discharge
- Increases due to increased blood flow to the vagina and cervix.
- Should be white/clear and mucoid;
  - offensive, coloured, or itchy may indicate an infection
  - profuse and watery may indicate ruptured membranes.
- Management:
  - exclude ruptured membranes
  - exclude STI and candidiasis (common in pregnancy)
  - reassurance.

Itching and rashes
- Skin changes and itching are common in pregnancy.
- Rashes are usually self-limiting and not serious.
- Management:
  - full history and examination to exclude infectious causes (eg varicella, Chapter 4, p. 156) and obstetric cholestasis (see 📖 p. 210)
  - emollients and simple over-the-counter 'anti-itch creams'
  - reassurance—most will resolve after delivery
  - referral to dermatologist if severe.

Other common minor symptoms of pregnancy include:
- Breast enlargement and pain:
  - may be helped with supportive underwear.
- Mild breathlessness on exertion
  - important to exclude pulmonary embolus and anaemia.
- Headaches
  - important to exclude pre-eclampsia or (rare) neurological cause.
- Tiredness.
- Insomnia.
- Stretch marks.
- Labile mood.
- Calf cramps.
- Braxton Hicks contractions.

Antepartum haemorrhage: overview

Antepartum haemorrhage (APH) is bleeding from the genital tract in pregnancy at ≥24 weeks gestation before onset of labour.

Causes of antepartum haemorrhage
- Unexplained (~97%):
  - usually marginal placental bleeds (i.e. minor placental abruptions).
- Placenta praevia (~1%).
- Placental abruption (~1%).
- Others (~1%), including:
- Maternal
  - incidental (cervical erosion/ectropion)
  - local infection of cervix/vagina
  - a 'show'
  - genital tract tumours
  - varicosities
  - trauma.
- Fetal
  - vasa praevia.

Women with placenta praevia or placental abruption may present with typical symptoms and signs and with recognized risk factors. However, there may be minimal or no PV loss in a large abruption and an abruption is usually, but not always, painful.

⚠ There may be rapid and severe haemorrhage from a placenta praevia.

⚠ Most bleeding from an abruption is concealed.

Vasa praevia
- This occurs when the fetal vessels run in membranes below the presenting fetal part, unsupported by placental tissue or umbilical cord.
- Incidence is believed to be 1:2500 to 1:2700.
- May present with PV bleeding after rupture of fetal membranes followed by rapid fetal distress (from exsanguination).
- Reported fetal mortality ranges between 33% and 100%.
- Risk factors include:
  - low-lying placenta
  - multiple pregnancy
  - IVF pregnancy
  - bilobed and especially succenturiate lobed placentas.

Antepartum haemorrhage: assessment

Initial assessment

Rapid assessment of maternal and fetal condition is a vital first step as it may prove to be an obstetric emergency.

History

A basic clinical history should establish:
- Gestational age.
- Amount of bleeding (but don't forget concealed abruption).
- Associated or initiating factors (coitus/trauma).
- Abdominal pain.
- Fetal movements.
- Date of last smear.
- Previous episodes of PV bleeding in this pregnancy.
- Leakage of fluid PV.
- Previous uterine surgery (including CS).
- Smoking and use of illegal drugs (especially cocaine).
- Blood group and rhesus status (will she need anti-D?).
- Previous obstetric history (placental abruption/IUGR, placenta praevia).
- Position of placenta, if known from previous scan.

Maternal assessment

This should include:
- Blood pressure.
- Pulse.
- Other signs of haemodynamic compromise (e.g. peripheral vaso-constriction or central cyanosis).
- Uterine palpation for size, tenderness, fetal lie, presenting part (if it is engaged, it is not a placenta praevia).

⚠ Remember, never perform a vaginal examination (VE) in presence of PV bleeding without first excluding a placenta praevia ('No PV until no PP').

Once a placenta praevia is excluded, a speculum examination should be undertaken to assess degree of bleeding, possible local causes of bleeding (trauma, polyps, ectropion), and to determine if membranes ruptured. A digital examination will ascertain cervical changes indicative of labour.

Fetal assessment
- Establish whether a fetal heart can be heard.
- Ensure that it is fetal and not maternal (remember, the mother may be very tachycardic).
- If fetal heart is heard and gestation is estimated to be 26 weeks or more, FHR monitoring should be commenced.

Placenta praevia (PP): see Fig. 2.1

Definition
- When the placenta is inserted, wholly or in part, into the lower segment of the uterus.

Major (grade III or IV)
The placenta lies over the cervical os.

⚠ Cervical effacement and dilatation would result in catastrophic bleeding and potential maternal and therefore fetal death.

Minor (grade I or II)
The placenta lies in the lower segment, close to or encroaching on, the cervical os

Incidence
About 0.5% of pregnancies at term

Diagnosis
Transvaginal USS is safe and is more accurate than transabdominal USS in locating the placenta.

Management
- Women with major PP who have previously bled should be admitted from 34 weeks gestation.
- Women with asymptomatic major PP may remain at home if they:
  - are close to the hospital
  - are fully aware of the risks to themselves and their baby
  - have a constant companion
  - have telecommunication and transport.

Delivery is likely to be by CS if the placental edge is <2 cm from the internal os, especially if it is posterior or thick.

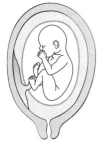
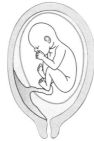
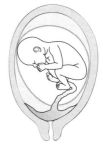

Normal placenta   Minor placenta praevia   Major placenta praevia

Fig. 2.1 Placenta praevia.

Antepartum haemorrhage: management

Following assessment, women will fall into one of two categories:
- Bleeding is heavy and continuing, and mother or fetus is, or soon will be, compromised (see 📖 Chapter 10: Massive obstetric haemorrhage, p. 377).
- Bleeding minor, or settling, and neither mother nor fetus compromised: see below.

Limited APH

If the bleeding was minor, is settling and there are no signs of compromise, the following investigations should be undertaken:

Maternal:
- FBC.
- Kleihauer testing, if woman known to be RhD negative, to determine extent of feto-maternal haemorrhage and if more anti-D is required.
- Group and save serum.
- Coagulation screen may be useful in cases of suspected abruption.

▶ In the event of APH, all RhD negative women require 500 IU of anti-D immunoglobulin, unless they are already sensitized.
More anti-D may be required based on the result of the Kleihauer test.

Fetal
- Ultrasound to establish fetal well-being (growth/volume of amniotic fluid) and to confirm placental location.
- Umbilical artery Doppler measurement (the function of the placenta may be compromised by small abruptions).
- Ongoing antenatal management after a limited APH.
- Most units admit women who have had an APH for 24 hours, as the risk of further bleeding is estimated to be greatest during that time.
- If the bleeding settles and mother is discharged, a clear plan for remaining pregnancy should be made including extra fetal surveillance of growth and well-being.
- If all remains well, induction at term is not usually indicated.
- Surveillance after due date may need to be increased.

▶ Management must be individualized according to suspected cause of bleeding, gestation, fetal assessment and continuing maternal risk factors.

💕 Management of women with a minor placenta praevia and minimal or no ongoing PV bleeding at an early gestation is controversial.

📖 RCOG Guideline 27. Placenta praevia and placenta accreta: Diagnosis and management. www. rcog.org.uk

⚠ All women who have had an APH are high-risk and surveillance of both mother and fetus needs to be ↑.
⚠ History of APH ↑ risk of bleeding at delivery 'APH=PPH'.

Placental abruption

Definition
When the placenta separates from the uterus before delivery of the fetus. Blood accumulates behind the placenta, in the uterine cavity or is lost through the cervix.

Types
• Concealed: no external bleeding evident (<20%).
• Revealed: vaginal bleeding.

Presentation
• Usually present with abdominal pain.
• Typically sudden onset, constant and severe.
• Posterior placentas may give rise to severe backache.
• The uterus is tender on palpation.
• Uterine activity is common.
• The uterus may later become hard (often described as 'woody').
• Many will be in labour (up to 50% on presentation).
• Bleeding is very variable, often dark.
• Maternal hypovolaemia is evident with large abruptions.
• Maternal signs of shock.
• Fetal distress is common and precedes fetal death.

⚠ Remember the extent of the maternal haemorrhage may be much greater then the apparent vaginal loss

Incidence
0.5–1.0% of pregnancies.

Diagnosis
The diagnosis is made clinically. Ultrasound is of use to confirm fetal well-being and exclude placenta praevia.

Management
• Admit all women with vaginal bleeding or unexplained abdominal pain.
• Establish immediate fetal well-being with cardiotocography (CTG) and USS ASAP.
• If fetal distress or maternal compromise, resuscitate and deliver (see 📖 Chapter 10: Massive obstetric haemorrhage, p. 377)
• If no fetal distress, and bleeding and pain cease, consider delivery by term.

Blood pressure in pregnancy: physiology

Basic physiology

Blood pressure (BP) is directly related to systemic vascular resistance and cardiac output and follows a distinct course during pregnancy:

- ↓ in early pregnancy until 24 weeks due to a ↓ in vascular resistance.
- ↑ after 24 weeks until delivery via an ↑ in stroke volume.
- ↓ after delivery but may peak again 3–4 days postpartum.

⚠ Most women book in the 1st or 2nd trimester, so be aware of the pregnant woman with a high booking BP; she may have previously undetected chronic hypertension. This is especially important in older pregnant women.

Blood pressure measurement

- BP must be measured correctly to avoid falsely high or low readings that may influence clinical management.
- BP should be measured sitting or in the supine position with a left sided tilt (to avoid compression of the inferior vena cava by the pregnant uterus which reduces blood flow to the heart and consequently stroke volume and leads to falsely low BP) with the upper arm at the level of the heart.
- Use the correct cuff size (a normal adult cuff is usually for an upper arm of 34 cm or less). A cuff too small may lead to a falsely high reading.
- The diastolic BP should be taken as Korotkoff V (the absence of sound) rather than Korotkoff IV (muffling of sound), which was previously used, unless the sound is heard all the way down to zero.

⚠ Be aware of the use of automated BP monitors. They may under-record the BP especially in pre-eclampsia. If unsure, check with a sphygmomanometer.

Blood pressure in pregnancy: hypertension

Pre-eclampsia
See 📖 p. 62.

Pregnancy-induced hypertension (PIH)

- Defined as hypertension in the second half of pregnancy in the absence of proteinuria or other markers of pre-eclampsia.
- Affects 6–7% of pregnancies
- At ↑ risk of going on to develop pre-eclampsia (15–26%).
- The risk ↑ with earlier onset of hypertension.
- Delivery should be aimed at the time of the EDD.
- BP usually returns to pre-pregnancy limits within 6 weeks of delivery.

Chronic hypertension
- It complicates 3–5% of pregnancies.
- Pregnant women who have a high booking BP (130–140/80–90 or more) are likely to have chronic hypertension.
- Increased risk of developing pre-eclampsia.
- Delivery should be planned at around the time of the EDD.

▶ Now more common because of an older pregnant population.

⚠ If BP is very high it is important to exclude a secondary cause rather than attributing it to essential hypertension.

Postpartum hypertension
- New hypertension may arise in the postpartum period.
- It is important to determine whether this is physiological, pre-existing chronic hypertension or new onset pre-eclampsia.

▶ Remember BP peaks on the 3rd to 4th day postpartum.

⚠ Symptoms such as epigastric pain or visual disturbance and new-onset proteinuria are more suggestive of postpartum pre-eclampsia.

Postnatal management of hypertension
- Postnatally methyldopa should be changed to a β-blocker because of the risk of postnatal depression (see Table 2.1).
- Captopril can be used (up to 25 mg PO tds).
- Nifedipine (10 mg PO bd up to 30 mg PO qds) may also be used.

▶ Women should be told that breast-feeding is safe with these drugs.

- The GP can follow up the BP in the community and titrate the medication to the BP.
- Women on medication should be offered a postnatal follow up appointment 6 weeks postnatally.
- The BP may stay raised for up to 6 months.
- If still raised after this it is important to look for secondary causes of hypertension.

Secondary causes of hypertension

- Renal disease.
- Cardiac disease, e.g. coarctation of the aorta.
- Endocrine causes, e.g. Cushing's syndrome, Conn's syndrome, or rarely a phaeochromocytoma.

Women with chronic hypertension are at risk of:

- Superimposed pre-eclampsia.
- Fetal growth restriction.
- Placental abruption.

Table 2.1 Antihypertensive medications

Medication	Dose	Side effects	Breast-feeding
Methyldopa	250 mg bd up to 1 g tds	Depression change postnatally	Yes
Nifedipine	10 mg bd up to 30 mg tds	Tachycardia, flushing headache	Yes
Hydralazine	25 mg tds up to 75 mg qds	Tachycardia and pounding heartbeat headache, diarrhoea	Yes
Atenolol	50–100 mg od	Avoid in asthma	Yes
Oxprenolol	80 mg tds to 120 mg tds	Avoid in asthma May cause nightmares	Yes
Labetalol	100 mg bd up to 600 mg qds	Avoid in asthma	
	IV Infusion for severe refractory hypertension		Yes
ACE inhibitors	Postpartum only, as fetotoxic		captopril safe

Pre-eclampsia: overview

Pre-eclampsia is a multisystem disorder characterized by hypertension and proteinuria and is thought to arise from the placenta. However, it can present in a wide variety of ways and not always in the classical fashion. It has a wide spectrum of severity ranging form mild to severe (eclampsia). It is a leading cause of maternal morbidity and mortality in the UK. It is a common cause of prematurity and hospital admission and has huge economic implications.

Definition of pre-eclampsia

Due to its heterogeneous nature it can be difficult to define clinically.
- It is usually taken to be a BP ≥140/90 AND ≥300 mg proteinuria in a 24-hour collection.
- In those women who are already hypertensive a rise in the systolic BP ≥ 30 mmHg or diastolic BP ≥ 15 mmHg is used.
- There may be other clues such as abnormal biochemistry or fetal growth restriction.

▶ Several individual features may add up to a diagnosis of pre-eclampsia.

Incidence
- Pre-eclampsia affects up to 10% of pregnancies (usually in a mild form).
- Severe pre-eclampsia affects up to 1% of pregnancies.

Prediction of pre-eclampsia (see text box on p. 63)
History:
- There is an increased (×7) chance of pre-eclampsia in subsequent pregnancies in women who have had pre-eclampsia before.
- The risk increases with earlier onset, increasing severity, and HELLP syndrome (see 📖 p. 68).
- Presence of other risk factors such as medical disease, family history.
- **Blood tests**:
  - raised uric acid, low platelets and high Hb may help differentiate pre-eclampsia from PIH before proteinuria occurs
  - interest is growing in vascular endothelial growth factor (VEGF) and placental growth factor (PlGF) (↓ before pre-eclampsia develops), and soluble fms-like tyrosine kinase 1 (sFlt-1) (↑ before pre-eclampsia is manifest).
- **Ultrasound**:
  - uterine artery Dopplers at 22–24 weeks are predictive of early onset or severe pre-eclampsia.

Prevention of pre-eclampsia
Women who have had severe early-onset pre-eclampsia should be offered low-dose aspirin (75 mg po od) in the next pregnancy as it may reduce the incidence of repeat severe pre-eclampsia.

Risk factors for pre-eclampsia

- Previous severe/early onset pre-eclampsia ×7.
- Age >40 or teenager.
- Family history (mother or sister) ×4.
- Obesity (BMI > 30) ×2.
- Primiparity ×2–3.
- Multiple pregnancy ×2.
- Long birth interval (>10 years) ×2–3.
- Fetal hydrops.
- Hydatidiform mole.
- Pre-existing medical conditions:
  - hypertension
  - renal disease
  - diabetes
  - antiphospholipid antibodies
  - thrombophilias
  - connective tissue disease.

Pre-eclampsia: clinical features and investigations

Pre-eclampsia can present with a wide variety of signs and symptoms. It presents to the clinician a diagnostic dilemma and never ceases to surprise. Many women with pre-eclampsia are asymptomatic.

Symptoms
- Headache (esp. frontal).
- Visual disturbance (esp. flashing lights).
- Epigastric or RUQ pain.
- Nausea and vomiting.
- Rapid oedema (esp. face).

⚠ Symptoms usually occur only with severe disease.

Signs
- Hypertension (>140/90; severe if >170/110).
- Proteinuria (>300 mg in 24 hours).
- Facial oedema.
- Epigastric/RUQ tenderness is a sign of liver involvement and capsule distension.
- Confusion.
- Hyperreflexia and/or clonus (>3 beats) is a sign of cerebral irritability.
- Uterine tenderness or vaginal bleeding from a placental abruption.
- Fetal growth restriction on ultrasound, particularly if <36 weeks.

Laboratory investigations
FBC
- Relative high Hb due to haemoconcentration.
- Thrombocytopaenia.
- Anaemia if haemolysis (HELLP—see 📖 p. 68).

Coagulation profile
- Prolonged PT and APTT.

Biochemistry
- ↑ urate.
- ↑ urea and creatinine.
- Abnormal LFTs (↑ transaminases).
- ↑ LDH (a marker for haemolysis).
- ↑ proteinuria (>300 mg protein/24 hours).

Pre-eclampsia: management

Pre-eclampsia has a number of severe complications (see box). The cure is delivery of the placenta. Management depends on several issues including maternal and fetal well-being and gestational age.

Severe complications of pre-eclampsia

- Eclampsia.
- HELLP (haemolysis, elevated liver enzymes, and low platelets).
- Cerebral haemorrhage.
- Disseminated intravascular coagulation (DIC).
- Renal failure.
- Placental abruption.

Outpatient management of pre-eclampsia

- Appropriate if:
  - BP <160 systolic and <110 diastolic and can be controlled
  - no or low (≤1+/ <300 mg per 24 hours) proteinuria
  - asymptomatic.
- Difficult to distinguish from gestational hypertension.
- Warn about development of symptoms.
- 1–2 per week review of BP and urine.
- Weekly review of blood biochemistry.

Mild–moderate pre-eclampsia:

- BP <160 systolic and <110 diastolic with significant proteinuria and no maternal complications.
- Once significant proteinuria occurs, admission is advised:
  - ≥ 2+ protein
  - >300 mg proteinuria/24 hours
  - a split protein:creatinine ratio can be a useful screening test for proteinuria—check with your lab for their normal values but in general >30 equates to >300 mg proteinuria/24 hours.
- 4 hourly BP.
- 24 hour urine collection for protein.
- Daily urinalysis.
- Daily fetal assessment with CTG.
- Regular blood tests (every 2–3 days unless symptoms or signs worsen).
- Regular ultrasound assessment (fortnightly growth and twice weekly Doppler/liquor volume depending on severity of pre-eclampsia).

▶ If BP increases (>160 systolic OR >110 diastolic) anti-hypertensive therapy should be started (see Table 2.1, p. 61). Medication does not cure the condition but its aim is to prevent the hypertensive complications of pre-eclampsia.

Severe pre-eclampsia: management

⚠ Defined as the occurrence of BP ≥160 systolic or ≥110 diastolic in the presence of significant proteinuria (≥1 g/24 hours or ≥2+ on dipstick), **or** if maternal complications occur.

▶ Senior obstetric, anaesthetic, and midwifery staff should be informed and be involved in the management of a woman with severe pre-eclampsia.

BP management

- ⚠ BP needs to be stabilized with antihypertensive medication (must aim for <160 systolic AND <110 diastolic).
- Initially use PO nifedipine 10 mg:
  - can be given twice half an hour apart.
- If BP remains high after nifedipine:
  - start IV labetalol infusion
  - ↑ infusion rate until BP is adequately controlled.
- IV hydralazine may be used in some units.

Other management

- Take bloods for FBC, U+Es, LFTs and clotting profile
- Strict fluid balance chart:
  - consider a catheter.
- CTG monitoring of fetus until condition stable.
- Ultrasound of the fetus:
  - evidence of IUGR
  - establish weight if severely preterm
  - assess condition using fetal and umbilical artery Doppler.

⚠ If <34 weeks steroids should be given and the pregnancy may be managed expectantly unless the maternal or fetal condition worsens.

Treatment

- The only treatment is delivery, but this can be delayed with intensive monitoring if <34 weeks
- Pre-eclampsia often worsens for 24 hours after delivery.

Indications for immediate delivery include:

- Worsening thrombocytopaenia or coaguloathy.
- Worsening liver or renal function.
- Severe maternal symptoms, especially epigastric pain.
- Fetal reasons such as fetal distress or reversed umbilical artery flow.
- HELLP syndrome or eclampsia.

Eclampsia and HELLP syndrome

Eclampsia

Eclampsia is defined as the occurrence of a tonic clonic seizure in association with a diagnosis of pre-eclampsia.

- It complicates approximately 1–2 % of pre-eclamptic pregnancies.
- It may be the initial presentation of pre-eclampsia and occur without hypertension or proteinuria.
- Fits may occur antenatally (38%), intrapartum (18%) or postnatally usually within the first 48 hours (44%).

⚠ Eclampsia is an obstetric emergency. Every hospital in the UK should have an eclampsia protocol and eclampsia box with all the drugs for treatment.

⚠ When new to a hospital go and familiarize yourself with the protocol and the whereabouts of the drug box.

⚠ Eclampsia is a sign of severe disease: most women who die with pre-eclampsia or eclampsia, do so from other complications such as blood loss, intracranial haemorrhage, or HELLP.

HELLP syndrome

Serious complication regarded by most as a variant of severe pre-eclampsia which manifests with haemolysis (H), elevated liver enzymes (EL) and low platelets (LP).

- Incidence is estimated at 5–20% of pre-eclamptic pregnancies.
- Maternal mortality is estimated at 1% with perinatal mortality estimates of 10–60%
- Commonly, liver enzymes ↑ and platelets ↓ before haemolysis occurs.
- Syndrome is usually self-limiting but permanent liver or renal damage may occur.
- Symptoms include:
  - epigastric or RUQ pain (65%)
  - nausea and vomiting (35%)
- Signs include
  - tenderness RUQ
  - ↑ BP and other features of pre-eclampsia.
- Eclampsia may coexist.
- Delivery is indicated.
- Treatment is supportive and as for eclampsia.
- Although platelet levels may be very low, platelet infusions are only required if bleeding, or for surgery and <40.

⚠ Beware of epigastric pain in pregnant and immediately postnatal women: always check the BP, urine, and liver enzymes.

Management of eclampsia

▶▶ Call for help—obstetric SpR, SHO and consultant, anaesthetic SpR and consultant, delivery suite coordinator.
- Basic principles of airway, breathing and circulation plus IV access.
- Most eclamptic fits are short lasting and terminate spontaneously.
- Magnesium ($MgSO_4$) is the drug of choice for both control of fits and preventing (further) seizures.
- A loading dose of 4 g should be given over 5–10 minutes followed by an infusion of 1 g/hour for 24 hours.
- If further fits another dose of 2 g can be given as a bolus (the therapeutic range for magnesium is 2–4 mmol/L).
- In repeated seizures use diazepam (if still fitting the patient may need intubation and ventilation and imaging of the head to rule out a cerebral haemorrhage).
- Strict monitoring of the patient is mandatory.
- Pulse, BP, respiration rate, and oxygen saturations every 15 minutes.
- A urometer and hourly urine.
- Assessment of reflexes every hour for Mg toxicity (usually knee reflexes, but use biceps if epidural in situ).
- Mg toxicity is characterized by confusion, loss of reflexes and respiratory depression.
- Half/stop infusion if oliguric (<20 mL/hour) or raised creatinine and seek senior/renal advice.
- If toxic give 1 g calcium gluconate over 10 minutes.
- If hypertensive (BP > 160/110) give BP-lowering drugs:
  - oral nifedipine
  - IV labetalol (avoid in asthmatics).
- Fluid restrict the patient to 80 mL/hour or 1 mL/kg/hour due to the risk of pulmonary oedema (even if oliguric the risk of renal failure is small), monitor the renal function with the creatinine.
- A CVP may be needed if there has been associated maternal haemorrhage and fluid balance is difficult or if the creatinine rises.
- The fetus should be continuously monitored with the CTG.
- Deliver the fetus once stable.
- Vaginal delivery is not contraindicated if the cervix is favourable.
- If HELLP syndrome coexists, consider high-dose steroids, involvement of renal and liver physicians.
- The 3rd stage should be managed with 5–10 units oxytocin rather than Syntometrine® or ergometrine because of the increase in BP.

Multiple pregnancy: overview

Incidence
- About 1 in 34 babies born in the UK is a twin or triplet. The incidence of multiple pregnancy had been rising but now appears to be stable at:
  - twins—15:1000
  - triplets—1:5000
  - quadruplets—1:360 000
- Higher multiples than this are extremely rare but do occur:
  - a surviving set of quintuplets was born in the UK in 2007.

📖 www.multiplebirths.org.uk

Aetiology
There are multiple predisposing factors including:
- Previous multiple pregnancy.
- Family history.
- Increasing parity.
- Increasing maternal age:
  - <20 years: 6:1000
  - >35 years: 22:1000
  - >45 years: 57:1000.
- Ethnicity:
  - Nigeria: 40:1000
  - Japan: 7:1000.
- Assisted reproduction—incidence of multiple pregnancy:
  - clomiphene—10%
  - intrauterine insemination (IUI)—10–20%
  - *in vitro* fertilization (IVF) with 2 embryo transfer—20–30%.

▶ In an attempt to decrease this complication, the Human Fertilisation and Embryology Authority (HFEA) recommend that no more than two embryos should be transferred per IVF cycle.

📖 www.hfea.gov.uk/cps/rde/xchg/hfea

Multiple pregnancy: types

Dizygotic twins

Dizygotic twins are a result of two separate ova being fertilized by different sperm and simultaneously implanting and developing. Consequently these fetuses will have separate amniotic membranes and placentas (dichorionic and diamniotic—DCDA). These twins may be of different sex. This mechanism accounts for two thirds of multiple pregnancies and it is this type that is most affected by predisposing factors such as age and ethnicity.

Monozygotic twins

Monozygotic twins result from the division into two of a single, already developing, embryo. These twins are genetically identical and are therefore always the same sex. Whether they share the same amniotic membrane and/or chorion depends on the stage of development when the embryo divides. About two thirds are monochorionic diamniotic.

See Fig. 2.2 for an explanation of the mechanism of twinning.

Timing of division in monozygotic twins
- <3 days → dichorionic, diamniotic (DCDA) 30%.
- 4–7 days → monochorionic, diamniotic (MCDA) 70%.
- 8–12 days → monochorionic, monoamniotic (MCMA) <1%.
- >12 days → conjoined twins (very rare).

The worldwide monozygotic twining rate appears to be constant at about 3.5 per 1000. However, the rate is slightly greater than expected with IVF treatment.

Diagnosis

There are several signs and symptoms associated with multiple pregnancy including:
- Hyperemesis gravidarum.
- Uterus is larger than expected for dates.
- Three or more fetal poles may be palpable >24 weeks.
- Two fetal hearts may be heard on auscultation.

However, the vast majority are diagnosed on ultrasound in the 1st trimester (at a dating or nuchal translucency scan). As most women in the UK now have an ultrasound scan at some stage in their pregnancy, the diagnosis is rarely missed.

Chorionicity

Determining chorionicity allows risk stratification for multiple pregnancy and is best done by ultrasound in the 1st trimester or early in the 2nd. The key indicators are:
- Obviously widely separated sacs or placentae—dichorionic.
- Membrane insertion showing the lambda sign—dichorionic.
- Absence of lambda sign <14 weeks diagnostic of monochorionic.
- Fetuses of different sex—dichorionic (dizygotic).

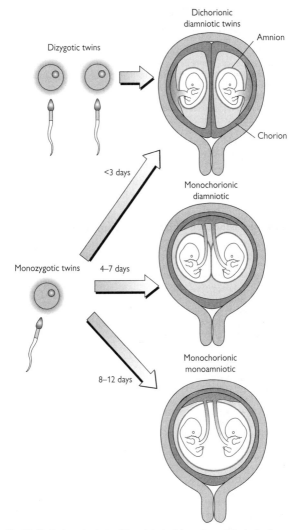

Fig. 2.2 Mechanism of twinning. Dizygotic twins (a) are always dichorionic, diamnoitic, but with monozygotic twins (a, b and c), the type will depend on the time of the division of the conceptus.

Multiple pregnancy: antenatal care

- All multiple pregnancies are by definition 'high risk' and the care should be consultant led.
- Establish chorionicity: this is most accurately diagnosed in the 1st trimester (absence of lambda sign diagnostic), so an early USS should be considered with any indications of multiple pregnancy (e.g. fundus palpable before 12 weeks or exaggerated symptoms of early pregnancy).
- Routine use of iron and folate supplements should be considered.
- A detailed anomaly scan should be undertaken.
- Serial growth scans at 28, 32, and 36 weeks for dichorionic twins.
- More frequent antenatal checks because of ↑ risk of pre-eclampsia.
- Discuss mode of delivery.
- Establish presentation of leading twin by 34 weeks.
- Consider delivery at 38 weeks: induction.

⚠ Surveillance needs to be more intensive for monochorionic twins particularly <24 weeks, or higher multiples, so referral to a specialist fetal medicine team is advisable.

Fetal risks associated with multiple pregnancy

- ↑ risk of miscarriage—especially with monochorionic twins.
- Congenital abnormalities more common in monochorionic twins including:
  - neural tube defects
  - cardiac abnormalities
  - gastrointestinal atresia.
- Intrauterine growth restriction (IUGR)—up to 25% of twins.
- Preterm labour—main cause of perinatal morbidity and mortality:
  - 40% twins deliver before 37 weeks
  - 10% twins deliver before 32 weeks.
- ↑ perinatal mortality:
  - singletons 5:1000
  - twins 18:1000
  - triplets 53:1000.
- ↑ risk of intrauterine death (stillbirth):
  - singletons 8:1000
  - twins 31:1000
  - triplets 84:1000.
- ↑ risk of disability (mainly, but not entirely, due to prematurity and low birth weight).
- ↑ incidence of cerebral palsy:
  - singletons 2:1000
  - twins 7:1000
  - triplets 27:1000.
- Vanishing twin syndrome—one twin apparently being reabsorbed at an early gestation (1st trimester).

Maternal risks associated with multiple pregnancy

The risks of pregnancy appear to be heightened with twins compared to singletons, leaving mothers at an increased risk of:
- Hyperemesis gravidarum.
- Anaemia.
- Pre-eclampsia (5× greater risk with twins than singletons).
- Gestational diabetes.
- Polyhydramnios.
- Placenta praevia.
- Antepartum and postpartum haemorrhage.
- Operative delivery.

Coping with more than one baby

There are significant financial implications arising from multiple births, as well as the time commitment involved in caring for more than one newborn baby.
- Breastfeeding may be psychologically as well as physically demanding.
- Unsurprisingly, the incidence of postnatal depression is higher among mothers of twins.
- There are several support groups available and their assistance must not be underestimated.

📖 Twins and multiple birth association www.tamba.org.uk

Twin-to-twin transfusion syndrome (TTTS)

This affects about 5–25% of monochorionic twin pregnancies and left untreated has an 80% mortality rate. It may occur acutely at any stage or more commonly take a chronic course, which at its worst, leads to severe fetal compromise at a gestation too early to consider delivery. It is caused by aberrant vascular anastamoses within the placenta which redistribute the fetal blood. Effectively, blood from the 'donor' twin is transfused to the 'recipient' twin.

Effects of twin-to-twin transfusion on the fetus

Donor twin:
- Hypovolaemic and anaemic.
- Oligohydramnios—appear 'stuck' to the placenta or uterine wall.
- Growth restriction.

Recipient twin:
- Hypervolaemic and polycythaemic.
- Large bladder and polyhydramnios.
- Evidence of fetal hydrops (ascites, pleural and pericardial effusions)
- This twin is often more at risk than the donor.

▶ Monochorionic twins require intensive monitoring for signs of twin-to-twin transfusion syndrome, usually in the form of serial USS at fortnightly intervals from 12 weeks. This is best performed in a specialist fetal medicine unit. The treatment options potentially available include:
- Laser ablation of the placental anastamoses. This method is associated with a lower risk of neonatal handicap.
- Selective feticide by cord occlusion is reserved for refractory disease.
- Serial amnioreductions: mainly symptomatic relief only.
- Septostomy—allows equilibration between the two amniotic sacs.

📖 www.eurofoetus.org

Intrauterine death of a twin

- **Dichorionic:** the death of one twin in the 1st trimester or early part of the 2nd does not appear to adversely affect the remaining fetus. Loss in the late part of the 2nd or 3rd trimester usually precipitates labour, with 90% having delivered within 3 weeks.
- **Monochorionic**: because of the shared circulation, subsequent death or severe damage from hypovolaemia follows in up to 25% where one of the pair dies. There is little evidence that immediate delivery decreases the risk of brain injury.

Multiple pregnancy: labour

- For all multiple pregnancies mode of delivery is debated and a RCT is in progress.
- The second twin is at increased risk of perinatal mortality but it is not currently the case that all twins should be delivered by CS.
- For labour, the leading twin should be cephalic (~80%), and there should be no absolute contraindication (e.g. two previous CS).
- Triplets and higher-order multiples are usually delivered by CS.
- Some authorities advise CS for monochorionic twins.

For management of labour and delivery see text box on p. 79.

Intrapartum risks associated with multiple pregnancy include:

- Malpresentation.
- Fetal hypoxia in second twin after delivery of the first.
- Cord prolapse.
- Operative delivery.
- Postpartum haemorrhage.
- Rare:
  - cord entanglement (MCMA twins only)
  - head entrapment with each other: 'locked twins'.

Management of labour and delivery for twins

- Twins are usually induced at ~38 weeks gestation but many will have delivered spontaneously before then.
- The woman should have IV access and a current G+S.
- Fetal distress is more common in twins; continuous fetal monitoring with CTG is important throughout labour.
- This becomes imperative after the first twin has delivered to avoid hypoxia in the second.
- It may be helpful to monitor the leading twin with a fetal scalp electrode and the other abdominally.
- An epidural may be helpful, especially if there are difficulties delivering the second twin, but is not essential.
- Many units choose to deliver twins in theatre as there is more space available and it provides immediate recourse to surgical intervention if required.
- The importance of support for the mother cannot be overestimated.
- The leading twin should be delivered as for a singleton but with care to ensure adequate monitoring of the second throughout.
- After delivery of the first baby, the lie of the second twin should be checked and gently 'stabilized' by abdominal palpation while a VE is performed to assess the station of the presenting part.
- It may be helpful to have an ultrasound scanner available in case of concerns about malpresentation of the second twin.
- Once the presenting part enters the pelvis the membranes can be broken and the second twin is usually delivered within 20 minutes of the first.
- Judicious use of oxytocin may help if the contractions diminish after delivery of the first twin.
- If fetal distress occurs in the second twin, delivery may be expedited with either forceps or ventouse.
- If this is inappropriate, the choice is between CS or breech extraction (often after internal podalic version).
- Breech extraction involves gentle and continuous traction on one or both feet and must only be performed by an experienced obstetrician.
- It is never used to deliver singleton breeches.
- As there is an increased risk of uterine atony, syntometrine and prophylactic oxytocin infusion is recommended.

Breech presentation: overview

Breech presentation occurs when the baby's buttocks lie over the maternal pelvis. The lie is longitudinal, and the head is found in the fundus. This becomes decreasingly common with gestation, such that breech presentation at term occurs with only 3–4% of fetuses, but is much more common preterm.

Types of breech

- Extended breeches (70%):
  - both legs extended with feet by head; presenting part is the buttocks.
- Flexed breeches (15%):
  - legs flexed at the knees so that both buttocks and feet are presenting.
- Footling breeches (15%):
  - one leg flexed and one extended.

Causes and associations of breech presentation

- Idiopathic (most common).
- Preterm delivery.
- Previous breech presentation.
- Uterine abnormalities e.g. fibroids and Mullerian duct abnormalities.
- Placenta praevia and obstructions to the pelvis.
- Fetal abnormalities.
- Multiple pregnancy.

Consequences of breech presentation

Fetal

- There is an increased risk of hypoxia and trauma in labour.
- Irrespective of the mode of delivery, neonatal and longer-term risks are increased. The reasons for this are incompletely understood but may be due in part to:
  - association with congenital abnormalities
  - many preterm babies are breech at the time of delivery.

Maternal

Most breeches are delivered by CS.

Diagnosis of breech presentation

- Before 36 weeks breech presentation is not important unless the woman is in labour.
- Breech presentation is commonly undiagnosed before labour (30%).
- On examination:
  - lie is longitudinal
  - the head can be palpated at the fundus
  - the presenting part is not hard
  - the fetal heart is best heard high up on the uterus
- Ultrasound confirms the diagnosis and should also assess growth and anatomy because of the association with fetal abnormalities.

External cephalic version (ECV)

- This is performed from 36 weeks in nulliparous women and 37 weeks in multiparous ones. The intention is to reduce the need for delivery by CS.
- **Method:** after USS, a forward roll technique is used. The breech is elevated from the pelvis, and pushed to the side where the back is; the head is then pushed forward and the roll completed. Excessive force must not be used. After the attempt, CTG is performed and anti-D given if the mother is Rh negative. See Fig. 2.3.
- **Efficacy:** the success rate is about 50%. Spontaneous reversion to breech presentation occurs in 3%. Attempting ECV halves the chance of non-cephalic presentation at delivery and greatly reduces the risk of CS. Nulliparity, difficulty palpating the head, high uterine tone, an engaged breech, less amniotic fluid, and white ethnicity are associated with more difficulty.
- **Facilitation:** success rates are increased by the use of tocolysis, such as salbutamol, given either electively or if a first attempt fails. Epidural or spinal analgesia are not usually used.
- **Safety:** approximately 0.5% will require immediate delivery by CS due to fetal heart rate abnormalities or vaginal bleeding. Theoretical and minor risks include pain, precipitation of labour, placental abruption, fetomaternal haemorrhage, and cord accidents. The chances of CS during labour are slightly higher than with a fetus that has always been cephalic.
- **Other methods:** So-called natural methods of version (postural methods, acupuncture, moxabustion) remain unproven.

Contraindications to ECV

Absolute
- Caesarean delivery already indicated.
- Antepartum haemorrhage.
- Fetal compromise.
- Oligohydramnios.
- Rhesus isoimmunization.
- Pre-eclampsia.

Relative
- One previous CS.
- Fetal abnormality.
- Maternal hypertension.

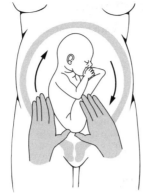

1. Gently disimpact the breech from the pelvis, guiding it towards the iliac fossa

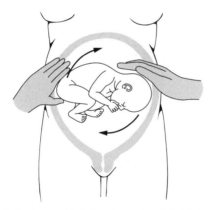

2. Continue to guide the breech upwards until the baby is transverse, then gentle pressure on the occiput helps to complete the forward roll.

Fig. 2.3 External cephalic version.

Breech presentation: delivery

Mode of delivery of breech presentation

- If ECV is declined or fails, or the breech is undiagnosed, the parents should be appraised of the evidence about breech birth.
- Most breech deliveries in the UK, USA, and Europe are by CS, because meta-analysis of RCTs has shown this to reduce neonatal mortality and short-term morbidity, although not longer-term morbidity.
- Elective CS appears protective even where the ideal conditions for vaginal delivery are present and the attendant is highly experienced.
- This policy does not increase maternal morbidity because attempting a vaginal delivery still carries a considerable risk of emergency CS, which is a more risky procedure
- These findings have been criticized because of the trials' methodology and the way that breech labours were managed; nevertheless this is the best evidence currently available.
- The breech in advanced labour, or who is a second twin, or preterm is not necessarily best delivered by CS.

Vaginal delivery of the breech fetus

Knowledge and experience of this remains important because breech delivery requires skill and will occasionally be inevitable because of diagnosis in advanced labour or because of the mother's wishes.

Ideal selection for vaginal breech delivery

- Fetus is not compromised.
- Estimated fetal weight is <4 kg.
- Spontaneous onset of labour.
- Extended breech presentation.

⚠ There is a risk of cord prolapse which is greatest in footling breeches (15%).

⚠ Oxytocin augmentation is not advised and failure of the buttocks to descend after full dilatation is a sign that delivery may be difficult.

📖 Hannah et al. Planned Caesarean section versus planned vaginal birth for breech presentation at term: a randomized multi-centre trial. *The Lancet*, 2000;356:1375–83.

Vaginal breech delivery technique

- Maternal effort should be delayed until the buttocks are visible.
- After delivery of the buttocks the baby is encouraged to remain back upwards but should not otherwise be touched until the scapula is visible.
- The arms are then hooked down by the index finger at the fetal elbow bringing them down its chest.
- The body is then allowed to hang.
- If the arms are stretched above the chest and cannot be reached, *Lovset's* manoeuvre is required.
  - This involves placing the hands around the body with the thumbs on the sacrum and rotating the baby clockwise 180° clockwise and then counterclockwise with gentle downward traction.
  - This allows the anterior shoulder and then the posterior shoulder to enter the pelvis and for the arm to be delivered from below the pubic arch.
- When the nape of the neck is visible, delivery is achieved by placing two fingers of the right hand over the maxilla and two fingers of the left at the back of the head to flex it (*Mauriceau–Smellie–Veit* manoeuvre) and maternal pushing is encouraged.
- If this fails to deliver the head, forceps should be applied before the next contraction.
- Delivery of the head should be gentle and controlled to avoid rapid decompression which could cause intracranial bleeding.
- The upright position for delivery is advocated by some experienced attendants but there is no proof that this makes delivery safer.

Transverse, oblique, and unstable lie

Definition

- A **transverse** or **oblique** lie occurs when the axis of the fetus is across the axis of the uterus. This is common before term, but occurs in only 1% of fetuses after 37 weeks.
- **Unstable** lie occurs when the lie is still changing, usually several times a day, and may be transverse or longitudinal lie, and cephalic or breech presentation. See Fig. 2.4.

Causes and associations of abnormal fetal lie

- Multiparity (particularly >para 2) with lax uterus (common).
- Polohydramnios.
- Uterine abnormalities, e.g. fibroids and Mullerian duct abnormalities.
- Placenta praevia and obstructions to the pelvis.
- Fetal abnormalities.
- Multiple pregnancy.

Assessment

- Ascertain stability from the history: has the presentation been changing?
- Ascertain fetal lie by palpation.
- Neither the head nor buttocks will be presenting.
- Also assess the laxity of the uterine wall.
- Does the presenting part move easily.
- Ultrasound should be performed to help ascertain the cause.

Risks of abnormal lie

- Labour with a non-longitudinal lie will result in obstructed labour and potential uterine rupture.
- Membrane rupture risks cord prolapse because with longitudinal lie, the presenting part usually prevents descent of the cord through the cervix.

Management of abnormal lie

- Admission to hospital from 37 weeks is usually recommended with unstable lie, so that CS can be carried out if labour starts or the membranes rupture and the lie is not longitudinal.
- Whilst the lie remains unstable, the woman should remain in hospital.
- With increasing gestation the lie will usually revert to longitudinal and in these circumstances she can be discharged.
- If the lie does not stabilize, a CS is usually performed at 41 weeks.
- Some advocate a stabilizing induction whereby the fetus is turned to cephalic and an amniotomy immediately performed. This requires expertise.
- If the lie is stable but not longitudinal, a CS should be considered at 39 weeks.

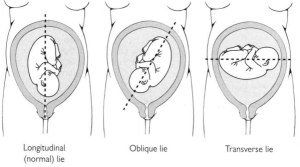

Longitudinal
(normal) lie

Oblique lie

Transverse lie

Fig 2.4 Longitudinal, oblique, and transverse fetal lie.

Abdominal pain in pregnancy: pregnancy related (<24 weeks)

The diagnosis of acute abdominal pain in pregnancy can be challenging. It is often difficult to differentiate between gynaecological, non-gynaecological, and pregnancy-related causes of abdominal pain. Some of the routine surgical investigations and procedures carry a risk to the fetus but this needs to be balanced against the risk of delayed diagnosis and treatment which would be harmful to both mother and child.

Miscarriage (see 📖 Chapter 15, p. 506)
- Can be associated with lower abdominal dull ache to severe continuous or colicky pain.
- Vaginal bleeding is present in most cases.
- Positive urine pregnancy test, pelvic examination, and USS are helpful in diagnosis.

Ectopic pregnancy (see 📖 Chapter 15, p. 510)
- Usually unilateral lower abdominal pain at <12 weeks gestation.
- Associated with brownish vaginal bleeding.
- Shoulder tip pain is suggestive of haemoperitoneum (bleeding ectopic).
- Serum hCG, USS, and laparoscopy are diagnostic.

Constipation
- Physiological changes in pregnancy results in the slowing of gut peristalsis.

Signs and symptoms
- Varied but colicky lower abdominal pain (L>R) is the most common.

Management
- High-fibre diet.
- Osmotic laxatives.
- Glycerine suppositories.

Round ligament pain
This pain is attributed to stretching of the round ligaments.

Incidence
- 20–30% pregnancies.

Signs and symptoms
- Commonly presents in 1st and 2nd trimester.
- Pain is often bilateral and located on the outer aspect of the uterus.
- Radiating to the groin.
- Aggravated by movement (especially getting up from a chair or turning over in bed).

Treatment
- Reassurance.
- Simple analgesia.
- Support belts may help.

Urinary tract infection

UTIs are more common in pregnancy and are an important cause of preterm labour.

Signs and symptoms
- Suprapubic/lower abdominal pain.
- Dysuria, nocturia, and frequency.

Investigations
- Urine dipstick:
  - nitrites confirm a UTI
  - blood, leucocytes, and protein raises index of suspicion.
- MSU.

Management
- Antibiotics.
- Analgesia.
- ↑ fluid intake.

Fibroids—red degeneration

Uterine fibroids occur in 20% of women of reproductive age. They may increase in size during pregnancy compromising blood supply to central areas causing pain. This is known as red degeneration.

Incidence
15% of pregnant women who have fibroids.

Symptoms and signs
- Usually occurs between the 12th and 22nd week of pregnancy.
- Constant pain localized to one area of the uterus coinciding with the site of the fibroid (may be severe pain).
- May have a low-grade pyrexia.

Investigations
- USS (identifies fibroids but cannot confirm red degeneration).
- FBC (may show leucocytosis).

Treatment
- Analgesia (pain should resolve in 4–7 days; however, it may be severe and prolonged, so advice from pain specialists should be sought).

▶ Placental abruption differs in that the fibroid uterus is soft except at the site of the fibroid and the FH is normal.

⚠ Myomectomy must not be performed in pregnancy as it will bleed ++ (the only exception being for a torted pedunculated fibroid).

Abdominal pain in pregnancy: pregnancy related (>24 weeks)

Labour

Signs and symptoms
- Usually presents with regular painful contractions.
- Pre-term labour may present with a history of vague abdominal pain which the woman may not associate with uterine activity.

⚠ Consider a VE in pregnant women with abdominal pain.

Braxton Hicks contractions

These are spontaneous contractions of the uterus, commonly occurring in the 3rd trimester. It may be difficult for the patient to differentiate between them and labour.

Signs and symptoms
- Painless and infrequent tightenings of the uterus.
- Vaginal examination reveals uneffaced and closed cervix.

Investigations
- Exclusion of precipitants of preterm labour (dipstick/MSU for UTI).

Treatment
- Reassurance.

Symphysis pubis dysfunction (see 📖 p. 49)

Signs and symptoms
  Pubic pain relating to upper thighs and perineum.
- Aggravated by movement.
- Difficulty walking resulting in a waddling gait.

Treatment
- Analgesia and physiotherapy.

Reflux oesophagitis

Relaxation of the oesophageal sphincter occurs in pregnancy and the pressure of the gravid uterus on the distal end of the oesophagus, results in an increased incidence of reflux oesophagitis. Gastric ulceration is less common due to decreased gastric acid secretion.

Incidence
60–70% of pregnant women.

Risk factors
Polyhydramnios.
Multiple pregnancy.

Signs and symptoms
Epigastric/retrosternal burning pain exacerbated by lying flat.

Management
- Exclude pre-eclampsia.
- Antacids, H_2 receptor antagonists.
- Dietary and lifestyle advice (avoidance of supine position).

Uterine rupture

This usually occurs during labour but has been reported antenatally.

Risk factors
- Previous CS or other uterine surgery.
- Congenital abnormalities of the uterus.
- Use of oxytocin in labour.
- Failure to recognize obstructed labour.

Signs and symptoms
- Tenderness over sites of previous uterine scars.
- Fetal parts may be easily palpable.
- Vaginal bleeding may be evident.
- Signs of maternal shock may be present.

△ CTG may show fetal distress and change in apparent uterine activity (contractions may seem to disappear on the tocograph).

Investigations
- FBC.
- Cross-match blood.

Management
- Maternal resuscitation.
- Urgent LSCS to deliver fetus and repair uterus.

Other causes of abdominal pain in pregnancy

- Placental abruption.
- Pre-eclampsia.
- HELLP.
- Acute fatty liver of pregnancy.

Abdominal pain in pregnancy: bowel related

Appendicitis

This is the most common surgical emergency in pregnant patients. Its incidence is 1:1500–2000 pregnancies with equal frequency in each trimester. Pregnant women have the same risk of appendicitis as non-pregnant women.

Signs and symptoms
- Classically periumbilical pain shifting to right lower quadrant.

⚠ Pain moves towards the right upper quadrant during the 2nd and 3rd trimesters due to displacement of the appendix by a gravid uterus.
- Nausea and vomiting.
- Anorexia
- Guarding and rebound tenderness present in 70% patients.

⚠ Rovsing's sign and fever are often absent in the pregnant patient.

Investigations
- WCC and CRP are often ↑
- USS: to exclude other causes of pain, CT/MRI may be considered.

Management
Diagnostic laparoscopy/laparotomy and appendicectomy.

⚠ Fetal loss is 3–5% with an unruptured appendix,↑ to 20% if ruptured.

Intestinal obstruction

It is the third most common non-obstetric reason for laparotomy during pregnancy. It complicates 1 in 1500–3000 pregnancies. Incidence increases as the pregnancy progresses. Adhesions are the commonest cause.

Signs and symptoms
- Acute abdominal pain.
- Vomiting.
- Constipation.
- Pyrexia.

Diagnosis
- Erect AXR showing gas-filled bowel with little gas in large intestine.
- USS (abdominal and pelvic).

Treatment
- Conservative treatment ('drip and suck').
- Surgery for any acute obstructive cause or when not responding to conservative management.

Causes of intestinal obstruction

- Adhesions.
- Volvulus.
- Intussusception.
- Hernia.
- Neoplasm.

Abdominal pain in pregnancy: other causes

Acute cholecystitis

The second most common surgical condition in pregnancy (progesterone diminishes smooth muscle tone and predisposes to cholestasis leading to gallstone formation). The incidence of gallstones is 7% in nulliparous and 19% in multiparous women. The incidence of acute cholecystitis is 1–8:10 000 pregnancies.

Signs and symptoms
- Colicky epigastric/right upper quadrant pain.
- Nausea and vomiting.
- Murphy's sign may be positive in acute cholecystits.
- Jaundice (indicating obstruction of the common bile duct).
- Signs of systemic infection (fever and tachycardia).

Investigations
- FBC, LFTs, CRP (WCC and alkaline phsphatase are ↑ in pregnancy).
- ↑ bilirubin (identify patients with concominant biliary tree obstruction).
- USS biliary tract (may demonstate calculi or a dilated biliary tree).

Management
- Conservative approach is the most common management.
- Analgesics and antiemetics.
- Hydration.
- Antibiotics.
- Cholecystectomy preferably by laparoscopic approach may be indicated in patients with recurrent biliary colic, acute cholecystitis and obstructive cholelithiasis (usually after delivery).

Adnexal torsion

This occurs when an enlarged ovary twists on its pedicle.

⚠ Torsion of the ovary and other adnexal structures is more common in pregnant than non-pregnant women.

Signs and symptoms
- Sudden onset unilateral colicky lower abdominal pain.
- Nausea, vomiting.
- There may be systemic symptoms such as fever.

Investigations
- WCC and CRP: may be elevated.
- USS pelvis may show an adnexal mass and Doppler studies may show impaired blood flow.

Management
If suspected, urgent laparotomy should be performed to either remove or untwist the adnexa. This may either preserve the ovary or present a non-viable ovary from becoming gangrenous.

Pancreatitis

Occurs more frequently in the 3rd trimester and immediate postpartum period. It can occur in early pregnancy associated with gallstones.

⚠ Although rare, it is more common in pregnancy than in non-pregnant women of a similar age.

Incidence
1 in 5000 pregnancies.

Risk factors
- Gallstone disease.
- High alcohol intake.
- Hyperlipidaemia.

Signs and symptoms
- Epigastric pain commonly radiating to the back.
- Pain exacerbated by lying flat and relieved by leaning forwards.
- Nausea and vomiting.

Investigations
- Serum amylase and lipase levels.
- USS to establish presence of gallstones.

Management
Conservative treatment is the mainstay:
- Intravenous fluids.
- Electrolyte replacement.
- Parenteral analgesics, e.g. morphine (pethidine is contraindicated).
- Bowel rest with or without nasogastric suction.

⚠ Early surgical intervention is recommended for gallstone pancreatitis in all trimesters as > 70% of patients will relapse before delivery.
- Laparoscopic/ open cholecystectomy.
- Endoscopic reterograde cholangio-pancreatography (ERCP) has a limited role in pregnancy because of radiation exposure to the fetus.

⚠ If pancreatitis is severe, liaise with HDU/ITU.

Non-abdominal causes of abdominal pain

Other conditions unrelated to abdominal structures may also present with abdominal pain:
- Lower lobe pneumonia
- Diabetic ketoacidosis
- Sickle cell crisis.

▶ Women with social problems and domestic abuse may repeatedly attend with undiagnosable pain and it is important to ask them about this directly but sympathetically.

Preterm labour: overview

Preterm birth is defined as delivery before 37 weeks.

- 1/3 is medically indicated (e.g. PET), and 2/3 spontaneous.
- Accounts for 5–10% of births but ~70% of perinatal deaths.
- It also causes long term handicap—blindness, deafness, and cerebral palsy.
- The incidence is ↑ over the years.
- >50% of women with painful preterm contractions will not deliver preterm: fetal fibronectin/transvaginal USS may help in diagnosis.

Risk factors for preterm delivery

Increased risk with:
- Previous preterm birth.
- Multiple pregnancy.
- Cervical surgery.
- Uterine anomalies.
- Medical conditions, e.g. renal disease.
- Pre-eclampsia and IUGR (spontaneous and iatrogenic).

Acute preterm labour

- Preterm labour associated with cervical weakness (avoid the term 'incompetence') classically presents with increased vaginal discharge, mild lower abdominal pain and bulging membranes on examination
- Preterm labour associated with factors such as infection, inflammation or abruption presents with lower abdominal pain, painful uterine contractions and vaginal loss.

▶ In practice it is often less clear cut than this, and infection and cervical weakness are related and often coexist.

History
- Ask about contractions—onset, frequency, duration, severity
- Constant pain
- Vaginal loss
- Fetal movements
- Obstetric history (check hand held notes)

Examination
- Maternal pulse, temperature, respiratory rate
- Uterine tenderness (suggests infection / abruption)
- Fetal presentation
- Speculum: look for blood, discharge, liquor
- Swabs (HVS, LVS/perianal)
- Gentle VE

Investigations
- FBC, CRP (raised WCC and CRP suggest infection)
- Swabs, MSU
- USS for fetal presentation (malpresentation common) and EFW
- Consider fetal fibronectin/transvaginal USS if available (see 📖 p. 98).

Management of preterm labour

- Establish whether threatened or 'real' preterm labour:
  - transvaginal cervical length scan (>15 mm unlikely to labour)
  - fibronectin assay: if negative, unlikely to labour.
- Admit if risk high.
- Inform SCBU.
- Arrange in-utero transfer if no suitable beds available.
- Check fetal presentation with USS.
- Steroids (12 mg betametasone IM—two doses 24 hours apart).

▶Antenatal steroids reduce rates of respiratory distress, intraventricular haemorrhage and neonatal death (RCOG grade A recommendation).

- Consider tocolysis (drug treatment to prevent labour and delivery).
  - Allows time for steroid administration and in-utero transfer.
  - Currently used tocolytics include nifedipine and atosiban IV.

◆ Aim should be not just prolongation of gestation (a surrogate measure) but improvement in perinatal morbidity and mortality. Trials of tocolysis have not shown improvement in these substantive outcome measures, so some prefer to avoid them.

- Liaison with senior obstetricians and neonatologists is essential, especially at the margins of viability (23–26 weeks). A clear plan needs to be made about:
  - mode of delivery
  - monitoring in labour
  - presence of pediatrician/appropriate intervention at delivery
- Give IV antibiotics in labour.

📖 Antenatal corticosteroids to prevent respiratory distress syndrome. RCOG guideline no.7 (2004). www.rcog.org

📖 Tocolytic drugs for women in preterm labour. RCOG guideline no. 1(B) (2002). www.rcog.org

Preterm labour: prediction and prevention

Prevention

Treatment of bacterial vaginosis (BV)

Some evidence suggests this may reduce the incidence of preterm prelabour rupture of membranes (PPROM) and low birth weight in women with previous preterm birth. Clindamycin rather than metronidazole is used.

Progesterone

🖝 Has been shown in two RCTs to be effective in reducing the incidence of preterm birth but some have called for further studies before its use becomes widespread.

Cervical sutures (cerclage)

🖝 May be of benefit in selected cases. Can be inserted vaginally or, in extreme cases, abdominally. Not thought to be useful in multiple pregnancies.
- Elective (women with previous loss from cervical weakness).
- Ultrasound-indicated (in response to shortening cervix on TVS).
- Rescue (in response to cervical dilatation).

Reduction of pregnancy number

Selective reduction of triplet or higher-order multiple pregnancies (to 2) reduces the risk of preterm labour while slightly increasing the risk of early miscarriage.

Methods for prediction of preterm labour

Transvaginal USS of cervix
- In asymptomatic women with a singleton pregnancy:
  - risk of delivering before 32 weeks is 4% if cervix is <15 mm long at 23 weeks
  - increasing exponentially to 78% if cervix is 5 mm.
- In symptomatic women with a singleton pregnancy:
  - cervix <15 mm, risk of delivery within 7 days is 49%
  - cervix >15 mm, risk of delivery within 7 days <1%.

Fetal fibronectin (FFN)
- FFN is a protein not usually present in cervicovaginal secretions at 22–36 weeks.
- Those with a positive FFN test are more likely to deliver (test for FFN with swab and commercially available kit).
- Predicts preterm birth within 7–10 days of testing (positive likelihood ratio of 5.42 and negative LR of 0.25).

Preterm prelabour rupture of membranes (PPROM)

- This complicates 1/3 of preterm deliveries.
- About 1/3 is associated with overt infection (more common at earlier gestations).

History
- Ask about vaginal loss.
  - Gush.
  - Constant trickle or dampness.

⚠ Look for chorioamnionitis as it is associated with significant neonatal morbidity and mortality.

> **Features suggestive of chorioamnionitis**
>
> History:
> - Fever/malaise.
> - Abdominal pain, including contractions.
> - Purulent/offensive vaginal discharge.
>
> Examination:
> - Maternal pyrexia and tachycardia.
> - Uterine tenderness.
> - Fetal tachycardia.
> - Speculum: offensive vaginal discharge—yellow/brown.
>
> ▶ Avoid VE as this increases the risk of introducing infection.

Investigations
- FBC, CRP (raised WCC and CRP indicate infection).
- Swabs (HVS, LVS).
- MSU.
- USS for fetal presentation, EFW, and liquor volume.

Preterm prelabour rupture of membranes (PPROM): management

- If evidence of chorioamnionitis:
  - steroids (betametasone 12 mg IM)
  - deliver
  - broad spectrum antibiotic cover
- If no evidence of chorioamnionitis, manage conservatively:
  - admit
  - inform SCBU and liaise with neonatologists
  - steroids (12 mg betametasone IM—two doses 24 hours apart)
  - antibiotics (erythromycin).

▶ Use of antibiotics reduces major markers of neonatal morbidity. The ORACLE trial showed erythromycin to be beneficial.

△ Co-amoxiclav is associated with an increased risk of NEC and should be avoided.

Prognosis

Depends on:
- Gestation at delivery.
- Gestation at PPROM:
  - PPROM at <20 weeks—few survivors
  - PPROM > 22 weeks—survival up to 50%.
- Reason for PPROM:
  - prognosis better if PPROM secondary to invasive procedure (e.g. amniocentesis) rather than spontaneous.

Risks to fetus from PPROM

- Prematurity.
- Infection.
- Pulmonary hypoplasia.
- Limb contractures.

Table 2.2 Data from EPICure study (cohort of babies born in UK and Ireland in 1995)

Gestation (weeks)	Survival to discharge (as % of live births)	Survival (severe disability) (as % of live births)
<23	1	50
23–23+6	11	31
24–24+6	26	24
25–25+6	44	22

📖 The EPICure Study: outcomes to discharge from hospital for babies born at the threshold of viability. *Pediatrics* 2000;106: 659–71.

Prolonged pregnancy: overview

Prolonged pregnancy is a cause of anxiety for both women and obstetricians. It is a common occurrence and is a recognized cause of increased fetal morbidity and mortality.

Definition of prolonged pregnancy

According to the International Federation of Gynaecology and Obstetrics (FIGO), prolonged pregnancy is defined as any pregnancy that exceeds 42 weeks (294 days) from the first day of the last menstrual period (LMP) in a woman with regular 28 day cycles. Different terminologies are used generally in day to day practice such as postdates, post-term and post-maturity.

Incidence

The incidence of pregnancy lasting 42 weeks or more is 3–10%. With one previous prolonged pregnancy there is a 30% chance of another one. With a history of two this rises to 40%. Incidence also varies depending on whether EDD is based on LMP or dating USS. Women who book in the 1st trimester and have an early dating scan have an incidence of prolonged pregnancy of <5%.

Dates cannot be relied upon in the following circumstances:
- Uncertainty of LMP (10–30% of women).
- Irregular periods.
- Recent use of combined oral contraceptive pill (COCP).
- Conception during lactational amenorrhea.

Fetal risks of prolonged pregnancy

Perinatal mortality ↑ after 42 weeks of gestation:
- Intrapartum deaths are 4 times more common.
- Early neonatal deaths are 3 times more common.

Other risks include:
- Meconium aspiration and assisted ventilation.
- Oligohydramnios.
- Macrosomia, shoulder dystocia, and fetal injury.
- Cephalhaematoma.
- Fetal distress in labour.
- Neonatal—hypothermia, hypoglycaemia, polycythaemia and growth restriction.

Maternal risks
- Maternal anxiety and psychological morbidity.
- Increased intervention:
  - induction of labour
  - operative delivery with ↑ risk of genital tract trauma.

Fetal postmaturity syndrome

- This is used to describe post-term infants who show signs of intrauterine malnutrition.
- The neonate has a scaphoid abdomen, little subcutaneous fat on the body or limbs, peeling skin over the palm and feet, overgrown nails, and an anxious, alert look.
- The baby's skin is also stained with meconium.
- This condition constitutes only a small proportion of babies born after 42 weeks.

⚠ These features can be seen at an earlier gestation in babies with IUGR. Hence, the term prolonged pregnancy is preferred to postmaturity for pregnancy beyond 42 weeks.

Prolonged pregnancy: management

- Attempt to confirm the EDD as accurately as possible:
  - EDD based on 1st trimester USS is accurate to within a week.
- Assess any other risk factors which may be an indication to induce close to the EDD:
  - pre-eclampsia
  - diabetes
  - antepartum haemorrhage
  - IUGR associated with placental insufficiency.
- Offer 'stretch and sweep' at 41 weeks.
- Offer induction of labour between 41 and 42 weeks:
  - this slightly reduces perinatal mortality
  - it also reduces the risk of CS
  - but it 'medicalizes' many labours
  - if declined, ensure adequate fetal surveillance.

Fetal monitoring

This should include an initial USS assessment of growth and amniotic fluid volume. Women should be offered daily CTGs after 42 weeks. They should also be advised to report any decrease in fetal movements.

(See Chapter 3: Monitoring the high-risk fetus, 📖 p. 148.)

Counselling

Most units in the UK advise induction of labour by 42 weeks because of the increased perinatal mortality and morbidity beyond this time. However, many women regard elective induction of labour as interference with the natural phenomenon of childbirth. It is therefore important to discuss the issue sensitively and respect the women's decision. Written information should be provided clearly outlining the arguments for and against induction to ensure the women is able make an informed decision. Any specific risk factors complicating her pregnancy, such as pre-eclampsia, should be clearly explained and the conversation carefully documented in the notes.

Those mothers who prefer to await spontaneous onset of labour should have appropriate counselling regarding increased fetal mortality and morbidity. They should also have adequate fetal surveillance, which should include a USS assessment of fetal growth and liquor volume.

📖 Department of Health (1993). Changing childbirth, report of the Expert Maternity Group, Cumberledge Report. HMSO, London.

Fetal medicine

Prenatal diagnosis: overview

Benefits

Congenital abnormalities affect approximately 2% of newborn babies in the UK, and account for around 21% of perinatal and infant deaths, as well as causing significant disability and morbidity later in life. Although some pregnancies are known to be at high risk, e.g. for mothers with type I diabetes or parents with a previously affected child, the vast majority of congenital defects occur unexpectedly in otherwise uncomplicated pregnancies. Prenatal identification in such situations can help in a multitude of ways:

- Enabling decision on timing, mode and place of delivery (e.g. in a unit which provides paediatric surgery).
- Preparing parents to cope with an affected child.
- Introducing parents to specialist neonatal services.
- Ensuring fetal surveillance, such as later ultrasound scans to monitor the condition and ensure the best possible outcome.
- Potentially allowing in-utero treatment (rarely available at present).
- Giving parents the option of terminating the pregnancy in severe cases.

Counselling

The news that there is a problem with their unborn child is often devastating for parents. How they respond to the situation will vary with such factors as age, social background, and religious belief. It is a mistake to think that parents will automatically wish to terminate the pregnancy. Many will choose to go on, even in the face of abnormalities incompatible with life. Some parents report that the opportunity to hold their child enabled them to grieve. Other parents will choose to terminate. Counselling must be supportive, informative, and non-directional. Care must also be taken to counsel adequately before any screening tests. If parents have no intention of having the riskier diagnostic tests performed then there is little benefit in screening and much anxiety may be generated. Detailed written information should always be provided beforehand.

Trisomy 21 (Down's syndrome)

Down's syndrome is the commonest identifiable cause of learning disability. It usually occurs as a result of non-disjunction of chromosome 21 at meiosis (95%) but may also be due to a balanced translocation in the parents (4%). An estimated 1% is due to mosaicism. It has variable penetrance, which explains the wide range of features and characteristics seen in people with Down's syndrome. Around 50% will have one or more serious congenital abnormality. Around 10% will die before the age of 5 years, and the current life expectancy is 50–55 years.

Risk of trisomy 21 ↑ with maternal age:

- <25 years   1:1500
- 30 years   1:910
- 35 years   1:380
- 40 years   1:110
- 45 years   1:30

- Natural prevalence 1:600 live births, but incidence is now 6:10 000 due to termination of pregnancy.
- Typical appearance:
  - flat nasal bridge
  - epicanthic folds
  - single palmar crease.
- Intellectual impairment:
  - 80% profound or severe
  - mean mental age at 21 years is 5 years
  - increased risk of early-onset dementia.
- Congenital malformations:
  - cardiac abnormalities (46%, e.g. VSD, ASD, and tetralogy of Fallot)
  - gastrointestinal atresias are common (e.g. duodenal atresia).
- Increased risk of other medical conditions, including:
  - leukaemia
  - thyroid disorders
  - epilepsy.

Genetic counselling after diagnosis of trisomy 21

- If the karyotype indicates straightforward trisomy 21 from non-disjunction, the risk of recurrence is ~1% above the risk from maternal age alone.
- If a chromosomal translocation is demonstrated, the recurrence risk is 1:10 for an affected mother and 1:50 if it is the father carrying the abnormality.

Support groups

Down Syndrome Association 📖 www.dsa-uk.com

Down Syndrome Medical Interest Group 📖 www.dsmig.org.uk

Other types of aneuploidy

Trisomy 18 (Edwards' syndrome)

The second most common autosomal trisomy. Most are due to non-disjunction at meiosis. The vast majority will die soon after birth.

- Incidence 1:6000 live births (prevalence estimated at 1:3000).
- Risk increases with increasing maternal age.
- Features:
  - craniofacial abnormalities including small facial features and low-set ears
  - rocker bottom feet
  - severe mental disability.
- Congenital malformations:
  - cardiac abnormalities in almost all fetuses (VSD, ASD, or PDA)
  - gastrointestinal abnormalities
  - urogenital abnormalities.

Trisomy 13 (Patau's syndrome)

The least common autosomal trisomy. Around 75% are due to non-disjunction. The vast majority will die soon after birth.

- Incidence 1:10 000 live births.
- Risk increases with increasing maternal age.
- Features:
  - craniofacial, including cyclopia with proboscis located on forehead.
  - microcephaly.
  - severe mental disability.
- Congenital malformations (midline):
  - holoprosencephaly (failure of cleavage of the embryonic forebrain)
  - gastrointestinal abnormalities, especially exomphalos
  - cleft lip and palate.

📖 www.rarechromo.org

Turner's syndrome (45 XO)

This affects only females and is due to the loss of an X chromosome. It is one of the few chromosomal abnormalities that does not result in mental impairment. Almost all women with Turner's syndrome will have short stature and loss of ovarian function, but the extent of the other features varies enormously.

- Incidence 1:2500 live female births.
- Features include:
  - short stature, webbed neck and wide carrying angle
  - non-functioning 'streak' ovaries
  - coarctation of the aorta.

📖 www.tss.org.uk

Klinefelter's syndrome (47 XXY)

This affects only males and is caused by non-disjunction of the X chromosomes. The individual is almost always sterile and may have hypogonadism. They are phenotypically tall with occasionally reduced IQ.

- Incidence 1:700 live male births.

Screening for chromosomal abnormalities

Ideally, screening should be offered to all women at the time of booking. In the UK, the National Screening Committee (NSC) has stated that by April 2007 all centres should offer a screening test that for Down's syndrome, the most common chromosomal abnormality, has a detection rate of 75% with a false positive rate of no more than 3%.

☞ Currently, not all centres can achieve this.

📖 www.nsc.nhs.uk/

Counselling

Detailed, unbiased, written information should be provided about the condition itself, types of test available, and the implications of the results. It is important for a woman to understand that a negative result does not guarantee that her baby does not have an abnormality.

Screening relies on the integration of different independent risk factors, such as maternal age, blood hormone levels, and scan findings. These findings are slightly dependent on factors including maternal weight, ethnicity, IVF pregnancies, smoking, multiple pregnancy, and diabetes, and calculations are modified according to these.

Screening versus diagnostic tests

Care must always be taken to explain the difference between the types of test available including their advantages, disadvantages, and limitations.

Screening tests
- Should be cheap and widely available.
- Non-invasive, safe, and acceptable.
- Have good sensitivity (high detection rate) and specificity (low false-positive rate).
- Provide a measure of the risk of being affected by a certain disorder (e.g. 1 in 100 risk of Down's syndrome).
- Must have a suitable diagnostic test for those identified as 'high risk'.

Diagnostic tests
- Needs to definitely confirm or reject the suspected diagnosis (e.g. the fetus does, or does not, have Down's syndrome).
- Must be as safe as possible.
- Must have high sensitivity and specificity.
- The implications of the disorder tested for must be serious enough to warrant an invasive test.

Combined and serum integrated tests

Combined test

When
- Scan and blood test at 11 to 13+6 weeks.

How
- Ultrasound (nuchal) scan measurement of the subcutaneous tissue between the skin and the soft tissue overlying the cervical spine with the fetus in the neutral position.
- A blood test measuring:
  - pregnancy associated plasma protein-A (PAPP-A)
  - β-human chorionic gonadotrophin (hCG).

Risk of trisomy 21 is calculated by multiplying the background maternal age and gestation-related risk by a likelihood ratio derived from the NT measurement and the two blood tests.

Combined test

Advantages
- Performance ~90% detection for 5% FPR (75% for 3%).
- May detect other abnormalities such as anencephaly.
- An increased NT is also a marker for structural defects, e.g. cardiac malformations.
- Result usually available in 1st trimester allowing surgical TOP.
- Acceptable detection of all trisomies.

Disadvantages
- Expensive and difficult to perform nuchal scan.

Serum integrated test

When
Blood test at 10 weeks, then again at 15 weeks.

How
- Dating scan (but not nuchal scan).
- PAPP-A at 10 weeks.
- Quadruple test at 15 weeks measuring:
  - oestriol
  - hCG
  - AFP
  - inhibin A.

Risk of trisomy 21 is calculated by multiplying the background maternal age and gestation related risk by a likelihood ratio derived from the two stages of blood tests.

Serum integrated test

Advantages
- Good detection rate.
- By not relying on a nuchal scan, may be cheaper and easier to perform.

Disadvantages
- Little experience in practice.
- Two-stage screen: result available only after 15 weeks.
- Not useful for multiple pregnancies.

Significance of raised serum AFP

An elevated level of maternal serum AFP (greater than 2.2 multiples of median, MoM) can also be used as a screening tool for open neural tube defects. It is also elevated in other conditions, including:
- Abdominal wall defects.
- Congenital nephrosis.
- Upper fetal bowel obstruction.
- Placental or umbilical cord tumours.
- Sacrococcygeal teratoma.
- Multiple pregnancy.
- After bleeding in early pregnancy.

An elevated AFP should trigger closer fetal and maternal surveillance as it is also a marker of adverse perinatal outcomes including:
- Fetal death.
- Intrauterine growth restriction (IUGR).
- Late pregnancy bleeding.
- Preterm delivery.

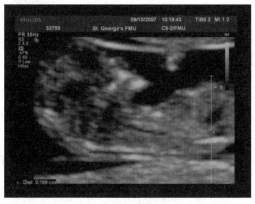

Fig. 3.1 Nuchal translucency at 11–14 weeks USS.

Integrated and other tests

Integrated test

When
- Nuchal scan and blood tests (10–13+6 weeks).
- Blood tests again at 15 weeks.

How
- Nuchal scan.
- PAPP-A at 10 weeks.
- Quadruple test at 15 weeks measuring:
  - oestriol
  - hCG
  - AFP
  - inhibin A.

Risk of trisomy 21 is calculated by multiplying the background maternal age and gestation related risk by a likelihood ratio derived from the nuchal scan and the two stages of blood tests.

Combined test

Advantages
- Most sensitive test in common usage.

Disadvantages
- Two-stage screen: result available only after 15 weeks.
- Expensive and difficult to perform nuchal scan.

Other tests available

Double test
- This uses AFP and hCG without AFP at 16 weeks.
- It does not meet NSC criteria (< 60% detection rate for 5% false positive rate).

Triple test
- This uses hCG, oestriol, and AFP only at 16 weeks.
- It does not meet NSC criteria (~70% detection rate for 5% false positive rate).

Quadruple test
- This uses oestriol, hCG, AFP, and inhibin A at 16 weeks.
- It does not meet NSC criteria (75% detection rate for 5% false positive rate).

Nasal bone or tricuspid regurgitation
- Fetuses with Down's syndrome are more likely to have an absent or hypoplastic nasal bone and have significant tricuspid regurgitation at 11–13+6 weeks.
- Only in conjunction with a nuchal scan can the presence or absence of these be used to modify the risk of a combined test.
- They may considerably increase the accuracy of the combined test.
- These are not commonly used because they require skill and time to detect accurately.

Table 3.1 Comparison of screening tests available for Down's syndrome

	Combined	Serum integrated test	Integrated test	Double test	Triple test	Quadruple test
Trimester	1st	1st & 2nd	1st & 2nd	2nd	2nd	2nd
Type	Scan & blood test	Two blood tests	Scan & two blood tests	Blood test	Blood test	Blood test
Detection rate	90%	85%	85%	<60%	71%	75%
For a given false positive rate	5%	2.7%	1.2%	5%	6%	5%

The SURUSS study

This was a large, multicentre trial aimed at identifying the most accurate, safe and cost-effective method of antenatal screening for Down's syndrome. The results from 47 053 singleton pregnancies showed that screening performance in the first trimester of pregnancy was similar to that in the second trimester. Screening which 'integrates' measurements from both trimesters into a single result is more effective than any available test performed in either trimester alone.

Specific recommendations from the SURUSS study

- Overall, the integrated test appears to offer the most effective and safest method of screening.
- If a nuchal translucency measurement is not available the preferred method is the serum integrated test.
- For women who do not attend for antenatal care until the 2nd trimester the quadruple test is best.
- For women who choose to have a screening test in the 1st trimester and accept the loss of efficacy and safety compared with the integrated test, the combined test is appropriate.

The performance of the serum integrated test in the SURUSS study was better than expected: most centres are introducing the combined test as a routine.

📖 www.wolfson.qmul.ac.uk/surusslink/

Diagnosis of structural abnormalities

This should be offered to all women in the UK at the time of booking and usually takes the form of the 'anomaly scan', a detailed ultrasound scan undertaken at around 20 weeks gestation. The aim is to identify specific structural malformations.

The detection of malformations may vary and is dependent on:
- The anatomical system affected.
- Gestational age at the time of the scan.
- Skill of the operator.
- Quality of the equipment.
- BMI of the mother.

Percentage of abnormalities detected by routine anomaly scan (These figures are better under optimum conditions)

- Central nervous system   76%
- Urinary tract   67%
- Pulmonary   50%
- Gastrointestinal   42%
- Skeletal   24%
- Cardiac   17%

📖 RCOG National evidence-based guidelines. Antenatal care Oct 2003 www.rcog.org.uk

RCOG minimum standards required for the 20 week anomaly scan

Fetal normality
- Head shape and internal structures:
  - cavum pellucidum
  - cerebellum
  - ventricular size at atrium <10 mm.
- Spine—longitudinal and transverse views.
- Abdominal shape and content at the level of:
  - stomach
  - kidneys
  - umbilicus.
- Renal pelvis (<5 mm AP measurement).
- Abdominal and thoracic appearance in the longitudinal axis:
  - diaphragm
  - bladder.
- Thorax at the level of the cardiac 'four chamber' view.
- Arms (three bones and hand).
- Legs (three bones and foot).

Optimal standard
- Cardiac outflow tracts.
- Face and lips.

Neural tube defects

These craniospinal defects occur early in development when the neural tube fails to close properly. The type and severity depends on the degree and site of the defect. There is growing evidence that the prevalence is declining, possibly due to the increased use of folate supplementation. Spina bifida and anencephaly make up over 95% of NTDs.
- Incidence 2:1000 in England (3:1000 in Scotland).

Anencephaly

Absence of the skull vault and cerebral cortex. It is incompatible with life, with babies rarely living more than a few hours if they are not stillborn.

Spina bifida

Incomplete fusion of vertebrae potentially allowing herniation of all or part of spinal cord. The malformation falls into three categories:
- Spina bifida occulta (mildest):
  - split in vertebrae with no herniation of spinal cord
  - varies from asymptomatic to mild neurological symptoms.
- Myelomeningocele (least common):
  - split in vertebrae with herniation of meninges and CSF
  - varies from normal neurological function to moderate symptoms.
- Meningocele (most severe):
  - split in vertebrae allows herniation of spinal cord and meninges
  - invariably have abnormal neurology at and below the lesion
  - usually have an abnormal cerebellum and hydocephalus, which may result in mental impairment.

⚠ Dietary supplementation with folic acid decreases the incidence of NTDs. Recommended doses are:
- 400 micrograms/day for 3 months before conception, continued to 12 weeks.
- 5 mg/day for women with a previously affected child or those who are taking anticonvulsants.

Specific USS findings with some neural tube defects
- Anencephaly:
  - absence of cranium and bulging eyes ('frog-like' appearance)
  - 99% will be detected by 20 weeks.
- Spina bifida—findings vary according to the severity of the lesion:
  - defect seen in the vertebral bodies or tissue overlying the spine
  - frontal bone scalloping ('lemon sign')
  - abnormal shaped cerebellum ('banana sign')
  - up to 95% detection rate for major defects

📖 Association for Spina Bifida and Hydrocephalus. www.asbah.org

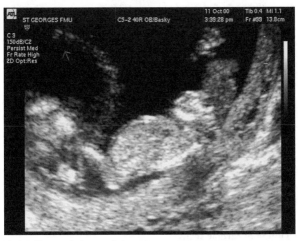

Fig. 3.2 Ultrasound of anencephaly.

Cardiac defects (congenital heart disease)

Cardiac defects are the most common major malformation in children with an estimated incidence of 6–8:1000. They may be associated with a chromosomal abnormality, commonly trisomy 21 or 18, and with many other congenital abnormalities. Where isolated, many can be surgically corrected at birth leading to a good quality of life. The most commonly seen abnormalities are ventricular septal defects (VSD) (Fig. 3.4).

Risk factors for cardiac abnormalities include:
- Family history of congenital heart disease (CHD) in 1st-degree relative (recurrence risk 3%).
- Previous affected child (risk depends on type).
- Drug exposure particularly anticonvulsants and lithium.
- Maternal diabetes mellitus.
- Other congenital abnormalities.
- Increased nuchal translucency (risk related to thickness).

Timing of cardiac scans
- In skilled hands many cardiac abnormalities can be seen at 12–13 weeks.
- Most cardiac abnormalities are missed at routine anomaly scans. The detection rate improves with training and specifically if 'three-vessel' and 'outflow tracts' views are found in addition to the four-chamber view (Fig 3.3).
- Cardiac abnormalities may be better detected at 22 weeks than at 20 weeks.
- Evolution of defects change and later scanning, e.g. at 32 weeks, may be beneficial.

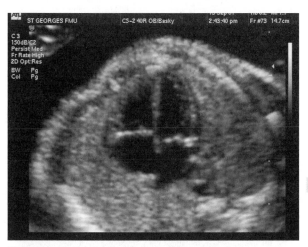

Fig. 3.3 USS of a normal cardiac four-chamber view.

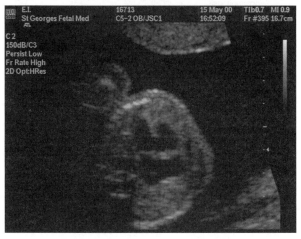

Fig. 3.4 USS of ventricular septal defect.

Urinary tract defects

Renal agenesis

Bilateral renal agenesis is lethal because of anhydramnios causing lung hypoplasia. It may not be evident until >16 weeks because amniotic fluid is not all urinary before this time.

Posterior urethral valve syndrome

This occurs in male fetuses where folds of mucosa block the bladder neck causing outflow obstruction. The severity is variable; back pressure may cause irreversible renal damage and oligohydramnios.

Hydronephrosis

Accounts for 75% of fetal renal abnormalities. At least 40% resolve spontaneously in the neonatal period. It is usually due to pelviueretric obstruction, vesicoureteric reflux, utereocele, or posterior urethral valves (Fig. 3.5). Most cases can be treated postnatally so the prognosis is excellent.

Specific USS findings with some urinary tract defects
- Posterior urethral valves:
  - thick walled dilated bladder with 'keyhole' sign of upper urethral dilatation
  - hydronephrosis
  - variable degrees of oligohydramnios according to severity.
- Ureterocele:
  - cystic area of prolapsed ureter in bladder.

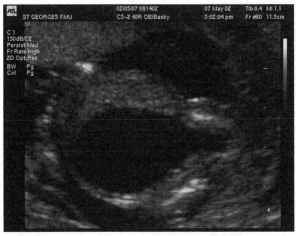

Fig. 3.5 Ultrasound of posterior urethral valve syndrome (keyhole bladder).

Lung defects

Lung hypoplasia

- Failure to develop sufficient alveoli to permit adequate gas exchange at delivery.
- Often due to mid-trimester oligohydramnios from very preterm rupture of membranes or renal anomalies.
- May be due to compression (e.g. diaphragmatic hernia).
- Severity is increased with:
  - preterm rupture of membranes at less than 25 weeks gestation
  - severe oligohydramnios (AFI <4) for more than 2 weeks
  - earlier delivery

⚠ Estimated mortality rate 71–95%.

Diaphragmatic hernia

- A defect in the diaphragm results in the abdominal contents herniating into the chest.
- There is a 30% incidence of aneuploidy and a strong association with other malformations.
- The degree of compromise is correlated to the amount of compression of the original chest contents; prognosis is worse if the liver is in the chest and if little contralateral lung tissue is visible.
- ~40% will die postnatally of lung hypoplasia; the others will require postnatal surgery.
- Experimental in-utero treatment for severe cases involves tracheal obstruction (FETO).

Congenital cystic adenomatoid malformation (CCAM)

- A rare form of lung disease where the normal alveolar tissue is replaced by a proliferation of cysts resembling bronchioles.
- The prognosis is good but occasional very severe cases may cause hydrops.

☛ Postnatal surgery in asymptomatic cases is contentious.

Specific ultrasound findings with some lung defects

- Diaphragmatic hernia:
  - stomach or liver is seen within chest cavity
  - with a left-sided hernia, the heart may be deviated to the right
  - abdominal circumference is often smaller than expected
  - usually detectable at 20 weeks.
- Congenital cystic adenomatoid malformation (CCAM):
  - cystic mass present within the lung parenchyma
  - usually detectable at 20 weeks (Fig. 3.6).

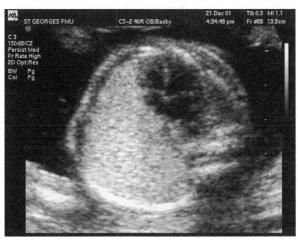

Fig. 3.6 USS of congenital cystic adenomatoid malformation (CCAM).

Gastrointestinal defects

Exomphalos (omphalocele)

- Failure of the gut to return into the abdominal cavity after the normal embryological extrusion and rotation; the bowel, and sometimes other viscera, are contained within a sac and the umbilical cord arises from the apex of this sac.
- Approximately 1/3 occur with chromosomal abnormalities and up to 50% of the remainder have other malformations (e.g. cardiac).
- Prognosis depends on karyotype, presence of coexisting malformations, and presence of bowel ischaemia.
- Require referral to a fetal medicine centre and postnatal surgery.
- Exomphalos alone is not an indication for delivery by CS.

Gastroschisis

- This involves protrusion of the gut through an anterior abdominal wall defect, usually to the right of the umbilical cord; the bowel is not covered by a sac and floats freely.
- Usually occurs in very young women: rare after 25 years.
- There is no increased risk of chromosomal abnormalities.
- The fetal gastrointestinal tract may become obstructed or atretic.
- ~1 in 10 will die in utero or postnatally, but in the remainder the prognosis is good.
- Require referral to a fetal medicine centre and postnatal surgery.
- Vaginal delivery is not necessarily contraindicated.

Gastrointestinal obstruction

- Duodenal atresia: 30% have trisomy 21.
- Oesophageal atresia: 15% have aneuploidy.
- Other atresias: may occur with syndromes or gastroschisis.
- Cystic fibrosis is common with bowel obstruction.

Specific USS findings with some gastrointestinal defects

- Anterior abdominal wall defects:
  - bowel is seen outside the abdominal wall
  - detection rates >95%.
- Duodenal atresia:
  - distension of stomach and proximal duodenum ('double bubble') (Fig 3.7)
  - may not be apparent by 20 weeks but usually seen by 25 weeks
  - polyhydramnios.
- Oesophageal atresia:
  - absence of stomach bubble and polyhydramnios
  - often not seen due to presence of a tracheo-oesophageal fistula.

Table 3.2 Comparison of the features of exomphalos and gastroschisis

	Exomphalos	Gastroschisis
Viscera contained within a sac	Yes, unless ruptured	No
Insertion of umbilical cord	At apex of sac	Next to the defect
Evisceration of:	Liver ± intestinal loops, spleen	Intestinal loops only
Chromosomal abnormalities	30%	<1%
Other malformations	50%	<5%
Mortality	40%	5–10%

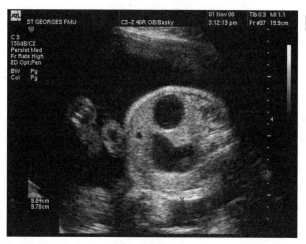

Fig. 3.7 USS of duodenal atresia ('double bubble').

Soft markers on ultrasound scan

Some ultrasound features seen at 20 weeks are called 'soft markers'. These may themselves be of little significance, but are nevertheless slightly more common in chromosomally abnormal fetuses. They can therefore be used (more commonly in the US than in Europe) to modify the risk of aneuploidy.

Unfortunately these features may cause considerable parental anxiety as they are often, mistakenly, seen as abnormalities.

Choroid plexus cysts (Fig 3.8)

- Small cysts in the choroid plexus, seen in about 1% of 20 week scans.
- Weakly associated with trisomy 18.
- In isolation minimally increase risk of chromosomal abnormalities.

Echogenic intracardiac foci

- 1 or more small echogenic foci ('golf balls') in the cardiac ventricles.
- No significance for cardiac defects.
- Slight increase (~1.5-fold) in risk of chromosomal abnormalities.

Mild renal pelvic dilatation

- Dilatation of ≥5 mm and ≤10 mm at 20 weeks.
- Slightly increased (~1.5-fold) risk of chromosomal abnormalities.
- Repeat scan in 3rd trimester (to ensure not enlarged) and neonatal follow-up is recommended.

Echogenic bowel

- Bowel with areas of echogenicity similar in brightness to bone.
- Moderate association (~5-fold increase) with chromosomal abnormalities.
- Although usually benign, occasionally associated with increased perinatal risk, cystic fibrosis, and bowel obstruction.
- Consider referral for expert opinion.

Two-vessel umbilical cord

- Cord contains only one umbilical artery.
- Slight increase in chromosomal abnormalities.
- Slight increase in perinatal risk, renal tract and cardiac abnormalities.

Increased nuchal fold (Fig 3.9)

- 20 week equivalent of nuchal translucency (>6 mm in transverse section).
- Increased risk of chromosomal abnormalities (~10-fold).
- Amniocentesis for chromosomal abnormalities is usually offered.
- Slight association with other structural abnormalities.
- Sign of early hydrops.

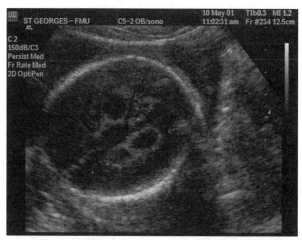

Fig. 3.8 USS of choroid plexus cysts.

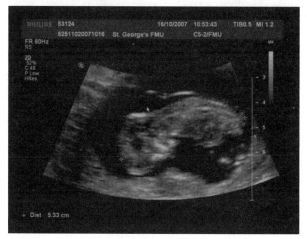

Fig. 3.9 USS of increased nuchal fold.

Diagnostic tests

Chorionic villus sampling (CVS) (Fig 3.10)

This diagnostic test is usually performed between 10 and 13 weeks and involves aspiration of some trophoblastic cells. The amount of tissue obtained is small but sufficient for karyotyping, and with the development of FISH and PCR, rapid analysis is possible. It requires ultrasound guidance, and can be performed either transabdominally or transcervically.

Indications
- For karyotyping if 1st trimester screening test suggests high risk for aneuploidy.
- For DNA analysis if parents are carriers of an identifiable gene mutation such as cystic fibrosis or thalassaemia.

Benefits
- Allows 1st trimester TOP if an abnormality is detected:
  - can be performed surgically
  - can be done before the pregnancy has become physically apparent.
- Rapid karyotyping as trophoblast cells are more easily cultured than the squames obtained by amniocentesis.

Risks
- Miscarriage as a result of CVS is estimated at 1%.
- Increases risk of vertical transmission of blood-borne viruses such as HIV and hepatitis B.
- False negative results (rare) from contamination with maternal cells—especially with DNA analysis requiring PCR.
- Placental mosaicism producing misleading results—estimated at <1%.

Amniocentesis (Fig 3.11)

This is usually undertaken from 15 weeks onwards. It involves aspiration of amniotic fluid which contains fetal cells shed from the skin and gut. It is performed transabdominally with ultrasound guidance.

Indications
- For karyotyping if screening tests suggest aneuploidy.
- For DNA analysis if parents are carriers of an identifiable gene mutation such as cystic fibrosis or thalassaemia.
- For enzyme assays looking for inborn errors of metabolism.
- For diagnosis of fetal infections such as CMV and toxoplasmosis.

Benefits
- Lower procedure attributed miscarriage rate than CVS ~1%.
- Less risk of maternal contamination or placental mosaicism.

Risks
- Miscarriage as a result of amniocentesis is estimated at 1%, although recent data suggests that the risk of miscarriage after amniocentesis is very little higher than would occur naturally.
- Failure to culture cells ~0.5%.
- Full karyotyping may take 3 weeks (results for certain chromosomal abnormalities may be available more rapidly using FISH or PCR).

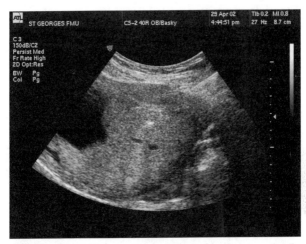

Fig. 3.10 Chorionic villus sampling.

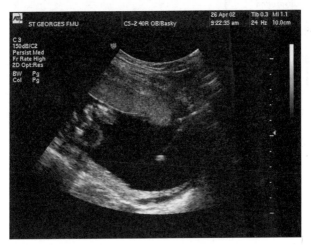

Fig. 3.11 Amniocentesis.

Fetal hydrops: overview

Definition
Fetal hydrops is the abnormal accumulation of serous fluid in two or more fetal compartments. This may be pleural or pericardial effusions, ascites, skin oedema, polyhydramnios, or placental oedema. It may be divided into non-immune and immune causes.

Pathophysiology
The mechanism for the development of hydrops appears to be due to an imbalance of interstitial fluid production and inadequate lymphatic return. This can result from congestive heart failure, obstructed lymphatic flow, or decreased plasma osmotic pressure.
- **Immune hydrops** results from fetal anaemia that is due to blood group incompatibility between the mother and the fetus.
- **Non-immune hydrops** results from other causes, including fetal anaemia that is due to other causes such as fetal infection.

Incidence
Occurs in ~1:2000 births.

Non-immune fetal hydrops: diagnosis and investigations
Ultrasound
- The diagnosis is made by an ultrasound scan.
- Associated structural abnormalities may be seen.
- Fetal echocardiography is required to diagnose cardiac lesions.
- Peak systolic velocity in the middle cerebral artery identifies fetal anaemia.

Fetal blood or amniotic fluid sampling
- Fetal blood sampling if anaemia is suspected (with blood ready for in-utero transfusion).
- Amniotic fluid or fetal blood for chromosome analysis ± virology.

Maternal blood testing
- Kleihauer test for feto-maternal haemorrhage.
- Antibody screen must be performed to exclude immune hydrops.
- Virology (initially for parvovirus).
- Consider haemoglobin electrophoresis for α-thalassaemia trait.

Non-immune fetal hydrops: principal causes

Severe anaemia
- Congenital parvovirus B19 infection.
- α-thalassaemia major (common in areas such as south-east Asia).
- Massive feto-maternal haemorrhage.
- Glucose-6-phosphate dehydrogenase deficiency.

Cardiac abnormalities, including:
- Structural abnormalities.
- Fetal tachyarrhythmia (SVT or atrial flutter).
- Congenital heart block.

Chromosomal abnormalities including:
- Trisomies 13, 18, and 21.
- Turner's syndrome (45X0).

Other genetic syndromes, including:
- Multiple other syndromes, e.g. achondrogenesis, Noonan's syndrome, Fryn's syndrome, myotonic dystrophy.

Other infections (see 📖 Chapter 4)
- Toxoplasmosis.
- Rubella.
- Cytomegalovirus (CMV).
- Varicella.

Other structural abnormalities, including:
- Congenital cystadenomatous malformation (CCAM).
- Diaphragmatic hernia.
- Pleural effusions.

Twin-to-twin transfusion syndrome (see 📖 Chapter 2, p. 76)
- Recipient from volume overload and donor from anaemia.

Placental
- Chorioangioma.

Non-immune hydrops: treatment

The prognosis depends on the underlying cause. Where treatment is not possible, the option of termination of pregnancy should be discussed. In the 3rd trimester, delivery may be a better alternative than in-utero treatment.

If severe polyhydramnios is present, removal of excess amniotic fluid (amnioreduction) may reduce the risk of preterm labour. Consider giving steroids before the procedure as it carries a small risk of triggering preterm labour.

Treatable causes of non-immune fetal hydrops

Fetal anaemia
- In-utero blood transfusion may be performed.

Pleural effusions or large CCAM
- In-utero percutaneous drainage and subsequent insertion of shunt into amniotic fluid may be possible.

Twin-to-twin transfusion syndrome
- Laser photocoagulation of placental anastomoses improves the prognosis.

Cardiac
- Tachyarrhythmias may be treated with maternal digoxin and flecainide.
- Stenting of stenotic cardiac valves is possible but is usually too late if hydrops has already developed.

Rhesus isoimmunisation (immune hydrops)

Definition

Rhesus isoimmunization occurs when a maternal antibody response is mounted against fetal red cells. These IgG antibodies cross the placenta and cause fetal red blood cell destruction. The ensuing anaemia, if severe, precipitates fetal hydrops which is often referred to as immune hydrops.

Rhesus blood groups

The rhesus system consists of three linked gene pairs; one allele of each pair is dominant to the other: C/c, D/d, and E/e. There are only five antigens as d is not an antigen, it merely implies the absence of D. Inheritance is Mendelian. The D gene is the most significant cause of isoimmunization, because about 16% of white mothers are rhesus D negative (d/d). The incidence is lower in Afro-Caribbean and Asian populations. Other significant antigens include c, E, and the atypical Kell antibody. Because of the success of anti-D prophylaxis, these now account for up to 1/2 of the cases of isoimmunisation.

Pathophysiology of rhesus disease

Fetal cells cross into the maternal circulation in normal pregnancy; the amount is increased during particular 'sensitizing events'.

The fetus may carry the gene for an antigen which the mother does not have—with rhesus D, the fetus may be D/d (rhesus D positive) whilst the mother is d/d (rhesus D negative).

Individuals exposed to a 'foreign' antigen mount an immune response (sensitization); initially this is IgM, which cannot cross the placenta so this pregnancy is not at risk.

Re-exposure in a subsequent pregnancy causes the primed memory B cells to produce IgG, which actively crosses into the fetal circulation.

IgG binds to fetal red cells, which are then destroyed in the reticuloendothelial system.

This causes a haemolytic anaemia (if erythropoesis is inadequate to compensate, severe anaemia causes high output cardiac failure, 'fetal hydrops' and ultimately, death).

In milder cases, haemolysis leads to neonatal anaemia, or jaundice from increased bilirubin levels.

Potential sensitizing events for rhesus disease

Termination of pregnancy or evacuation of retained prodcuts of conception (ERPC) after miscarriage.
Ectopic pregnancy.
Vaginal bleeding >12 weeks, or earlier if heavy.
External cephalic version (ECV).
Blunt abdominal trauma.
Invasive uterine procedure, e.g. amniocentesis or CVS.
Intrauterine death.
Delivery.

Rhesus disease: management

- All women should be checked for antibodies (rhesus and atypical) at booking, 28 and 34 weeks.
- If antibodies are detected, identifying the partner's status will help determine the potential fetal blood group and risk to the fetus.
- PCR of fetal cells in maternal blood may also determine the fetus's blood group, if the father is heterozygous or paternity is uncertain.
- Positive but low levels of antibodies (<10 IU/mL) should prompt repeat testing every 4 weeks.
- If levels are >10 IU/mL, assessment for fetal anaemia is required.

▶ Amniocentesis or fetal blood sampling based on antibody levels or history alone is now obsolete.

- The peak systolic velocity of the fetal middle cerebral artery (MCA) should be measured, looking for an indication of anaemia, about once a week.
- If it is increased (>1.5 multiples of median (MoM), normograms for gestation are available) fetal blood sampling is indicated, with blood available for transfusion.

Treatment

- If the fetal haemaotocrit is <30, irradiated, Rh-negative, CMV-negative packed red cells are transfused into the umbilical vein at the cord insertion, or into the hepatic vein.
- This can be performed from 18 weeks onwards (beyond 35 weeks, delivery is preferable).
- Haemolysis will continue and the transfusion is repeated either every 2 weeks or when the MCA becomes abnormal again.

⚠ The risk of fetal loss, or need for urgent delivery if >26 weeks, is 1–3% per transfusion in skilled hands.

Postnatal management

- Anaemia can be corrected by blood transfusion.
- Severe anaemia may be accompanied by a coagulopathy from decreased platelets and clotting factors.
- Hyperbilirubinaemia and jaundice occur because in utero the mother cleared this red blood cell breakdown product but the immature neonatal liver is unable to cope (this usually needs phototherapy but may require exchange transfusion)

⚠ Antibodies may persist for weeks, causing continued haemolysis in the neonate; this requires careful monitoring with haematocrit measurements.

Prevention of rhesus (D) disease

If sufficient anti-D immunoglobulin is given to the mother it will bind to any fetal red cells in her circulation carrying the D antigen. This prevents her own immune system from recognizing them and therefore becoming sensitized.

- Anti-D (500 IU) is given to all women who are rhesus negative (d/d):
  - routinely at 28 and 34 weeks
  - within 72 hours of any potentially sensitizing event
  - after delivery if the neonate is found to be rhesus positive (D/d).
- Occasionally, large feto-maternal haemorrhages occur during sensitizing events. If this is suspected a Kleihauer test should be performed as the standard dose of anti-D may not be sufficient. This should be routinely undertaken at delivery if the neonate is RhD positive.
- Other antibodies, particularly anti-kell and anti-c, now account for about half of all cases fetal haemolysis.
- The use of anti-D, together with smaller family sizes, mean that rhesus disease is now rare. Only about 2% of RhD negative women in the UK have been sensitized.

Oligohydramnios

Amniotic fluid after 20 weeks largely consists of fetal urine. The volume depends on urine production, fetal swallowing, and absorption. Normal volume varies with gestation, and is highest between 24 and 36 weeks. The volume is measured by ultrasound, either by measuring the deepest vertical pool, or by adding up the deepest pools in the four quadrants of the uterus (amniotic fluid index, AFI).

In oligohydramnios, the amniotic fluid volume is reduced. Normograms of both measures are available, but as a general rule, a deepest pool of <2 cm or an AFI of <8 cm is considered low.

Complications
- Related to cause:
  - preterm rupture of the membranes is commonly followed by delivery and/or intrauterine infection
  - IUGR is an important cause of fetal and neonatal mortality and long term morbidity.
- Related to reduced volume:
  - lung hypoplasia if occurs <22 weeks
  - limb abnormalities, e.g. talipes, if prolonged.
  - Oligohydramnios before 22 weeks has a very poor prognosis.

Investigations
- USS of fetus, including Doppler.
- Speculum examination to look for ruptured membranes.
- If suspected SROM: CRP, FBC, and vaginal swabs should be taken.

Management of oligohydramnios

If SROM at 37 or more weeks:
- Induce labour unless CS is indicated for another reason.

If SROM before 37 weeks:
- give prophylactic oral erythromycin
- monitor for signs of infection (4 hourly temperature and pulse)
- daily CTGs.

If IUGR:
- manage according to umbilical artery Doppler and CTG.

If apparently isolated oligohydramnios:
- reconsider cause
- intervention is not usual if umbilical artery Dopplers are normal.

If fetal renal tract abnormality:
- refer to fetal medicine centre.

Causes of oligohydramnios
- Leakage of amniotic fluid:
  - spontaneous rupture of the membranes (SROM).
- Reduced fetal urine production:
  - IUGR
  - fetal renal failure or abnormalities
  - post-dates pregnancy
- Obstruction to fetal urine output:
  - fetal abnormalities such as posterior urethral valves.

Polyhydramnios

The amniotic fluid is increased. In general a deepest pool of >8 cm or an AFI >22 is abnormal.

Causes of polyhydramnios

- Increased fetal urine production:
  - maternal diabetes
  - twin–twin transfusion syndrome (recipient twin).
  - fetal hydrops.
- Fetal inability to swallow or absorb amniotic fluid:
  - fetal GI tract obstruction (e.g. duodenal atresia, tracheo-oesophageal fistula)
  - fetal neurological or muscular abnormalities (e.g. myotonic dystrophy, anencephaly)
  - other rare abnormalities or syndromes (e.g. facial obstruction)
- Idiopathic (usually mild).

Complications

- Preterm delivery, probably because of uterine stretch.
- Of the cause: e.g. duodenal atresia is associated with trisomy 21.
- Malpresentation at delivery because of increased room for fetus.
- Maternal discomfort because of abdominal distension.

Investigations

- Exclude maternal diabetes with a glucose tolerance test (GTT).
- Ultrasound examination of fetus.

Polyhydramnios: management

- Severe polyhydramnios is usually associated with fetal abnormality, if massive (e.g. AFI >40), amnioreduction (drainage of excess fluid with a needle), or non-steroidals (NSAIDs).
- If fetal abnormality, refer to fetal medicine centre.
- Twin–twin transfusion syndrome is best managed in a fetal medicine centre, usually with laser ablation of placental anastomoses.
- If preterm, assess risk of delivery with cervical scan, and consider steroids.
- If unstable or transverse lie at term, admit to hospital:
  - CS if labour ensues with an abnormal lie.

⚠ NSAIDs cause fetal oliguria and can constrict the ductus arteriosus therefore close supervision is indicated.

Intrauterine growth restriction (IUGR): overview

The fetus is believed to have an inherent growth potential which under ideal conditions should produce a healthy baby of the appropriate size. Attaining this potential relies on such factors as a healthy mother, well-functioning placenta and the absence of pathology. If the in-utero circumstances are less than ideal, the fetus will fail to achieve its full potential growth and fetal well-being may be compromised. This problem is analogous to 'failure to thrive' in children and is termed intrauterine growth restriction (IUGR).

Definition

▶ The term IUGR implies a fetus that is pathologically small.

Most epidemiological studies use **small for gestational age** (SGA) as a surrogate marker. The most commonly used method of identification of SGA is where the estimated weight of the fetus is below the 10th percentile for its gestational age.

This method is imperfect because it includes small but healthy babies, and average-sized unhealthy babies that should have been born big.

Identifying inherent growth potential

To identify actual pathology and to improve detection of IUGR it is important to try to define the inherent growth potential of each individual fetus. Physiological factors known to affect growth and birthweight include:
• Maternal height and, to a lesser extent, paternal height.
• Maternal weight in early pregnancy.
• Parity.
• Ethnic origin.
• Gender of the fetus.

Some of these factors have been used to generate customized growth charts which aim to identify the optimal growth curve for an individual fetus. These are freely available at www.gestation.net. They appear to reduce the rate of constitutionally small babies being classed as IUGR (false positive rate) while helping to increase detection of pathologically small babies.

Defining expected growth also requires accurate dating of the pregnancy, ideally by USS in the 1st trimester between 8 and 13 weeks gestation.

📖 www.pi.nhs.uk/growth/index_growth.htm

📖 www.gestation.net

Importance of IUGR

For IUGR fetuses compared to the normally grown population:
- Perinatal mortality is 6–10 times greater.
- Incidence of cerebral palsy is 4 times greater.
- 30% of all stillborn infants are growth restricted.

IUGR fetuses are also more likely to have:
- Intrapartum fetal distress and asphyxia.
- Meconium aspiration.
- Emergency CS.
- Necrotizing enterocolitis.
- Hypoglycaemia and hypocalcaemia.

Intrauterine growth restriction (IUGR): causes

Causes of growth restriction may be grouped into maternal, utero-placental, and fetal.

⚠ By far the most common cause is utero-placental insufficiency.

Maternal causes of IUGR

- Chronic maternal disease, including:
  - hypertension
  - cardiac disease
  - chronic renal failure.
- Substance abuse:
  - alcohol
  - recreational drug use.
- Smoking.
- Autoimmune diseases, including:
  - antiphospholipid antibody syndrome.
- Genetic disorders, including:
  - Phenylketonuria.
- Poor nutrition.
- Low socio-economic status.

Placental causes of IUGR (placental insufficiency)

- Abnormal trophoblast invasion:
  - pre-eclampsia
  - placenta accreta.
- Infarction.
- Abruption.
- Placental location:
  - placenta praevia.
- Tumours:
  - chorioangiomas (placental haemangiomas).
- Abnormal umbilical cord or cord insertion:
  - two-vessel cord.

Fetal causes of IUGR

- Genetic abnormalities, including:
  - trisomy 13, 18, or 21
  - Turner's syndrome
  - Triploidy.
- Congenital abnormalities, including:
  - Cardiac, e.g. tetralogy of Fallot, transposition of the great vessels
  - Gastroschisis.
- Congenital infection, including:
  - CMV
  - rubella
  - toxoplasmosis.
- Multiple pregnancy.

Intrauterine growth restriction (IUGR): management and outcome

Symmetric and asymmetric IUGR

IUGR is often classified into symmetric and asymmetric, although the two groups overlap substantially:

- **Symmetric growth restriction** describes a fetus whose entire body is proportionately small and tends to be seen with very early onset IUGR, often due to chromosomal abnormalities.
- **Asymmetric growth restriction** is seen with an undernourished fetus who is compensating by directing most of its energy to maintaining the growth of vital organs such as the brain and heart at the expense of the liver, fat, and muscle. This 'head-sparing effect' results in a normal head size with small abdominal circumference and thin limbs. It is most often seen with IUGR secondary to placental insufficiency. If the insult is sustained long enough the fetus begins to lose the ability to compensate and head growth also becomes affected.

Management

Early identification and intensive fetal monitoring are the keys to managing IUGR. The aim is to continue the pregnancy safely for as long as possible, thereby decreasing the problems associated with prematurity, but deliver before the fetus becomes excessively compromised. This is covered in depth in Antenatal fetal surveillance, 📖 p. 144.

Long-term outcome

Most congenitally normal IUGR babies will go on to grow normally in infancy and childhood, but there may be more subtle long term consequences including up to 1/3 of children not reaching their predicted adult height, and childhood attention and performance deficits.

The effects appear to last into adulthood with a stimulus or insult at a critical, sensitive period of early life having permanent effects on structure, physiology, and metabolism. People who were small or disproportionate (thin or short) at birth have been found to have higher rates of coronary heart disease, high blood pressure, high cholesterol concentrations, and abnormal glucose-insulin metabolism. (Barker hypothesis).

📖 Godfrey KM, Barker DJ. Fetal nutrition and adult disease. *Am J Clin Nutr*. 2000;71(5 Suppl): 1344S–52S.

Antenatal fetal surveillance: overview

Facts

The fetus is vulnerable to any strain in the uteroplacental unit—its supply line for nutrition and gas exchange. Nearly 1/100 babies in developed countries are stillborn and 1/3 of all stillbirths occur in babies that are small for dates.

Any uteroplacental shortfall becomes more critical as the fetus gets bigger, and there is an extraordinary rate of growth during the last weeks of pregnancy. The stillbirth risk rises at the same stage.

▶ There are no treatments to reverse uteroplacental insufficiency but, potentially, delivering the baby at the right time can prevent death and disability.

⚠ The only intervention is delivery so monitoring is not useful if the fetus could not survive if it were delivered, i.e. if it is <24 weeks or <500 g.

Stages in fetal surveillance

Antepartum fetal monitoring is done in two stages.
- **Stage 1—assigning risk:**
  - finding normal babies developing in an abnormal situation.
- **Stage 2—timing delivery:**
  - after 37 weeks babies, at high risk should be delivered
  - preterm babies should be delivered only if they show signs of distress, ensuring maximum maturity while avoiding any harm.

Assigning risk (see Fig. 3.12)

- No method of antenatal monitoring is perfect—all 'miss' affected fetuses (false negatives) and 'pick up' normal fetuses (false positives).
- Potential problems with such screening include increasing the rate of major interventions (such as CS) without benefit.
- Given the low prevalence of fetal compromise, the positive predictive value of all tests when applied to low-risk populations is poor, but they perform better when applied to high-risk populations and therefore an estimation of the background risk must be made.
- Risk is assigned considering the mother's health (e.g. pre-eclampsia) and the outcome of any previous pregnancy.

✦ In the future, formal assessment of placental function using serum markers and ultrasound could establish itself as a routine test, in the same way as screening for Down's syndrome.

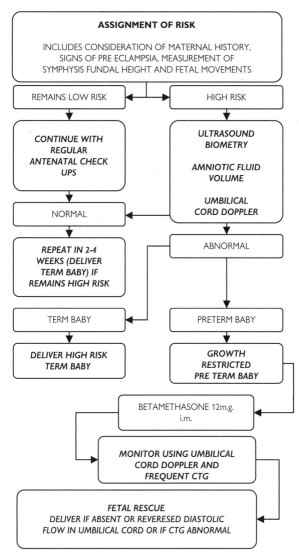

Fig. 3.12 Assigning risk in antenatal monitoring.

Identifying the high-risk fetus

Symphysis–fundal height
- Measurement of the symphysis–fundal height (cm).
- Sequential measurements can reveal changes in fetal growth.
- The detection rate of small for gestational age babies is improved by using 'customized' fundal height charts displaying curves that are specific to the mother's height, weight, parity, and ethnic group (see IUGR, 📖 p. 140)
- If the growth is suspected to be abnormal, a USS should be organized.

Routine monitoring of fetal movement
- The positive predictive value of maternal perception of reduced fetal movements is low.
- The 'count to ten' method monitoring of fetal movement involves asking the mother to record on a chart the time interval each day required to feel ten movements.
- This is not effective in reducing the incidence of antenatal fetal death. Mothers should simply be advised to contact their midwife or the hospital for further assessment if there is a reduction in fetal movement.

Auscultation of the fetal heart
- Auscultation of the fetal heart is done (using either a hand-held Doppler or a Pinard stethoscope) as part of a standard antenatal examination.
- It confirms that the fetus is alive but provides very little predictive information and, therefore, does not have a value beyond reassuring the mother that the fetus is alive at the time.

Ultrasound assessment of fetal growth
Accurate knowledge of the age of the fetus is required. The fetal head circumference (HC) and abdominal circumference (AC) are measured together with the deepest pool of amniotic fluid using ultrasound and the results are charted against gestational age. The position of the baby and the placenta are noted. Serial measurements are useful to assess the pattern of the fetal growth.

Late ultrasound aims to detect:
- Growth problems in the baby.
- Abnormalities in the amount of fluid around the baby.
- Problems with the placenta.
- Problems with the baby's position.

It should be used only where growth abnormality is suspected (SFH outside the normal range) or the patient is at high risk of uteroplacental insufficiency, because it does not improve outcome in unselected patients.

Monitoring the high-risk fetus: Doppler ultrasound

Doppler ultrasound uses sound waves to study blood circulation in the baby, uterus and placenta.

Uterine artery Doppler

- Resistance within the placenta can be measured from the maternal side, usually as a screening test at 23 weeks.
- High resistance in the uterine artery indicates that the mother is at increased risk of developing early onset pre-eclampsia or having a baby with IUGR, therefore she should be offered extra monitoring in pregnancy.

Umbilical artery Doppler

- Increasing resistance in the umbilical artery is an indicator of placental failure. Using this in high-risk pregnancies reduces the risk of fetal death and the need for interventions around birth, such as CS.
- Diagnostic:
  - a high resistance can help to differentiate a normal baby from one that is not reaching its full growth potential
  - abnormal waveforms in the umbilical artery are an early sign of fetal impairment and tend to precede changes in CTG.
- Monitoring:
  - in very preterm babies Doppler can be used to time fetal rescue.

Understanding umbilical artery Dopplers

- When the placenta is functioning normally, flow through the umbilical artery is not impeded by end organ resistance, therefore, blood continues to flow forwards (away from the heart) during cardiac diastole, seen on Doppler wave form as 'end diastolic flow' (Fig. 3.13).
- As the uteroplacental unit begins to fail, the vascular resistance rises and the forward flow in diastole begins to be reduced (this can be numerically quantified and used for monitoring).
- When the resistance is very high, blood no longer flows forwards in diastole, this is called 'absent end diastolic flow' (AEDF) (Fig 3.14).
- When the situation is critical, the resistance is so great that blood may flow back towards the heart during diastole, this is called 'reversed end diastolic flow' (REDF) (Fig. 3.15).

△ These signs are used to differentiate those fetuses that are coping in an adverse situation from those that need immediate delivery

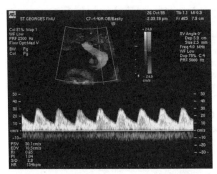

Fig. 3.13 Example of normal umbilical artery Doppler waveform.

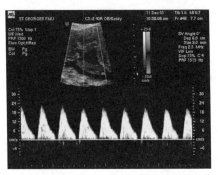

Fig 3.14 Example of umbilical artery Doppler waveform with absent end diastolic flow (AEDF).

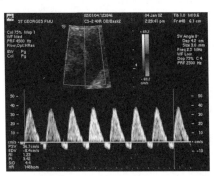

Fig 3.15 Example of umbilical artery Doppler waveform with reversed end diastolic flow (REDF).

Monitoring the high risk fetus: cardiotocography (CTG)

(See Chapter 6, 📖 p. 280)

- CTG is the output of electronic monitoring of the fetal heart rate, cor-related with any uterine contractions.
- Analysis by inspecting the CTG is difficult but it is more reproducible when done by computer systems, e.g. Oxford Sonicaid.

Normal CTG

- The baseline fetal heart rate between 110–160 beats/minute and varying from that baseline by 5–25 beats/minute.
- The heart rate should speed up by at least 15 beats/minute for at least 15 seconds (accelerations). Two accelerations should be seen in 20 minutes (reactive).
- There should be no slowing of the fetal heart rate from the baseline (decelerations).

▶ The most useful features in assessing the fetus' health are the variability and presence or absence of accelerations.

Abnormal CTG

- ⚠ Caused by a failure of autonomic regulation of the heart rate. This is an end-stage event, so the lead-time between uteroplacental insuf-ficiency causing an abnormal CTG and fetal death or long-term damage is short, and this limits its usefulness in antenatal screening.
- ☙ CTG has not been found to be useful in low-risk populations.

CTG is used to exclude current compromise in:

- Acute conditions known to cause fetal compromise e.g. abruption and in women reporting reduced fetal movements.
- Daily in the surveillance of chronic conditions that are associated with uteroplacental insufficiency such as pre-eclampsia and IUGR.

📖 Antenatal care for the healthy pregnant woman. Chapter 12: Fetal growth and wellbeing. NICE, 2003. www.nice.org.uk/guidance/CG6

Infectious diseases in pregnancy

nent (including
ction. However,
indicated, with

Rubella (German measles)

Epidemiology
- RNA togavirus.
- Spread by respiratory droplets—person to person.
- Incubation 14–21 days.
- Infectious for 7 days before and after appearance of rash.
- Re-infection can occur mostly with vaccine-induced immunity.

Symptoms
- Mild, febrile illness.
- Maculopapular rash.
- Arthralgia.
- Lymphadenopathy.
- Symptoms only present in 50–75% of cases.

Diagnosis
Requires serological confirmation with paired samples; acute and convalescent phase (21–28 days later). Recent infection is confirmed by:
- Appearance of IgM antibodies
- ≥Fourfold ↑ in IgG antibody titres.

Rubella-associated congenital defects

The virus disrupts mitosis, retarding cellular division and causing vascular damage. Major malformations are most likely during organogenesis with severity decreasing with advancing gestation. Defects include:
- Sensorineural deafness.
- Cardiac abnormalities including VSD, PDA.
- Eye lesions (congenital cataracts, microphthalmia, and glaucoma).
- Microcephaly and mental retardation.

Late-developing sequelae include:
- Diabetes.
- Thyroid disorders.
- Progressive panencephalitis.

Prevention
- 'Herd immunity' is maintained by widespread childhood vaccination, although the recent concerns over the safety of the MMR vaccine has decreased the uptake in the UK. Ideally, women should be tested before pregnancy to ensure immunity, but routine screening at booking identifies those at risk and in need of postnatal vaccination.

⚠ The vaccine is a live attenuated virus and therefore contraindicated in pregnancy. Women are counselled to avoid pregnancy for 10–12 weeks after vaccination although there is little evidence of association with congenital infection.

Table 4.1 Risk of congenital defects by gestation in primary rubella infection

Gestation	Risk of transmission	Risk of congenital abnormality	Treatment
<13 weeks	80%	Almost all infected fetuses	TOP may be offered without invasive prenatal diagnosis
13–16 weeks	50%	About 35% of those infected (mainly deafness)	Fetal blood sampling may be later offered to confirm infection
>16 weeks	25%	Rarely causes defects	Reassurance

Cytomegalovirus (CMV)

Epidemiology
- Herpes virus.
- Transmitted in bodily fluids—low infectivity.
- Can remain dormant within host for life making reactivation common.
- Seroprevelence ~50% of UK women.
- Incidence of primary infection in pregnancy ~1:100.

Symptoms
Asymptomatic in 95% of cases. May present with:
- Fever.
- Malaise.
- Lymphadenopathy and atypical lymphocytosis.

Diagnosis

Maternal infection
Usually requires serological confirmation with paired samples; acute and convalescent phase (14 days later). Recent infection is confirmed by:
- Significant ↑ in IgM antibodies (may persist for up to 8 months).
- ↑ IgG antibody titres.
- Culture/PCR of maternal urine (not widely available).

Fetal infection
- Culture/PCR of amniotic fluid (after 20 weeks).

CMV-associated congenital defects

- IUGR.
- Microcephaly.
- Hepatosplenamegaly and thrombocytopenia.
- Jaundice.
- Chorioretinitis.
- Later-developing sequelae include:
  - psychomotor retardation—reported to account for as much as 10% of mental retardation in children <6 years old
  - sensorineural hearing loss

Outcome
- With a primary maternal infection 40% of fetuses will be infected, irrespective of gestation. Of these:
- 90% are normal at birth, of which:
  - 20% will develop late, usually minor sequelae.
- 10% are symptomatic, of which:
  - 33% will die
  - 67% will have long-term problems.

Management
As most fetuses will be unaffected, counselling about managem TOP) is very difficult even in the face of confirmed fetal infe close monitoring of fetal growth and well-being is clearly appropriate paediatric follow-up.

Varicella (chickenpox)

Epidemiology
- Varicella zoster virus (VZV)—DNA virus.
- Spread by respiratory droplets and contact with vesicle fluid.
- Incubation 10–21 days.
- Infectious from 2 days before rash until all vesicles are crusted.
- Seroprevalence ~90% of UK women immune.
- Incidence of primary infection in pregnancy ~3:1000.

Symptoms
- Fever.
- Malaise.
- Maculopapular rash which becomes vesicular then crusts over.

Diagnosis
If there has been exposure without a good history of previous infection, serum should be tested for VZV IgG antibodies. If antibodies are detected within 10 days of contact, immunity can be assumed and reassurance given. If not, varicella immunoglobulin (VZIG) should be given as soon as possible. Diagnosis of varicella itself is usually made on the history of contact and appearance of the typical rash.

> **Maternal risks**
>
> ⚠ Varicella in pregnancy is often more severe and may be life-threatening as a consequence of:
> - Varicella pneumonia.
> - Hepatitis.
> - Encephalitis.

Fetal risks
Fetal infection rate is thought to be ~25% in all trimesters: if <20 weeks there is a 2% risk of fetal varicella syndrome with congenital defects including:
- Skin scarring.
- Limb hypoplasia.
- Eye lesions (congenital cataracts, microphthalmia, and chorioretinitis).
- Neurological abnormalities (mental retardation, microcephaly, cortical atrophy, and dysfunction of bladder and bowel sphincters).

Neonatal risks
▶ Neonatal varicella is seen in babies whose mothers contracted it in the last 4 weeks of pregnancy. Severe infection, which may be fatal, is most likely to occur if the rash appears 5 days before delivery or 2 days after. These babies should all receive VZIG as soon as possible.

Treatment
Oral aciclovir reduces the duration of symptoms if given within 24 hours of the rash appearing. Its effect on the incidence of serious sequelae is unknown.

Table 4.2 Risk to fetus from primary maternal varicella infection by gestation

Gestation	Risk to fetus	Management
<20 weeks	2% will develop fetal varicella syndrome (FVS)	Detailed ultrasound examination at 16–20 weeks, may consider TOP if evidence of FVS seen. Neonatal ophthalmic examination
>20 weeks	Not associated with congenital abnormality	Fetal and neonatal surveillance
Within 4 weeks of delivery	About 20% will develop neonatal varicella infection	VZIG as soon as possible, 14 days monitoring for signs of infection and aciclovir if varicella develops

📖 Green Top Guidelines. www.rcog.org.uk

Parvovirus B19

Epidemiology
- DNA virus.
- Spread by respiratory droplets—person to person.
- Incubation 4–20 days.
- Seroprevalence ~50% of UK women immune.
- Incidence of primary infection in pregnancy < 1:100.

Symptoms
- Often asymptomatic.
- Typical 'slapped cheek' rash (erythema infectiosum).
- Fever.
- Arthralgia.

Diagnosis
Requires serological confirmation with paired samples; acute and convalescent phase (>10 days later). Recent infection is confirmed by:
- Appearance of IgM antibodies
- ↑ IgG antibodies.

Maternal risks
Minimal in fit and healthy women. However, immunocompromised individuals are at risk of sudden haemolysis potentially severe enough to require blood transfusion.

Fetal risks
- Fetal infection rate is thought to be ~30%.
- The virus causes suppression of erythropoesis sometimes with thrombocytopenia and direct cardiac toxicity, eventually resulting in cardiac failure and hydrops fetalis.
- There are no congenital defects associated with parvovirus infection.

⚠ About 10% of fetuses infected at <20 weeks gestation will die.

Management
Serial ultrasound scans, measuring the peak systolic velocity of the fetal middle cerebral artery, are required to monitor for anaemia as this may develop many weeks after the initial infection. In-utero blood transfusion may be possible to prevent fetal demise in severely anaemic, hydropic fetuses. These patients should be cared for in a specialist fetal medicine unit.

Toxoplasmosis

Epidemiology
- Protozoan parasite *Toxoplasma gondii*.
- Spread by contact with cat faeces and eating undercooked meat.
- Incubation <2 days.
- Seroprevalence: ~20% of UK women immune.
- Incidence of primary infection in pregnancy ~1:500. Rare in UK.

Symptoms
Asymptomatic in about 80% of cases. May present with:
- Fever.
- Lymphadenopathy.

Diagnosis
Maternal infection
Requires serological confirmation with paired samples; acute and convalescent phase (>28 days later). Recent infection is confirmed by:
- Isolated very high titres of IgM antibodies (may persist for up to 1 year).
- Concurrent high IgM and IgG antibodies.
- Fourfold ↑ IgG antibodies.

Fetal infection
May be diagnosed by the presence of IgM antibodies in amniotic fluid or fetal blood. Amniocentesis is accurate only after 20 weeks. Although ultrasound signs such as cerebral ventriculomegaly can occur most affected fetuses have a normal scan.

Maternal risks
Minimal in fit and healthy women. However, immunocompromised individuals are at risk of severe disseminated illness with chorioretinitis and encephalitis.

Fetal risks
Spontaneous miscarriage is common with infection in the first trimester. Defects associated with primary infection include:
- Chorioretinitis.
- Microcephaly and hydrocephalus.
- Intracranial calcification.
- Mental retardation.

Management
Starting spiramycin on diagnosis of maternal infection may decrease the risk of fetal infection. If vertical transmission occurs combination anti-toxoplasmosis therapy is used. Neonatal follow-up should include an ophthalmic review and cranial radiological studies. It is usually recommended that future pregnancies are delayed until maternal IgM antibodies have been cleared.

Table 4.3 Risk of congenital defects by gestation in toxoplasmosis infection

Gestation	Risk of transmission	Risk of congenital abnormality in infected fetuses
<12 weeks	~17%	75%
12–28 weeks	~25%	25%
>28 weeks	65%	<10%

Herpes simplex

Epidemiology

- Herpes simplex virus (HSV)—type 2 causes >70% genital infections.
- Spread by sexual contact.
- Incubation ~2–7 days.
- An individual may be infectious even when apparently asymptomatic.
- Seroprevalence of HSV 2: ~20% of UK women.

Symptoms

Primary HSV infection is the most severe and usually results in:

- Mild flu-like illness.
- Inguinal lymphadenopathy.
- Vulvitis and pain sometimes severe enough to cause urinary retention.
- Small, characteristic vesicles on the vulva.

Diagnosis

Usually made on the history appearance of the typical rash, but viral culture of vesicle fluid is the gold standard. Acute and convalescent antibody levels may sometimes be helpful.

Maternal risks

In pregnancy a primary attack may be severe with complications including:

- Meningitis.
- Sacral radiculopathy—causing urinary retention and constipation.
- Transverse myelitis.
- Disseminated infection.

Fetal risks

Primary infection may lead to miscarriage or preterm labour, but no related congenital defects have been identified.

Neonatal risks

Transmission rate from vaginal delivery during primary maternal infection may be as high as 50% but is relatively uncommon during a recurrent attack (<5%). Neonatal herpes appears during the first 2 weeks of life.

- 25% limited to eyes and mouth only.
- 75% widely disseminated, of which:
  - ~70% will die
  - many of the survivors will have long-term problems including mental retardation.

Management

Aciclovir may decrease severity and duration of the primary attack if given within 5 days of onset of symptoms. If labour is within 6 weeks of primary infection then delivery by CS is recommended provided the membranes have not been ruptured for >4 hours. With active vesicles from a recurrent attack, the risk of surgery must be carefully weighed against the very small risk of neonatal infection.

Hepatitis B

Epidemiology
- Hepatitis B virus (HBV)—DNA virus.
- Spread by infected blood, blood products or sexual contact.
- Incubation 2–6 months.
- Incidence of carrier status in UK women is ~1:100.

Symptoms
Prodrome of non-specific systemic and gastrointestinal symptoms followed by an episode of jaundice.

Diagnosis
Based on clinical picture and serological detection of:
- HB surface antigen (HBsAg) → current infection.
- HB e antigen (HBeAg) → active viral replication.
- Anti-HBsAg antibodies → indicates immunity either from infection or vaccination.

Maternal risks
In the developed world, hepatitis B infection in pregnancy has a similar course to that seen in the non-pregnant individual:
- 65% subclinical disease with full recovery.
- 25% develop acute hepatitis.
- 10% become chronic carriers.
- <0.5% develop fulminant hepatitis which has a significant mortality rate.

Fetal risks
Severe acute infection may lead to miscarriage or preterm labour but no related congenital defects have been identified.

Neonatal risks

Transmission usually occurs at delivery but <5% may be due to transplacental bleeding in utero. Neonatal infection may be fatal, and usually results in chronic carrier status with significant lifelong risks of cirrhosis and hepatocellular carcinoma. The carrier status of the mother at delivery determines the risk of vertical transmission:
- HBsAg and HBeAg positive: ~95% risk.
- HbsAg positive and HBeAg negative: <15% risk.

Management
▶ In the UK all women should be routinely screened for HBV at booking.

▶ High-risk women (e.g. commercial sex workers and IV drug users) should be counselled and vaccinated before pregnancy.

⚠ Babies whose mothers have acute or chronic HBV should receive HBV IgG and HBV vaccination within 24 hours of delivery. This is thought to be up to 95% effective at preventing neonatal HBV infection.

Group B streptococcus (GBS)

Epidemiology
- Streptococcus agalactiae.
- Common bowel commensal.
- Up to 20% women carry it vaginally.

Symptoms
- None.

Diagnosis
- Culture from a lower vaginal (LVS) and perianal swab.

Fetal risks
Associated with preterm prelabour rupture of membranes and preterm delivery.

Neonatal risks

Most frequent cause of early onset, severe neonatal infection (incidence 1:2000 live births). Up to 70% of babies whose mothers carry GBS will themselves be colonized at delivery, but only 1% of these will develop symptoms of sepsis. Early-onset GBS infection (<4 days from delivery) has about a 20% mortality rate and may present with:
- Pneumonia.
- Septicaemia.
- Meningitis.

Late-onset infection (>7 days) is not associated with maternal GBS carriage.

⚠ This carries a mortality rate of about 20%. Of those surviving, 50% will have serious neurological sequelae such as cortical blindness and deafness

Management
The RCOG does not recommend routine antenatal screening for GBS. However, intrapartum antibiotic prophylaxis should be offered to women with a history of previous neonatal GBS infection. Prophylaxis should also be considered if GBS is discovered incidentally in either the vagina or in urine but there is no benefit to be gained from attempting to eradicate it antenatally. Intrapartum prophylaxis should be considered with the following risk factors:
- Prematurity (<37 weeks).
- Prolonged rupture of membranes (>18 hours).
- Pyrexia in labour.

Antibiotics
The recommended prophylaxis in labour is IV benzylpenicillin started as soon as possible after onset of labour and at least 2 hours before delivery (3 g initially then 1.5 g every 4 hours throughout labour). In case of penicillin allergy, IV clindamycin should be used (900 mg every 8 hours).

📖 Green Top Guidelines www.rcog.org.uk

Other infections

Syphilis (see Chapter 16, 📖 p. 526)
- Currently relatively rare in the UK but reported to be increasing.
- Routinely screened for at booking but care must be taken when interpreting the results as biological false positives are common.
- The spirochaete can cross the placenta and is associated with pre-term delivery, still birth, and congenital syphilis defects which includes:
  - 8th nerve deafness
  - Hutchinson's teeth
  - saddle nose
  - sabre shins.
- Treatment with penicillin
  - <16 weeks—prevents virtually all congenital infection
  - >16 weeks—still effective in most cases.

Listeria monocytogenes

- Rare, affecting about 1:10 000 pregnancies in the UK.
- Found in soft cheese, pate, and undercooked meat and shellfish.
- Produces gastroenteritis often accompanied by flu-like symptoms.
- Crosses the placenta causing:
  - amnionitis
  - miscarriage or preterm labour.
- Neonatal infection may be:
  - generalized septicaemia
  - pneumonia
  - meningitis.
- Treatment is with high dose amoxicillin or erythromycin.

Malaria
- Protazoan infection, usually *Plasmodium falciparum*.
- Rare in the UK but must be considered if a history of travel to endemic areas.
- Major cause of pregnancy loss in tropical climates.
- Pregnancy increases the risk of developing severe disease.
- Symptoms include:
  - fever
  - rigors
  - abdominal pain
  - headache.
- Diagnosis is made from blood films.
- Effects on pregnancy:
  - miscarriage or pre-term delivery
  - stillbirth
  - congenital malaria
  - low birth weight ($2°$ to prematurity or IUGR).
- Proguanil and chloroquine are probably the safest drugs for malarial prophylaxis in pregnancy.

HIV and pregnancy

Facts
- Around 50 000 adults in the UK are infected with HIV (mainly HIV1).
- Over 1/2 have acquired their infection via heterosexual contact.
- The majority are of sub-Saharan African ethnicity.
- Highly active antiretroviral therapy (HAART) has ↑ life expectancy.
- In 2005 1091 babies were born to HIV-positive mothers.
- The risk of mother-to-child transmission (MTCT) is estimated to be 15–20% in non-breast-feeding mothers compared to 24–40% for breast-feeding mothers.
- MTCT can be reduced to 1% using antenatal HAART and CS, and avoiding breast-feeding.
- Pregnancy does not alter the course of the infection.
- High viral loads and low CD4 counts indicate the likelihood of the risk of MTCT and the need for the mother to receive therapy for her own health.

Prepregnancy counselling
⚠ Counselling of couples already known to be discordant with regard to HIV infection is important, as the risk of HIV transmission is estimated to be 0.03–1% for each act of unprotected intercourse.
- Where the mother is positive and the partner negative, self insemination with the partner's sperm is recommended.
- Sperm washing is recommended if the male is positive and the women negative.
- An alternative is donor insemination if the male partner is positive.
- IVF should take account of the parents' viral load, CD4 counts, and any AIDS defining illness.
- Consideration should be given to current therapy (HAART) as there is the possibility of teratogenicity with some drug combinations or taking folate antagonists for PCP prophylaxis.
- If the mother has already commenced on HAART she should continue this during pregnancy.

Antenatal screening

Routine antenatal screening was introduced in 1999 as part of the antenatal booking investigations. This is an opt-out policy and has increased the rate of HIV diagnosis significantly.

Confidentiality

⚠ It is estimated that 30–75% of the partners of HIV-positive mothers are unaware of the diagnosis.

▶ It is important to establish the need for health-care workers and partners to be aware of the diagnosis early so that an effective care plan can be put in place. This may require establishing a local mechanism to flag notes to indicate that additional information is available on a need-to-know basis should the mother be admitted as an emergency.

▶ Women should be encouraged to have all relevant information recorded in their hand-held notes.

HIV: antenatal care

Social and ethical issues

- Antenatal care should be delivered (See Fig. 4.1) by a multidisciplinary team which should include an obstetrician, HIV physician, paediatrician, and midwife.
- As there may be social, housing, or immigration issues, the involvement of social services should be considered.
- Other support groups may be required if there are issues with regard to drug addiction.
- Testing of other children is recommended.

⚠ Failure to engage with the antenatal care plan may require the involvement of legal services to address child protection issues.

▶ Local guidelines may exist for the eligibility for free NHS care; however, it is considered unethical to deny treatment to an HIV-positive mother as this treatment would protect her unborn child and potentially her own health.

Additional antenatal investigations

- Screening for STIs should be performed at presentation and repeated in the 3rd trimester.
- Hepatitis C screening should be performed as part of the initial assessment.
- Cervical cytology should be performed at presentation if this has not recently been performed.
- Syphilis serology should be repeated in the 3rd trimester.
- Viral load and CD4 count should be repeated every 3 months and specifically at 36 weeks to inform neonatal therapy.

Special considerations

- Increased fetal surveillance as there may be an ↑ risk of
  - miscarriage
  - stillbirth
  - IUGR
  - pre-eclampsia.
- If admitted with symptoms of pre-eclampsia, cholestasis of pregnancy, or 'unwell', consideration should be given to complications of antiretroviral therapy.
- Resistance testing should be considered if viral load remains high on therapy.
- There is no data with regard to viral transmission during invasive prenatal tests such as amniocentesis or CVS.

⚠ This should not exclude HIV-positive mothers from prenatal screening but consideration should be given to covering any procedure with antiretroviral therapy.

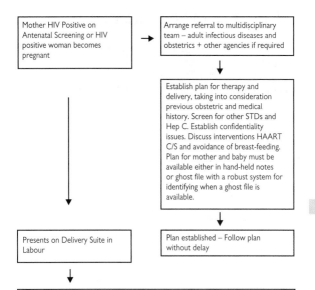

Mother HIV Positive on Antenatal Screening or HIV positive woman becomes pregnant

→

Arrange referral to multidisciplinary team – adult infectious diseases and obstetrics + other agencies if required

Establish plan for therapy and delivery, taking into consideration previous obstetric and medical history. Screen for other STDs and Hep C. Establish confidentiality issues. Discuss interventions HAART C/S and avoidance of breast-feeding. Plan for mother and baby must be available either in hand-held notes or ghost file with a robust system for identifying when a ghost file is available.

Presents on Delivery Suite in Labour

Plan established – Follow plan without delay

No Plan Available

Call the duty GU/ID Team (ask the patient which GU/ID consultant sees them to establish if there is a specific plan available) but do not delay in proceeding to:
- Intravenous ZDV during labour or caesarean section (load with 2mg/kg over 1 hour followed by continuous infusion of 1mg/kg/hour until delivery)
- Planned C/S if possible. If emergency C/S expedite delivery within 4 hours of rupture of membranes
- If vaginal delivery then avoid fetal scalp electrodes and FBS
- Recommend that the baby is not breast fed

Fig. 4.1 Flow chart for antenatal care of babies with HIV-positive mothers. Data courtsey of A Pollard, S Segal, J Seward, A Edwards, M Antony, T Peto, M Snelling and P Hurley of the Neonatal, Obstetric and GUM Departments of the John Radcliffe Hospital, Oxford.

HIV: mother-to-child transmission

There is a close linear relationship between maternal plasma viral load and the risk of transmission to the child. However, there is no level of viral load at which transmission has not occurred, as plasma viral load may not necessarily reflect genital viral load.

Effective prevention of MTCT can be achieved by:

• Antenatal highly active antiretroviral therapy (HAART).
• Delivery by CS.
• Avoidance of breast-feeding.

Risk factors for increased rate of MTCT

• Delivery is before 34 weeks gestation.
• Prolonged rupture of the membranes.
• Invasive procedures during labour such as the application of fetal scalp electrodes (FSE) or fetal blood sampling.

HAART (see Table 4.4)

• Monotherapy (usually with ZDV) is not recommended if the mother requires therapy for her own health.
• The use of montherapy which does not suppress viraemia may allow the emergence of resistant strains.
• Women requiring treatment for themselves (CD 4 count<350) should commence on combinations of three or more antiretroviral drugs at presentation.
• Women not requiring treatment outside pregnancy should commence HAART between 28 and 32 weeks gestation (referred to as START—short-term ART).
• Earlier commencement of START may be required depending on any history of preterm labour.
• Choice of HAART should be the responsibility of the HIV physician.

Table 4.4 Neonatal therapy (Oxford guidelines)

Clinical presentation	Suggested therapy	Duration
Mother commenced on HAART during pregnancy with ZDV containing combination AND last viral load <50 copies/mL	ZDV	4 weeks
Mother treated with HAART before pregnancy or on non-ZDV containing combination AND viral load <50 copies/mL	ZDV	4 weeks
Mother has had no ART and presents in labour or after delivery OR treated in pregnancy but last viral load >50 copies/mL	Triple Therapy NVP for 2 weeks, ZDV for 4 weeks 3TC for 4 weeks	Total 4 weeks
Baby born prematurely and not likely to be able to feed orally	Refer to paediatric ID as therapy will depend on maternal viral load	

Data courtesy of A Pollard, S Segal, J Serrard, A Edwards, M Anthony, T Peto, M Snelling and P Hurley of the Neonatal, Paediatric, Obstetric and GUM departments of the John Radcliffe Hospital, Oxford

HIV: perinatal and postnatal concerns

Delivery

Caesarean section
- There is clear benefit to women not taking HAART, or with a significant viral load.
- There may be some benefit from elective delivery at 38 rather than 39 weeks gestation (avoiding the spontaneous onset of labour).
- Should be performed within 4 hours of SROM.
- An IV infusion of ZDV should be commenced 4 hours before delivery and stopped after the cord is clamped.
- Early clamping of the cord is recommended.
- 'Bloodless' CS may be of benefit but is not routinely practised.

Vaginal delivery
- Women may choose not to be delivered by CS and this wish should be respected.
- Artificial rupture of the membranes (ROM) should be avoided.
- In the presence of ROM and no contractions augmentation of labour should take place immediately.
- The application of fetal scalp electrodes should be avoided.
- Fetal scalp blood sampling should not be performed.
- Delivery in water is not advised.
- Intravenous ZDV should be administered during labour even if there is no detectable viral load.

Neonatal management
- All infants born to HIV-positive mothers require ART for 4–6 weeks.
- The choice of monotherapy or combination therapy will depend on the mothers viral load (see Table 4.5).
- Neonates require testing at birth, 3 weeks, 6 weeks, and 6 months.
- The definitive test is an HIV antibody test at 18 months—a negative result at this time confirms that the child is not infected.
- Outcomes are given in Table 4.6.

☛ Whether the baby needs to be bathed immediately following delivery remains controversial.

Postnatal management and follow-up
- Women requiring therapy for their own health should continue HAART after delivery.
- Women who required START for prevention of MTCT may discontinue therapy on the advice of their HIV physician.
- All mothers and children require long-term follow-up.

▶ All cases of HIV in pregnancy (whether diagnosed before or during pregnancy) should be reported to The National Study of HIV in Pregnancy and Childhood at the RCOG even if the pregnancy is not continued to term. Email: nshpc@ich.uci.ac.uk

📖 Guidelines for the management of HIV infection in pregnant women and the prevention of mother-to-child transmission of HIV (2005) http://www.bhiva.org

Table 4.5 Classes of antiretroviral drugs

Class of drug	Examples	Potential problems
NRTIs Nucleoside analogue reverse transcriptase inhibitors	Zidovudine (ZDV—previously AZT) Lamivudine (3TC) Didanosine (ddl) Stavudine (d4T) Abacavir (ABC)	All are generally well tolerated, but there are reported case of anaemia, nausea and vomiting, elevated transaminases and hyperglycaemia. Lactic acidosis is a possibility when d4t and ddl are combined
NNRTIs Non-nucleoside analogue reverse transcriptase	Nevirapine (NVP) Delaviridine Efavirenz inhibitors	The greatest experience is with NVP, but although well tolerated there is an association with deranged liver function in women with good CD4 counts. Rash is also reported
PIs Protease inhibitors	Ritinovir Indinavir Nelfinavir Saquinavir	Hyperglycaemia is a risk with new onset diabetes or exacerbation of existing diabetes Diarrhoea, with nausea, vomiting and altered taste Altered liver function reported

Table 4.6 Neonatal Outcome Data. (National Study of HIV in Pregnancy and Childhood (NSHPC)—data to end of December 2006). Children born in the UK to women diagnosed before delivery*: year of birth and infection status. Data from RCOG, 2006

Year of birth	Total number of cases reported	Infected*	Indeter-minate +	Uninfected	Known to have died (infected and indeterminate only)
Total 1989–2006	6187	158	1472	4557	66
Example years					
2002	615	12	58	545	4
2005	1091	10	428	653	4

* An additional 633 infected children born to women who were undiagnosed at the time of delivery have also been reported.

+ Those currently described as indeterminate have results pending; most were born to diagnosed women and uninfected. Transmission rates should not be derived from these data because of reporting bias.

Vaccination and travel

Vaccination

- Live attenuated vaccines such as rubella, polio, or MMR are contraindicated in pregnancy.
- Passive immunization with specific human immunoglobulin is safe and may provide important protection (e.g. VZIG).
- Women who are HbsAg negative but considered at high risk should be offered HBV vaccination in pregnancy.
- Vaccinations for travel should be considered on an individual basis, and the small risk from the vaccine compared with the risk from contracting the disease:
  - cholera—limited efficacy therefore not recommended
  - hepatitis A—low risk, but consider human normal immunoglobulin (HNIG) for short periods
  - meningococcus—safety unknown, consider if high risk
  - rabies—consider immunoglobulin for post-exposure prophylaxis
  - tetanus—safe in pregnancy
  - yellow fever—safety unknown, consider if high risk.

Travel—general advice

Food

Avoid foodstuffs which may pose a potential risk of infection:
- Unwashed fruit and vegetables.
- Raw eggs.
- Undercooked meat.
- Tap water in countries with poor sanitation (beware of ice cubes).
- Shellfish in hepatitis A endemic areas.

Malaria

Appropriate antimalarials should be taken, accompanied by avoidance of exposure to mosquito bites:
- Mosquito nets.
- Long sleeves and trousers (tucked into socks).
- Insect repellents.

⚠ Recommend that she checks that her travel insurance will cover any health or pregnancy-related problems abroad. They may class pregnancy as a 'pre-existing condition' and therefore not cover it.

Flying in pregnancy

- Most airlines will allow pregnant women to fly up to 36 weeks gestation:
  - ~32 with multiple pregnancy
  - >28 weeks, many will request medical certification of fitness to fly.
- The risk of VTE significantly ↑ with flights of >8 hours.
- Simple measures should be recommended to ↓ the risk of VTE:
  - avoiding dehydration(and alcohol!)
  - regular short walks around the plane
  - graduated compression hosiery

☞ Consider low dose aspirin.

⚠ Women with other risk factors for DVT (such as factor V Leiden carriers) may require low-molecular weight heparin for flights of 5 hours or more.

Medical disorders in pregnancy

Epilepsy

- 0.6% of pregnancies occur in women with epilepsy.
- Most women have been diagnosed before conception.
- If the first seizure occurs in pregnancy there is a wide differential diagnosis (see box, p. 179).
- Seizure frequency can ↑(37%), ↓(13%) or remain unchanged (50%).
- Poorly controlled epileptics and those who stop medication are at the highest risk of ↑seizure frequency.

⚠ The fetus usually tolerates seizures without long-term sequelae but there is ↑ risk of fetal demise with status epilepticus.

Fetal risks

There is an increased risk of major congenital anomalies (5–10%) in women with epilepsy. Most of this risk is due to anticonvulsant medication; however, women not on antiepileptic drugs still have a higher risk than the general population. The use of multiple drugs carries a higher risk to the fetus than monotherapy. Higher doses lead to increased risk. Dividing doses and reducing peak blood levels may be beneficial. Any change in anticonvulsant therapy should be undertaken before pregnancy. Once pregnancy is diagnosed the woman should continue on her anticonvulsant drugs, and not change, as teratogenic risk exposure has already occurred. Folic acid (5 mg) reduces the risk of some anomalies.

> **Fetal risks of anticonvulsant therapy**
>
> - Teratogenicity: congenital anomalies or fetal anticonvulsant syndrome.
> - Neonatal withdrawal.
> - Vitamin K deficiency (enzyme inducers) → haemorrhagic disease of newborn.
> - Developmental delay and behavioural problems.

Drugs used in treatment of epilepsy

These have varying risks of congenital anomalies and can be divided according to their ability to induce liver enzymes.

Enzyme-inducing anticonvulsants

- Carbamazepine.
- Phenobarbital.
- Phenytoin.
- Primidone.

Non-enzyme-inducing anticonvulsants

- Valproate.
- Lamotrigine.
- Gabapentin.
- Ethosuximide.

Differential diagnosis of first seizure in pregnancy

- Eclampsia.
- Epilepsy.
- Infection:
  - meningitis
  - encephalitis
  - abscess.
- Metabolic:
  - drug or alcohol withdrawal
  - drug toxicity
  - hypoglycaemia
  - electrolyte imbalance (↓Na, ↑Na, ↓Ca).
- Severe hypoxia.
- Space-occupying lesion.
- Vascular:
  - cerebral vein thrombosis
  - thrombotic thrombocytopaenic purpura
  - cerebral infarction or haemorrhage.

☛ All patients who present with their first seizure in pregnancy should have imaging of the brain with CT or, preferably, MRI and be reviewed by a neurologist.

Main teratogenic risks of commonly used anticonvulsants

Valproate
- Neural tube defects: ↑ 10-fold (1–2%).
- Genitourinary anomalies (hypospadias).
- Cardiac anomalies.
- Facial clefts.
- Neurodevelopmental delay: ↑ 3.5-fold.

Carbamazepine
- Neural tube defects (0.5–1%).
- Cardiac anomalies.
- Facial clefts.

Phenytoin
- Facial clefts: ↑ 5 fold.
- Cardiac anomalies.

Epilepsy: management in pregnancy

Prepregnancy counselling
- Involve a neurologist to confirm diagnosis is epilepsy.
- Optimize treatment, achieve seizure control, and educate patient.
- Use the least number of drugs at the lowest dose to control seizures to minimize risk of congenital anomalies.
- Consider stopping drugs if seizure free for >2 years (warn of risk of seizures and implications for driving).
- All women should take folic acid 5 mg for at least 12 weeks before conception and continue until delivery (↓ risk of neural tube defects).
- Risk of epilepsy in the child (4% if one parent affected, 15% if both parents affected).

Antenatal care
- Do not change medication in pregnancy if well controlled, and stress the importance of compliance with medication.
- Prenatal screening:
  - α-fetoprotein (neural tube defects)
  - detailed anomaly scan (facial clefts and cardiac abnormalities).
- Consider fetal echocardiography at 22–24 weeks.
- Vitamin K 10 mg/day for the last 4 weeks of pregnancy (hepatic enzyme-inducing drugs may lead to neonatal coagulopathy).
- General advice (showers rather than baths, avoid sleep deprivation).

✒ There is no role for routine monitoring of drug levels (it may be useful in women with increased seizure frequency, suspected non-compliance, concern over toxic side effects, or polypharmacy).

Intrapartum care
- Aim for vaginal delivery (CS should be for obstetric indications; seizures are not an indication unless in status epilepticus).
- Labour is associated with increased risk of seizures due to sleep deprivation, reduced absorption of drugs and hyperventilation.
- Control seizures with benzodiazepines.
- Ensure usual anticonvulsants are taken.

Postnatal care
- The baby should be given vitamin K to reduce the risk of haemorrhagic disease of the newborn.
- Breast-feeding is not contraindicated (anticonvulsants reach breast milk and thus slow withdrawal occurs, although phenobarbital and benzodiazepines may cause sedation in the baby).
- If the anticonvulsant dose was increased in pregnancy it should be reduced back to prepregnancy levels slowly postpartum.
- Contraception with enzyme-inducing drugs:
  - COCP containing 50 mcg oestrogen with a shorter pill-free interval
  - POP is less effective
  - An IUCD is ideal.
- General advice (bathing and feeding) to minimize risk of harm to baby from seizures.

Cerebrovascular accident (CVA)

CVAs are rare in women of reproductive age but there is an increased risk in the postpartum period, especially the 1st week. There is a 9-fold increased risk for infarcts and 28-fold for haemorrhagic stroke in the first 6 weeks postpartum compared with non-pregnant women. Most of these CVAs occur in the carotid artery territory. Symptoms include:
• Abrupt onset of weakness.
• Sensory loss.
• Dysphasia.
Common risk factors for strokes at all ages include:
• Smoking.
• Diabetes.
• Hypertension.
• Hypercholesterolaemia.

There are other causes, often leading to emboli, in pregnancy. Frequently, no cause is found. Patients who have previously had a stroke are unlikely to have a further event in pregnancy.

Management
• Treatment depends on the cause.
• Anticoagulation may be appropriate.

Subarachnoid haemorrhage (SAH)
Outside pregnancy the commonest cause is a ruptured berry aneurysm, but arteriovenous malformations (AVM) may dilate in pregnancy due to the effect of oestrogen, resulting in a similar incidence.

Presentation
• Headache.
• Vomiting.
• Loss of/or impaired consciousness.
• Neck stiffness.
• Focal neurological signs.

Management
• Early treatment is recommended to reduce the chance of subsequent bleeding (the risk is high for AVM).
• Surgery is usually recommended—excision of the AVM or clipping of the aneurysm.
• Interventional radiology is associated with exposure of the fetus to large doses of radiation.
• Nimodipine is used to decrease vasospasm.
• Delivery:
  • labour is a high-risk time for bleeding, so elective CS should be recommended if the lesion is inoperable.
  • Epidural anaesthesia is contraindicated with a recent SAH due to raised intracranial pressure.
  • If the lesion has been successfully treated, vaginal delivery is recommended (a longer passive 2nd stage with early use of assisted delivery may reduce the risk of re-bleeding).

Causes of CVAs in pregnancy

Infarcts
- Pre-eclampsia/eclampsia.
- CNS vasculitis.
- Carotid artery dissection.
- Emboli:
  - mitral valve prolapse
  - peripartum cardiomyopathy
  - endocarditis
  - paradoxical emboli.
- Coagulopathies:
  - thrombophilia
  - antiphospholipid syndrome.
- Thrombotic thrombocytopaenic purpura (TTP).

Haemorrhagic
- Pre-eclampsia/eclampsia.
- Disseminated intravascular coagulation (DIC).
- Arteriovenous malformation (AVM).
- Ruptured berry aneurysm.
- CNS vasculitis.

Investigations

A neurologist should be involved in the investigation and management.
- MRI or CT scan of head.
- Cerebral angiography.
- Echocardiogram.
- Thrombophilia screen and antiphospholipid antibodies.

Cardiac disease: management in pregnancy

The pattern of heart disease in pregnancy has changed over the past few decades. Congenital heart disease is now more common than rheumatic heart disease. 0.9% of all pregnancies are complicated by cardiac problems.

⚠ Normal pregnancy is associated with significant haemodynamic changes. These may not be tolerated in women with heart disease.

Antenatal management

- Multidisciplinary management with an obstetrician, cardiologist, anaesthetist and, occasionally, cardiothoracic surgeon.
- Preconception counseling should be offered to:
  - optimize maternal cardiovascular status (may involve surgery)
  - modify medication
  - discuss maternal and fetal risks of pregnancy.
- The ability of a woman to tolerate pregnancy depends on:
  - exercise tolerance (New York Heart Association class)
  - presence of pulmonary hypertension or left heart obstruction
  - presence of cyanosis.
- Decide if termination recommended (e.g. in pulmonary hypertension).
- Correct factors that may lead to decompensation (anaemia, infection, hypertension, and arrhythmias).
- Monitor for signs of heart failure and consider maternal echo.
- Monitor fetal growth by serial ultrasound as risk of IUGR and death in utero, especially with maternal cyanosis.

⚠ Risk of congenital heart disease in fetus is 3–5% if either parent is affected. Some conditions carry higher risk. It is higher if mother rather than father is affected. Arrange for fetal echocardiography at 22 weeks.

Intrapartum and postpartum management

- A clear intrapartum care plan should be agreed before labour.
- Aim for a vaginal delivery with a short 2nd stage (CS is indicated if aortic root >4 cm, aortic dissection. or aneurysm).
- In labour maternal cardiac ± invasive monitoring may be required (the fetus should be continuously monitored).
- Avoid aortocaval compression.
- Decide on need for endocarditis prophylaxis.
- Blood loss should be minimized but avoid ergometrine (it causes tonic uterine contraction, expelling ~500 mL of blood into circulation; likewise, an infusion of oxytocin has fewer complications than a bolus).
- Epidural analgesia may reduce changes in heart rate and blood pressure associated with pain (low-dose epidural is usually well tolerated but may cause serious complications with restricted cardiac output)
- Pulmonary oedema can occur due to significant fluid changes in the first 3 days postpartum.
- Discuss contraception before discharge.

Haemodynamic changes in normal pregnancy

- Peripheral vasodilatation leads to a fall in systemic vascular resistance.
- Cardiac output increases by:
  - 40% during pregnancy (↑ heart rate and ↑ stroke volume)
  - 15% in the 1st stage of labour
  - 50% in the 2nd stage of labour.
- Following delivery there is further increased cardiac output due to increased venous return from:
  - relief of vena caval obstruction
  - tonic uterine contraction (expels blood into systemic circulation).
- Blood pressure falls in pregnancy and reaches a nadir around 24 weeks.
- Colloid osmotic pressure falls leading to increased susceptibility to pulmonary oedema.
- Hypercoagulability.

▶ These changes start in early pregnancy

---

❶ Risk of maternal mortality

High risk (25–50%)
- Pulmonary hypertension.
- Complicated aortic coarctation.
- Marfan's syndrome with aortic root involvement.
- Myocardial infarction.

Moderate risk (5–15%)
- Mitral Stenosis NYHA class 3 or 4.
- Aortic stenosis.
- Mechanical heart valves.

Minimal risk (<1%)
- ASD.
- VSD.
- PDA.
- Corrected tetralogy of Fallot.
- Tissue valve prosthesis.
- Pulmonary and tricuspid valve disease.
- Mitral stenosis NYHA class 1 or 2.
- Arrhythmias.

Artificial heart valves

Women with artificial heat valves usually have near-normal cardiac function and tolerate pregnancy well. The main maternal and fetal risk is from anti-coagulation which must be continued throughout pregnancy as without it there is a high mortality (valve thrombosis) and morbidity (stroke). The choice of anticoagulant should be made after discussion with the patient. Warfarin is safer for the mother but heparin is better for the fetus.

⚠There is a 25% risk of an embolic event per pregnancy.

Anticoagulant drugs and risks

Low molecular weight heparin (LMWH)
- Less maternal bleeding.
- No risk to fetus (does not cross the placenta).
- Increased risk of embolic events.
- Increased risk of valve thrombosis—may require emergency valve replacement and has a high mortality.
- Osteoporosis and heparin-induced thrombocytopenia.

Warfarin
- Increased risk of miscarriage.
- Risk of warfarin embryopathy (risk dose dependent: ↑ if >5 mg/day)
- Maternal and neonatal bleeding.
- Long half-life.

Management
- Antenatally there are 2 options:
  - continue warfarin throughout pregnancy—aim for INR of 3.0
  - conceive on warfarin, change to LMWH from 6–12 weeks to mini-mize risk of warfarin embryopathy, then use warfarin from 12 weeks to 37 weeks.
- Risk of bleeding in labour with warfarin (mother and baby) is high:
  - all patients should be changed to LMWH at 37 weeks
  - LMWH should be stopped in labour and restarted after delivery
  - warfarin should be re-started 3 days postpartum.
- Reversal in the event of life-threatening bleeding:
  - warfarin—fresh frozen plasma and vitamin K
  - LMWH—protamine sulphate.
- Heparin and warfarin can safely be given to breast-feeding mothers.
- Low-dose aspirin should be given with LMWH because of its anti-thrombotic effects and relative safety.

Tissue valves
- Bio-prosthetic or homograft valves do not require anticoagulation.
- They have a shorter life expectancy than mechanical valves, so struc-tural deterioration may occur in pregnancy (especially the mitral valve).
- Anticoagulation would still be required with arrhythmias, e.g. atrial fibrillation.

Endocarditis prophylaxis

Endocarditis prophylaxis should be given to the following 2 groups:

High risk
- Prosthetic heart valves (mechanical or tissue).
- Previous bacterial endocarditis.
- Complex cyanotic heart disease (Fallot's tetralogy, transposition).
- Surgically constructed systemic/pulmonary shunts.

Moderate risk
- Hypertrophic cardiomyopathy.
- Acquired valvular lesions.
- Mitral valve prolapse with regurgitation.
- Other congenital cardiac malformations.

Prophylaxis is not recommended for:
- Isolated secundum ASD.
- Surgically repaired ASD or VSD.
- Cardiac pacemakers.
- Mitral valve prolapse without regurgitation.

▶ Recommended antibiotics
- Amoxycillin 1 g IV plus gentamicin 120 mg IV at onset of labour or rupture of membranes then amoxicillin 500 mg orally 6 hours later.
- Vancomycin 1g IV or teicoplanin 400 mg IV if penicillin allergy with gentamicin 120 mg IV.

Acquired heart disease

Mitral stenosis

- This is the most common lesion of rheumatic heart disease (90%).
- ↑ risk of pulmonary oedema in pregnancy, greatest in labour
  - The ↑ in heart rate in pregnancy ↓ ventricular filling time and ↑ pulmonary blood volume leading to pulmonary oedema.
  - First line treatment for pulmonary oedema in pregnancy should be β-blockers, which slow the heart rate and improve left atrial emptying, and diuretics (add digoxin if in atrial fibrillation (AF)).
- Mitral stenosis is the most likely lesion to require treatment for pulmonary oedema, heart failure or surgery in pregnancy.
- With severe mitral stenosis, consider surgery before pregnancy.
- The risk of thromboembolism is ~1.5% in pregnancy, higher with left atrial enlargement and AF (treat with LMWH).

Mitral regurgitation

- It is well tolerated in pregnancy; heart failure is rare and pulmonary hypertension is a late event but endocarditis is more common.
- Mitral valve prolapse needs endocarditis prophylaxis only if associated mitral regurgitation.

Aortic stenosis

- Aortic valve disease is less common than mitral valve disease (it is less likely to be secondary to rheumatic disease, more likely to be due to a congenital bicuspid valve).
- The severity and risk of complications is dependent on the gradient across the valve: >100 mmHg in the non-pregnant state is severe.

⚠ Associated symptoms are chest pain, syncope, and sudden death.

Pulmonary hypertension and Eisenmenger's syndrome

- Primary pulmonary hypertension is an idiopathic abnormality of the pulmonary vasculature. In Eisenmenger's syndrome there is pulmonary hypertension with reversal of the initial left-to-right shunt and consequent cyanosis. There is a fixed high pulmonary vascular resistance and inability to increase pulmonary blood flow. This leads to slowly worsening hypoxaemia.

⚠ Maternal mortality is high, especially in the puerperium (40%).

- Women should be advised to avoid getting pregnant and termination recommended if pregnancy occurs.
- If termination is declined pregnancy should be managed with multidisciplinary care from cardiologists, obstetricians, and anaesthetists.
- Antenatal care includes anticoagulation, oxygen, bed rest, and serial assessment of fetal growth.
- Avoid manoeuvres that suddenly increase venous return, e.g. ergometrine and vagal tone (with resultant bradycardia).
- Delivery should be in a high dependency unit with tight control of blood pressure, fluid balance and oxygen saturations.

✒ Mode of delivery and epidural use are controversial.

Myocardial infarction and cardiomyopathy

Myocardial infarction (MI)

Is rare in pregnancy but has an increasing incidence due to increased age at pregnancy.

⚠ Mortality is high (20% immediate and 32% overall); it is highest in the puerperium.

- Risk factors include smoking, hypertension, diabetes, hypercholesterolaemia, family history, and obesity.
- There may be an atypical mechanism e.g. coronary spasm, arteritis, or coronary artery dissection.
- Diagnosis is based on history, ECG changes, and elevated cardiac enzymes (Troponin T or I).
- The patient should be managed on a coronary care unit by cardiologists.
- Angioplasty is more likely to precipitate a coronary artery dissection in pregnant women but should still be considered.
- Thrombolysis is relatively contraindicated.
- Delivery: Aim for a vaginal delivery with a short 2nd stage (avoid ergometrine as it can cause coronary artery spasm).
- Women with a past history of MI should have a prepregnancy assessment of cardiac function (echo and exercise test) with counselling on the basis of the results, and aspirin should be continued in pregnancy.

Peripartum cardiomyopathy

- This is a rare condition—incidence <1:5000.
- It occurs between 32 weeks and 6 months after delivery, but most commonly presents in the 1st month postpartum.
- Risk factors:
  - increasing maternal age
  - multiparity
  - multiple pregnancy
  - Afro-Caribbean ethnicity
  - poor socio-economic class
  - hypertension in pregnancy.
- Presentation is with breathlessness, palpitations, oedema, poor exercise tolerance, and embolic phenomena.
- Diagnosis involves global dilatation of all four chambers of the heart (seen on echo) with exclusion of other causes of cardiomyopathy.
- Management is supportive and should include ACE inhibitors and anticoagulation (☛ immunosuppression has been tried).
- If the diagnosis is made antenatally, delivery is indicated.
- Consider heart transplantation if there is heart failure despite optimal medical therapy.

⚠ Mortality is 25–50% (long-term survival is likely if the initial episode survived).

⚠ Recurrence risk is high (up to 50%). Avoid further pregnancies.

Congenital heart disease

The most common congenital heart diseases in pregnancy are patent ductus arteriosus, atrial septal defect, and ventricular septal defect. They are well tolerated in pregnancy.

Marfan's syndrome

This is an autosomal dominant condition (chromosome 15) caused by a defect in fibrillin synthesis (genetic testing is available). The main risk is of aortic dissection and rupture. This risk is related to a family history of rupture and degree of aortic root dilatation.

Management

- Monthly maternal echo for aortic dimensions until 8 weeks postpartum
- β-blockers should be given for hypertension or if aortic dilatation as they reduce progression and complications.
- Aim for vaginal delivery with a short 2nd stage (if aortic root dilatation is present, deliver by CS).

△ Mortality:
- <1% if aortic root <4 cm.
- >25% if aortic root >4 cm.
- Pregnancy is contraindicated with an aortic root >4.5 cm until aortic root replacement.

Coarctation of aorta

- This has usually been corrected before pregnancy. The main risk is of aortic dissection, this risk is highest if there is hypertension present (usually treated with β-blockers). The condition is also associated with berry aneurysms which can bleed in pregnancy causing cerebral haemorrhage.
- If uncorrected or recurrent, coarctation risks include:
  - hypertension
  - heart failure
  - angina.
- Avoid balloon angioplasty in pregnancy (↑ risk of dissection).
- Deliver by CS if there is associated aortic dilatation.

Fallot's tetralogy

- There are two main risks in pregnancy:
  - paradoxical emboli can pass from right-to-left through the shunt causing strokes
  - cyanosis affects the fetus leading to increased risk of miscarriage, IUGR, prematurity, and death in utero.
- Risks are minimized by anticoagulation (prophylactic dose LMWH), bed rest, and oxygen.

Anaemia

Physiological adaptation in pregnancy
- Plasma volume expansion (50%) is greater than ↑ in red cell mass (25%)
- This leads to physiological dilution with ↓ Hb and haematocrit.
- Anaemia is diagnosed if haemoglobin <10.5 g/dL in pregnancy.
- There should be no change in MCV or MCHC in normal pregnancies
- Normally pregnancy has:
  - 2–3-fold increase in iron requirements
  - 10–20-fold increase in folate requirements in pregnancy.

Iron-deficiency anaemia
- The most common cause of anaemia in pregnancy (90% of cases).
- Diagnosis: ↓MCV, ↓MCHC, and ↓ferritin.
- Often asymptomatic and detected on screening.
- Treat by oral iron supplementation:
  - the choice of preparation should be based on patient tolerance
  - vitamin C (orange juice) ↑ absorption, tea ↓ absorption.
- Parenteral iron should be considered in those who do not tolerate the oral preparations (corrects the anaemia more rapidly).
- The expected improvement in haemoglobin is ~1 g/dL/week.
- In situations such as multiple pregnancy or known depletion of iron stores, consider prophylactic supplementation even if no anaemia.
- If severe iron-deficiency anaemia (Hb<7 g/dL) is diagnosed near term, blood transfusion may be considered.

Folate deficiency
- Also common in pregnancy (5% of cases of anaemia).
- Risk factors include:
  - poor nutritional status
  - haematological problems with a rapid turnover of blood cells, e.g. haemolytic anaemia and haemoglobinopathies
  - drug interaction with folate metabolism, e.g. antiepileptics.
- Diagnosis: ↑MCV and ↓serum and ↓red cell folate.
- Folic acid is given preconception and in early pregnancy to reduce risk of neural tube defects (400 micrograms/day for general population).
- Women with high risk of neural tube defects should take 5 mg folic acid daily. The high-risk group includes:
  - patients on anticonvulsants
  - previous child affected with a neural tube defect
  - women with haematological disorders.

Vitamin B$_{12}$ deficiency
- Occurs in pernicious anaemia, terminal ileum disease, and strict vegans; associated with subfertility. It is uncommon to make a new diagnosis in pregnancy.
- Women with a previous diagnosis should continue treatment throughout pregnancy.

Sickle cell disease

Inheritance is autosomal recessive. Most commonly seen in people of Afro-Caribbean origin, but also occurs in those from the Middle East, Mediterranean, and Indian subcontinent. As diagnosis has usually been made in childhood, it is rare to make a new diagnosis in pregnancy.

Pathophysiology

Results in distortion of the shape of red cells into a rigid sickle shape. This leads to microvascular blockage, stasis, and infarction in any organ in the body. Crises can be precipitated by infection, dehydration, hypoxia, and cold.

Risks in pregnancy

- Crises are more common during pregnancy.
- ↑ risk of pre-eclampsia.
- ↑ risk of delivery by CS secondary to fetal distress.

Clinical features of sickle cell disease

- Haemolytic anaemia.
- Painful crises.
- Hyposplenism (chronic damage to the spleen results in atrophy).
- Increased risk of infection (UTI, pyelonephritis, pneumonia, puerperal sepsis).
- Avascular necrosis of bone.
- Increased risk of thromboembolic disease (PE, stroke).
- Acute chest syndrome (fever, chest pain, tachypnoea, ↑WCC, pulmonary infiltrates).
- Iron overload: leads to cardiomyopathy.
- Maternal mortality 2%.

Management

- Multidisciplinary care with an obstetrician and haematologist.
- Prepregnancy counselling should involve screening of the partner (if the partner is a carrier consider prenatal diagnosis).
- Stop iron-chelating agents before pregnancy.
- If there is a history of iron overload, arrange a maternal echo.
- Give folic acid 5 mg/day and penicillin prophylaxis for hyposplenism.
- Monitor Hb and HbS percentage and arrange transfusion if necessary (may have red cell antibodies from multiple transfusions).
- Screen for urine infection each visit.
- Treatment of a crisis involves adequate analgesia, oxygen, rehydration, and antibiotics if infection suspected (exchange transfusion may be required in severe crises).
- Regular assessment of fetal growth with ultrasound, including Doppler.
- Aim for vaginal delivery ensuring adequate hydration and avoiding hypoxia (continuous fetal monitoring as increased risk of fetal distress).
- Consider postnatal thromboprophylaxis.

☛ The use of prophylactic antibiotics is controversial.

Fetal risks in sickle cell disease

- Miscarriage.
- IUGR.
- Prematurity.
- Stillbirth.

⚠ Perinatal mortality is increased 4–6-fold compared to the general population.

Thalassaemia

Adult haemoglobin is made up from 2 α- and 2 β- globin chains associated with a haem complex. There are 4 genes for α-globin and 2 for β-globin chain production. An adult's blood is normally made up of HbA ($\alpha_2\beta_2$, 97%), HbA_2 ($\alpha_2\delta_2$, 1.5–3.5%) and HbF ($\alpha_2\gamma_2$, <1%). Thalassaemia is a group of genetic conditions leading to impaired production of these globin chains and resulting in red cells with inadequate haemoglobin content. Fetal haemoglobin consists of 2α and 2γ chains, so a fetus can not be affected by β-thalassaemia.

α-Thalassaemia

- Caused by defects in 1–4 of the α-globin genes.
- Most common in individuals from south-east Asia.
- A-thalassaemia trait has 2 (α0) or 3 (α+) normal genes:
  - women are usually asymptomatic but may become anaemic in pregnancy.
- In HbH there are 3 defective genes:
  - unstable haemoglobin is formed by tetramers of the β chain
  - chronic haemolysis results and iron overload is common
  - offspring will have either α0 or α+ thalassaemia.
- A-thalassaemia major (Hb Barts) has no functional α genes and is incompatible with life:
  - fetuses are often hydropic and born prematurely.
  - severe early onset pre-eclampsia often complicates the pregnancy.

β-Thalassaemia

- B-thalassaemia trait has one defective gene and women are asymptomatic but may become anaemic in pregnancy.
- It is most common in individuals form Cyprus and Asia.
- Incidence of β-thalassaemia minor is 1:10 000 in the UK compared to 1:7 in Cyprus:
  - offspring have a 1:4 chance of β-thalassaemia major.
- B-Thalassaemia major has two defective genes and women are often transfusion dependent:
  - iron overload can occur
  - puberty is often delayed
  - there is subfertility and only very few pregnancies have been reported.
- Repeated transfusions cause iron overload, leading to endocrine, hepatic, and cardiac dysfunction:
  - heart failure is the most common cause of death
  - iron-chelating therapy can reduce the incidence of iron overload
  - the condition can be cured by bone marrow transplant.

Management of pregnancy with thalassaemia

- Check ferritin in early pregnancy:
  - give iron supplements only if iron deficient.
- Women need folic acid 5 mg daily:
  - if failure to respond to folate PO then IM (and oral iron if needed), a blood transfusion may be required
  - parenteral iron should be avoided.
- If the woman has thalassaemia the partner needs screening:
  - if positive the couple needs counselling of the risk of pregnancy with thalassaemia major
  - prenatal diagnosis should be offered.

Screening for thalassaemia in pregnancy

- Screen all women of Mediterranean, Middle Eastern, Indian, Asian, African, or West Indian ethnic origin by haemoglobin electrophoresis at booking.
- In $\alpha 0$ and $\alpha +$ thalassaemia no abnormal haemoglobin made and there is no excess in HbA_2 or HbF:
  - Hb electrophoresis is normal
  - the diagnosis can be confirmed by globin chain synthesis studies or DNA analysis of nucleated cells.
- In α-thalassaemia there is a raised concentration of HbA_2 and/or HbF.
- Suspect the diagnosis of thalassaemia in the presence of:
  - low MCV
  - low MCHC
  - microcytic anaemia with normal MCHC (which differs from iron deficiency where the MCHC is also low).

Haemophilia

X-linked inherited deficiency of clotting factor VIII and IX that causes problems with bleeding. Haemophilia A (factor VIII deficiency) is 4 times more common than haemophilia B (factor IX deficiency). Can vary in severity depending on the clotting factor levels: mild (>5% to <40%), moderate (1–5%), or severe (<1%). Severity tends to be similar within members of one family. The use of prophylactic recombinant factor replacement from childhood has now drastically changed the outlook and life expectancy for affected children.

Incidence

- 15:100 000 males.
- Female carriers have one abnormal gene and do not usually have significant bleeding problems but the clotting factor level is around 1/2 normal (occasionally clotting factors may be much lower because of lyonization).
- Female carriers have a 50% chance of having an affected son and a 50% chance of having carrier daughters.
- An affected male will produce carrier daughters and unaffected sons.
- 1/3 of newly diagnosed infants have no family history and are the result of a new mutation.

Prenatal diagnosis and antenatal care

- Manage jointly with haematologist.
- Genetic counselling and prenatal diagnosis (if the mutation is known by DNA-based family studies) should be offered to affected families.
- Fetal sexing can be done if the mutation is not known with fetal blood sampling of males after 18 weeks.
- Check hepatitis serology as previous exposure to blood products.
- Maternal coagulation factor activity should be checked at booking, 28 and 34 weeks, and when clinically indicated (e.g. bleeding, before surgery).
- There is increase risk of postpartum haemorrhage (clotting factor levels increase in pregnancy in normal women and haemophilia carriers but fall rapidly to prepregnancy levels after delivery).

Intrapartum and postpartum care

- Aim for vaginal delivery.
- Check maternal coagulation factor activity aiming for levels >50 IU/L (give appropriate clotting factors if lower than this).
- Also send FBC, clotting screen, and group and save when in labour.
- Avoid fetal scalp electrodes, fetal blood sampling, ventouse, and rotational forceps deliveries in affected or unknown fetal status.
- Epidural anaesthesia can be used if normal coagulation screen, platelet count >100 × 10^9/L, normal bleeding time, and clotting factor >50 IU/L.
- Maintain clotting factors >50 IU/L for 5 days postpartum to reduce risk of postpartum haemorrhage.
- Avoid IM injections in neonate with possible clotting disorder.
- Send cord blood of males for clotting factor VIII or IX levels (refer to haemophilia centre if diagnosis is confirmed).

Von Willebrand's disease

- Autosomal dominant (types 1 and 2).
- Autosomal recessive (type 3)—more uncommon and severe.
- Stabilizes factor VIII and helps adherence of platelets to vessel wall.
- Diagnosis by measuring:
  - vWF antigen
  - factor VIII
  - ristocetin cofactor activity
- Levels of vWF and factor VIII increase in pregnancy and fall rapidly postpartum.
- Main risk is postpartum haemorrhage.
- desmopressin can be used in some type1 cases (it stimulates the release of vWF from endothelial cells).

Autoimmune idiopathic thrombocytopenic purpura (ITP)

- Caused by antibodies to surface antigens on platelets, leading to platelet destruction.
- Incidence 1–3:1000 pregnancies.
- Diagnosis is by exclusion of other causes of thrombocytopenia.
- Pregnancy does not affect the disease.

Fetal risks

- IgG antiplatlet antibodies can cross the placenta and cause fetal thrombocytopenia.
- Difficult to predict which fetus will be affected (it has no relation to maternal platelet count).
- Can lead to antenatal and intrapartum intracranial haemorrhage:
  - the overall risk is 2%
  - <2% with a history of ITP before pregnancy
  - risk is highest if there has been a previously affected child.

Management

- FBC every 2–4 weeks.
- Bleeding is unlikely if platelet count is >50 × 10^9/L (treatment is not required at this level).
- Patients with bleeding or platelet count <50 × 10^9/L should be started on oral steroids, >75% respond within 3 weeks.
- Patients who fail to respond to steroids can be treated with IV immunoglobulin.
- Splenectomy is rarely performed in pregnancy.
- Platelet transfusions may be required if rapid response is needed.
- In labour, avoid:
  - fetal scalp electrodes
  - fetal blood sampling
  - ventouse delivery
  - rotational forceps delivery.
- No fetal benefit from delivery by CS, but ↑ maternal risks.
- Cord platelet count should be taken at birth:
  - the count reaches a nadir at around day 4
  - the neonate may require intravenous immunoglobulin.

Causes of thrombocytopaenia in pregnancy

- Spurious.
- Gestational thrombocytopaenia.
- Pre-eclampsia.
- Idiopathic thrombocytopaenic purpura.
- Thrombotic thrombocytopaenic purpura.
- Disseminated intravascular coagulopathy.
- Systemic lupus erythematosus.
- Bone marrow suppression.

Asthma

This is the most common respiratory disease encountered in pregnancy and affects 1–4% of women of childbearing age. It is caused by reversible bronchoconstriction of smooth muscle in the airways, with inflammation and excess mucus production. Diagnosis is based on recurrent episodes of wheeze, shortness of breath, chest tightness or cough, and variation in peak expiratory flow rate (PFR) of >15% after treatment with bronchodilators. Pregnancy outcomes in women with asthma are usually good.

Effect of pregnancy on asthma

There is no consistent effect: 1/3 show no change in their asthma, 1/3 show improvement, and 1/3 deteriorate. Deterioration occurs most often between 24 and 36 weeks. There may be a different effect in different pregnancies. Deterioration may be caused by cessation of maintenance therapy.

Effect of asthma on pregnancy

Usually there is no effect on the fetus or course of the pregnancy, but poorly controlled asthma may be associated with low birth weight and preterm labour.

Management

- Current therapy should continue in pregnancy, women educated and reassured of the safety of the medication and warned not to stop their treatment.
- Women should continue to monitor their PFR (↑diurnal variation with ↓PFR in the night or early morning may be an early sign of worsening of asthma).
- Chronic and acute severe asthma should be treated as in the non-pregnant state (aim for oxygen saturation >95% and administer oxygen if required).
- Advise cessation of smoking.
- CXR should be considered to exclude pneumothorax.
- There is increased risk of gestational diabetes in women on long-term oral steroids.
- Asthma attacks are rare during labour; inhaled β-agonists can be used (there is no evidence that they interfere with uterine activity).
- Women on long-term oral steroids (prednisolone >7.5 mg/day for >2 weeks) are at risk of Addisonian collapse during labour—give hydrocortisone 100 mg every 8 hours.
- Prostaglandin F2α should only be used in cases of life-threatening postpartum haemorrhage because of its bronchoconstriction action.
- Breast-feeding should be encouraged as it may give the child some protection against developing allergies in later life.

✒ The fetus is at greater risk from under-treated asthma than from the drugs used in its treatment.

Asthma care: British Thoracic Society recommendations

- **Step 1:** inhaled short-acting β-agonists:
  - salbutamol or terbutaline.
- **Step 2:** inhaled steroids(up to 800 micrograms/day)
  - beclometasone, budesonide.
- **Step 3:** long acting beta-agonist
  - salmeterol or formoterol
- **Step 4:** high-dose inhaled steroid (up to 2000 micrograms/day) ± oral slow-release theophylline, leukotriene antagonists.
- **Step 5:** oral steroids:
  - review by respiratory physician if oral steroids commenced.

⚠ Leukotriene receptor antagonists should not be commenced in pregnancy but can be continued in women who have demonstrated significant improvement in asthma control that was not achievable by other medication

Acute severe asthma: management

- Medication:
  - nebulized bronchodilators
  - IV steroids
  - nebulized ipratropium
  - IV aminophylline or IV salbutamol
  - ± antibiotics if evidence of infection.
- Clinical findings:
  - heart rate >110 bpm
  - respiratory rate >25/min
  - pulsus paradoxus >20 mmHg
  - PFR <50% predicted
  - accessory muscle use
  - unable to complete sentences.

▶▶ Silent chest with very little wheeze may be a sign of life-threatening asthma.

Cystic fibrosis (CF)

This is one of the commonest genetic conditions, affecting 1:2000 people of European origin with a gene frequency of around 1:25. Transmission is autosomal recessive and disease is caused by defective function of the CF transmembrane conductance regulation (CFTR) chloride channel. The condition affects the lungs, gastrointestinal tract, pancreas, hepatobiliary system, and reproductive organs. Recurrent chest infections lead to bronchial damage and respiratory failure.

Life expectancy is improving (currently 36 years) and women with CF are now having families. However, most men are infertile owing to congenital absence of the vas deferens and women are subfertile because of unfavourable mucus, reduced BMI, and anovulation.

Prenatal counselling

The offspring will definitely receive one affected gene from the mother, so paternal status should be ascertained. There are many different gene mutations but screening will detect ~90% of mutations. The risk of an affected child is 2–2.5% for unknown paternal carrier status. If the father's screen is negative the risk of an affected child falls to 1:500. If the father is a carrier the chance of an affected child is 1:2. Chorionic villus sampling can then be performed to check the fetus for affected genes.

Management of pregnancy with CF

- Care involves a multidisciplinary team with chest physician (CF unit), obstetrician, dietitian, and physiotherapist.
- Principles of care involve control of respiratory infections, avoidance of hypoxia, maintaining nutrition and fetal surveillance.
- Chest physiotherapy should continue as in the non-pregnant state.
- Watch for signs of chest infection, which should be aggressively treated with antibiotics, tailored according to sputum culture results.

✦ Avoid tetracyclines and parenteral aminoglycosides; may cause ototoxicity in high doses

- Cardiac status should be checked by echocardiography.
- In the later stages of pregnancy patients can become breathless even without infections (if oxygen saturations are ≤90% at rest hospital admission for oxygen therapy is indicated).
- High calorie intake with pancreatic enzyme supplementation is required.
- 20% of adults with CF have diabetes and a further 15% have impaired glucose tolerance with ↑ risk of gestational diabetes.
- Fetal monitoring with regular growth scans (fetal risks are IUGR due to maternal hypoxaemia and preterm labour).
- Aim for a vaginal delivery (limit the 2nd stage, as pneumothoraces can occur with prolonged or repeated Valsalva manoevures).
- Avoid general anaesthesia and inhalational analgesia if possible
- Breast-feeding is recommended (ensure continued nutritional supplementation).

Predictors of poor maternal or fetal outcomes in CF

- Hypoxaemia: PaO2 <60 mmHg free from infection.
- Cyanosis.
- Pulmonary hypertension.
- Poor pre-pregnancy lung function: FEV_1 <50% predicted.
- Pancreatic insufficiency (especially diabetes) and malnutrition.
- Lung colonization with *Burkholderia cepacia*.

Respiratory infections

Pneumonia

This has the same incidence as in the non-pregnant population: 1–2:1000 pregnancies.
- Risk factors include smoking, chronic lung disease, immunosuppression.
- Clinical features are fever, cough, purulent sputum, chest pain, and breathlessness.
- Investigations: FBC, CRP, CXR, sputum culture, serology (mycoplasma, Legionella, and viral titres) and arterial blood gases.
- Fetal risks are preterm labour and possibly IUGR.
- Treatment involves physiotherapy, adequate oxygenation, hydration and appropriate antibiotics.

⚠Varicella infection (chickenpox) causes pneumonia in 10% of cases in pregnancy. Mortality is ~10% and is highest in the latter stages of pregnancy. Women who develop varicella in pregnancy should be treated with aciclovir; they should be hospitalized if respiratory signs develop (on a non-obstetric ward with barrier nursing).

Antibiotic recommendations for pneumonia

- Amoxycillin for community-acquired pneumonia. Use higher dose in pregnancy because of increased renal clearance (500 mg tds).
- Erythromycin if penicillin allergy.
- Add erythromycin or clarithromycin if atypical organisms suspected.
- Cephalosporin for hospital-acquired pneumonia.

Tuberculosis

- The incidence of TB is increasing in the UK, especially in the immuno-suppressed (HIV) and immigrant population. It is uncommon in pregnancy but does not adversely affect the outcome if it is diagnosed and treated appropriately in the first 20 weeks or so.
- Clinical features: cough, haemoptysis, fever, weight loss, chest pain and night sweats.

⚠ Diagnosis may be delayed by an unnecessary reluctance to perform investigations such as CXR in pregnancy.
- Investigations: CXR (classically calcification and upper lobe abnormalities), sputum microscopy with a Ziehl–Nielsen stain, sputum culture (can take 6 weeks), bronchoscopy if no sputum and tissue biopsies for extrapulmonary TB. A Mantoux test cannot distinguish active disease from previous disease or vaccination.
- There is increased risk of prematurity and IUGR if treatment is inadequate or delayed (transplacental spread of infection is rare).

Neonatal considerations

Transmission from mother to baby after delivery (or to other care givers) can occur if the mother remains infective (smear positive). Women usually become non-infectious (smear negative) within 2 weeks of starting treatment. The baby should be given BCG vaccination and, if smear positive, prophylaxis with isoniazid for 3 months.

Aetiological agent in pneumonia

- No cause found in substantial proportion of patients.
- *Streptococcus pneumoniae* (>50% of cases).
- *Haemophilus influenzae.*
- *Staphylococcus aureus* (often after a viral infection).
- *Klebsiella* (more common with chronic lung disease).
- *Pseudomonas aeruginosa* (more common with chronic lung disease).
- *Mycoplasma pneumoniae* (atypical organism).
- *Leigonella pneumoniae* (atypical organism).
- *Chlamydia psittaci* (atypical organism).
- Gram negative organisms (secondary to aspiration).
- *Pneumocystis carinii* (immunosuppressed).
- Fungal.
- Viral: influenza, varicella-zoster.

Management of TB in pregnancy

- Respiratory physician and microbiologist involvement is essential.
- Treatment should be supervised to encourage and confirm compliance.
- A minimum of 6 month course of treatment is required.
- A typical treatment regime for pulmonary TB would involve an initial phase of therapy with isoniazid, rifampicin, ethambutol ± pyrazinamide for 2 months, followed by a continuation phase of 4 months of isoniazid and rifampicin (and based on drug sensitivities)
  - **Isoniazid**: can cause demyelination and peripheral neuropathy. If given with pyridoxine considered safe in pregnancy. The risk of hepatitis is increased in pregnancy—monitor liver function monthly
  - **Rifampicin:** can be safely used in pregnancy. It is a liver enzyme inducer, therefore give vitamin K to the mother in the last 4 weeks of pregnancy to prevent haemorrhagic disease of the newborn
  - **Ethambutol**: is safe in pregnancy
  - **Streptomycin**: 10% risk of deafness in fetus due to damage to the 8th cranial nerve. It should not be used in pregnancy
  - **Pyrazinamide**: considered safe after the 1st trimester, occasionally used before 14 weeks.

Inflammatory bowel disease (IBD)

The incidence of IBD has been increasing over the past four decades. It usually affects young adults. Ulcerative colitis (UC) affects women more than men but Crohn's disease is equally distributed between the sexes. White people are more commonly affected than Afro-Caribbeans. The clinical features are diarrhoea, abdominal pain, rectal bleeding, and weight loss.

Effect of IBD on pregnancy

- Fertility, miscarriage, stillbirth, and fetal anomaly rates are not affected in women with quiescent or well-controlled disease.
- Active disease at conception, first presentation in pregnancy, colonic rather than small bowel disease alone, active disease after resection, and severe disease treated by surgery are all associated with increased risk of miscarriage, stillbirth, prematurity and low birth weight.
- Women with previous surgery and ileostomy usually tolerate pregnancy well, especially if disease quiescent but there is a risk of intestinal obstruction from the 2nd trimester.

Effect of pregnancy on IBD

Relapses frequently occur and can happen at any time in the pregnancy but tend to be particularly common in the first trimester (UC) and puerperium (Crohn's). The risk of exacerbation is not increased but similar to that of non-pregnant women.

Management of IBD in pregnancy

- Women should be encouraged to conceive during times of disease remission.
- High-dose folic acid (5 mg/day) should be given before conception to women on sulfasalazine, to protect against neural tube defects, as the drug impairs the metabolism of folate.
- Management is similar to the non-pregnant state. Maintenance therapy usually includes sulfasalazine, other 5-aminosalicylic acid derivatives and/or steroids (available orally or rectally).
- Active disease should be investigated by stool culture to exclude infection (including parasites), inflammatory markers and sigmoidoscopy to assess disease activity in colitis (manage by rehydration and drug therapy with sulfasalazine or steroids).
- If the active disease is refractory to steroids then azathioprine or ciclosporin may be used (cyclosporin is associated with IUGR).

⚠ Methotrexate and 6-mercaptopurine should be avoided in pregnancy

- Surgery is occasionally required in pregnancy when complications occur such as intestinal obstruction, haemorrhage, perforation, fistula, abscess formation, or toxic megacolon.
- Caesarean section is usually reserved for obstetric reasons but should be considered with severe perianal Crohn's disease, as a scarred perineum is inelastic and tears or episiotomy may result in fistula formation.
- Breast-feeding is safe in women on steroids and sulfasalazine.

Obstetric cholestasis

Obstetric cholestasis affects 0.7% of pregnancies in the UK. It is more common in women of Asian ethnicity and there is geographical variation in prevalence. 1/3 of patients have a family history of the condition. It usually occurs in the 3rd trimester and resolves spontaneously after delivery.

Symptoms
- Pruritus of the trunk and limbs, without a skin rash (often worst at night).
- Anorexia and malaise.
- Epigastric discomfort, steatorrhoea, and dark urine (less common).

Diagnosis
- Full investigation is required as it is a diagnosis of exclusion, but is usually made on the history, abnormal LFTs, and raised bile acids in the absence of any other cause for hepatic dysfunction.

Risks
Maternal risks
- Vitamin K deficiency (potentially leading to postpartum haemorrhage).

Fetal risks
- Preterm labour.
- Stillbirth.

Management of obstetric cholestasis
- Send LFTs and bile acids for all woman itching, without a rash
- If normal, they should be repeated every 1–2 weeks if symptoms persist, as itching can predate abnormal LFTs.
- Exclude other causes of pruritus and liver dysfunction.
- Water-soluble vitamin K should be commenced from diagnosis.
- Symptoms may be alleviated by topical emollients (antihistamines cause sedation but do not improve pruritus).
- Ursodeoxycholic acid (8–12 mg/kg daily in two divided doses) may reduce the pruritus between 1 and 7 days after starting treatment, but there is no proven benefit for fetal adverse effects.
- Fetal surveillance with ultrasound and CTG monitoring are commonly used but of no proven benefit.
- Postnatal resolution of symptoms and LFTs should be established.
- Recurrence risk in subsequent pregnancy is 45–70% (it can also recur with the combined contraceptive pill)

△ Intrauterine death is usually sudden and there is no evidence of placental insufficiency therefore CTG and USS may not be predictive.

△ Fetal death does not correlate with symptoms or blood results.

☛ As there is no way of detecting a fetus at risk, delivery is often recommended by 37–38 weeks but this is controversial.

Differential diagnosis of obstetric cholestasis

- Gallstones.
- Acute or chronic viral hepatitis.
- Primary biliary cirrhosis (anti-mitochondrial antibody +ve).
- Chronic active hepatitis (anti-smooth muscle antibody +ve).

Investigations for obstetric cholestasis

- Liver function tests:
  - 2–3-fold ↑ in ALT, AST, γGT or alkaline phosphatase
  - use pregnancy-specific reference ranges.
- Clotting screen.
- Bile acids.
- Ultrasound of the liver and biliary tree.
- Viral serology (hepatitis A, B,C, CMV, EBV).
- Autoimmune screen (anti-mitochondrial and anti-smooth muscle antibodies).

Causes of jaundice in pregnancy

- Causes not specific to pregnancy:
  - haemolysis
  - Gilbert's syndrome
  - viral hepatitis (hepatitis A, B, C, E EBV, CMV)
  - autoimmune hepatitis (primary biliary cirrhosis, chronic active hepatitis, sclerosing cholangitis)
  - gallstones
  - cirrhosis
  - drug-induced hepatotoxicity
  - malignancy.
- Causes specific to pregnancy (10% of cases):
  - hyperemesis gravidarum
  - pre-eclampsia/HELLP syndrome
  - acute fatty liver of pregnancy
  - obstetric cholestasis.

Acute fatty liver of pregnancy (AFLP)

This is a rare condition affecting 1:10 000 pregnancies. It typically presents in obese women in the third trimester and can occur at any parity. It is associated with twin pregnancy (9–25%), a male fetus (♂: ♀ ratio 3:1) and mild pre-eclampsia (30–60%).

⚠ AFLP has a maternal mortality of 18%, higher if diagnosis is delayed, and fetal mortality of 23%.

Clinical features of AFLP

- Abdominal pain.
- Nausea and vomiting.
- Jaundice.
- Headache.
- Fever.
- Confusion.
- Coma.

- Symptoms can progress rapidly to fulminant liver failure, DIC, and renal failure.
- Hypoglycaemia is common.
- Some women have polyuria secondary to transient diabetes insipidus.
- Investigations: FBC and film, clotting, U&E, urate, LFT, blood gases.

Differentiating AFLP from HELLP syndrome

Distinctive features of AFLP:
- Mild hypertension and proteinuria only.
- Profound and persistent hypoglycaemia.
- Marked hyperuricaemia.
- Fatty infiltration on imaging the liver (may also be normal).

Management of AFLP

- This should be in a high dependency or intensive care setting with a multidisciplinary team.
- Management should involve:
  - treatment of hypoglycaemia
  - correction of coagulopathy with IV vitamin K and fresh frozen plasma
  - strict control of blood pressure and fluid balance.
- Delivery should follow stabilization (regional anaesthesia is contra-indicated in presence of thrombocytopaenia or deranged clotting).
- Bleeding complications are common.
- Fluid balance may require central line or even Swan–Ganz catheters.
- Following delivery care is supportive, most women improve rapidly after delivery with no long-term liver damage.
- Some patients with fulminant hepatic failure may require transfer to a specialist liver unit.
- It is uncommon for recurrence to occur in subsequent pregnancies in the absence of the genetic condition long chain 3-hydroxyacyl-CoA dehydrogenase (LCHAD) deficiency.

Renal tract infections

More common in pregnancy because of dilatation of upper renal tract and urinary stasis. Asymptomatic bacteriuria affects 5–10% of pregnant women; untreated it can lead to symptomatic infection in 40% of cases.

- Cystitis complicates 1% of pregnancies.
- Pyelonephritis occurs in 1–2% of pregnant women and is associated with preterm labour.

▶ Women should be screened for asymptomatic bacteriuria with a MSU at booking. If this is negative the chance of developing a urinary infection in pregnancy is <2%.

Symptoms

- Cystitis: urinary frequency, urgency, dysuria, haematuria, proteinuria, and suprapubic pain.
- Pyelonephritis: fever, rigors, vomiting, loin and abdominal pain.

⚠ Consider the diagnosis of pyelonephritis in women presenting with hyperemesis or threatened preterm labour.

Investigations

- Urinalysis: the most useful markers are nitrites and leukocytes but they may be poor predictors of positive culture in asymptomatic bacteriuria.
- MSU: a positive result is confirmed with a culture of >100 000 organisms/mL. Mixed growth or non-significant culture—repeat MSU.
- Bloods: blood cultures, FBC, U&E, and CRP in a pyrexial patient.
- Renal USS: after a single episode of pyelonephritis or ≥ 2 UTI, to exclude hydronephrosis, congenital abnormality and calculi. 20% of pregnant women with pyelonephritis have an abnormal renal tract.

⚠ Monthly MSU should be sent in women with culture-proven urinary infection to prove eradication. 15% develop recurrent bacteriuria and require further treatment.

Treatment

- Oral antibiotics are recommended in asymptomatic bacteriuria and cystitis to prevent pyelonephritis and preterm labour.
- Pyelonephritis should be treated with intravenous antibiotics until the pyrexia settles and vomiting stopped, IV fluids, and antipyretics should also be given (manage in hospital because of risk of preterm labour).

Duration of treatment

- Asymptomatic bacteriuria: 3 days.
- Cystitis: 7 days.
- Pyelonephritis: 10–14 days.

Prevention

- Increase fluid intake.
- Double voiding and emptying bladder after sexual intercourse.
- Cranberry juice: proven in non-pregnant population to ↓ bacteriuria.
- Prophylactic antibiotics: if ≥ 2 culture positive urine infections + 1 risk factor.

Risk factors for urinary tract infection

- Antenatal:
    - previous infection (in previous pregnancy or outside pregnancy)
    - renal stones
    - diabetes mellitus
    - immunosuppression
    - polycystic kidneys
    - congenital anomalies of renal tract (e.g. duplex system)
    - neuropathic bladder.
- Postpartum (risk mainly associated with catheterization):
    - prolonged labour
    - prolonged 2nd stage
    - CS
    - pre-eclampsia.

Antibiotic options for renal tract infections

- Drug of choice depends on antibiotic sensitivities. Options include:
    - penicillin
    - cephalosporin
    - gentamicin—monitor levels to minimize risk of ototoxicity
    - trimethoprim—avoid in 1st trimester as it is a folate antagonist
    - nitrofurantoin—avoid in 3rd trimester as risk of haemolytic anaemia in neonate with glucose-6-phosphate dehydrogenase deficiency
    - sulphonamides—avoid in 3rd trimester as risk of kernicterus in neonate due to displacement of protein binding of bilirubin.
- Contra-indicated antibiotics:
    - Tetracyclines—causes permanent staining of teeth and problems with skeletal development
    - Ciprofloxacin—causes skeletal problems.

Renal stones

Incidence 1–4 per 1000, not ↑ in pregnancy. Common cause of abdominal pain severe enough to need hospital admission in pregnancy.
- May be asymptomatic or cause spasmodic loin pain, nausea + vomiting.
- MSU: microscopy may reveal crystals. Culture to exclude infection.
- USS, MRI, or CT urogram may demonstrate obstruction ± stone.
- Renal function should be checked.

Management:
- Analgesia, ↑ fluid intake, antibiotics if infection suspected.
- Most stones pass spontaneously.
- Urgent urology advise if signs of obstruction or infection.
- Cystoscopic, percutaneous or open stone removal or stenting.
- Lithotripsy is avoided in pregnancy.

Chronic renal disease

There are increased maternal and fetal risks to pregnancy with renal disease. This is dependent upon:
- The underlying cause of the renal impairment.
- The degree of renal impairment.
- The presence and control of hypertension.
- The amount of proteinuria.
  - As renal function deteriorates, so does the ability to conceive and sustain a pregnancy. Successful pregnancies are rare with a serum creatinine >275 μmol/L.

> ### Maternal risks
> - Accelerated, and possibly permanent, deterioration in renal function—this is more likely if there is also hypertension and proteinuria.
> - Hypertension.
> - Proteinuria.
> - Pre-eclampsia.
> - Venous thromboembolism (if nephritic level of proteinuria).
> - Urinary tract infection.
>
> ### Fetal risks
> - Miscarriage.
> - IUGR.
> - Spontaneous and iatrogenic preterm delivery.
> - Fetal death.

Management of pregnancy with chronic renal impairment
- Multidisciplinary care involving a renal physician.
- Baseline investigations, ideally before conception, include FBC, U&E, urate, 24 hour protein and creatinine clearance.
- Prepregnancy counselling (genetic counselling if a familial disorder)
- Antenatal care: early and regular attendance is advised (minimum of every 2 weeks). Aims of care are:
  - control BP: tight control lessens chance of renal function declining
  - monitor renal function and proteinuria
  - assess fetal size and well-being with serial growth scans + Doppler
  - early detection of complications: anaemia, UTI, pre-eclampsia, IUGR.
- Medication should be reviewed in pregnancy and may need altering. ACE inhibitors should be stopped as soon as pregnancy is confirmed.
- Prophylactic low-dose aspirin may reduce the risk of pre-eclampsia.
- Hospital admission should be considered in women with increasing proteinuria or hypertension, deteriorating renal function, or symptoms of pre-eclampsia.

⚠ Look for an underlying cause of deterioration in renal function: UTI, obstruction, dehydration, pre-eclampsia, renal vein thrombosis.

⚠ It can be difficult to differentiate between pre-eclampsia and deterioration of renal impairment. Thrombocytopaenia, IUGR, and ↑ urate suggest the former diagnosis.

- Aim for vaginal delivery, but rates of CS are increased.

Commonest causes of chronic renal impairment in pregnancy

- Reflux nephropathy.*
- Diabetes.
- Lupus nephritis.
- Chronic glomerulonephritides.
- Polycystic kidneys.*

* Condition may be familial. Adult polycystic kidney disease is inherited in an autosomal dominant manner.

Outcomes in pregnancy dependent on renal function

Mild renal impairment (creatinine <125 μmol/L)
- A successful outcome is achieved in 90% of cases
- Increasing proteinuria is common (>50% of pregnancies) and can be in nephrotic range.

Moderate renal impairment (creatinine 125–250 μmol/L)
- 25% of women experience an accelerated decline in renal function.
- Preterm delivery rate is up to 50%, one third have IUGR.
- A successful outcome is achieved in 60–90% of cases.

Severe renal impairment (creatinine >250 μmol/L)
- The risk of maternal complications is significantly higher than the chance of successful pregnancy, therefore advise against pregnancy.
- There is reduced fertility due to amenorrhoea.
- Permanent deterioration in renal function can occur in up to 25%.
- Preterm delivery rate is >70%, the rate of IUGR is 30%.

⚠ Creatinine level is dependent on muscle mass as well as renal function so patients may have significantly different creatinine clearance on 24 hour urine collection despite similar blood results. The latter is a more accurate reflection of renal function.

☙ Hypertension is an important predictor of outcome regardless of renal function.

Pregnancy after renal transplantation

Menstruation, ovulation, and fertility return after transplantation. Women should be informed of this and contraception discussed. Those who wish to conceive should be advised to wait 2 years after transplantation, until stabilization of renal function has been achieved and immunosuppression is at maintenance levels. The best outcomes are seen with:

- Well-controlled blood pressure.
- No proteinuria.
- No evidence of graft rejection.
- Plasma creatinine <180, preferably <125 μmol/L.

Maternal risks

- Increased risk of ectopic pregnancy: as a result of pelvic adhesions secondary to surgery, peritoneal dialysis, and pelvic infection.
- 15% develop significant deterioration in renal function, which may be permanent.
- In most cases pregnancy has no effect on graft survival or function
- Graft rejection ~5%: same as in non-pregnant women.
- Hypertension, proteinuria and pre-eclampsia: 30–40%.
- Infections, especially urinary tract: up to 40%.

Fetal risks

- Miscarriage and congenital anomaly rates are unchanged.
- IUGR 30%, higher if the mother is on cyclosporin.
- Preterm delivery 45–60%: may be iatrogenic, spontaneous, or secondary to preterm rupture of membranes.

⚠ If maternal complications occur before 28 weeks the chance of a successful pregnancy outcome falls from 95% to 75%.

Management of pregnancy in a transplant recipient

- Multidisciplinary management with a renal physician.
- Antenatal care should be at fortnightly intervals. The aim is:
  - serial assessment of renal function: deterioration may be caused by infection, dehydration, pre-eclampsia, drug toxicity or rejection
  - diagnosis and treatment of graft rejection
  - BP control (avoid ACE inhibitors and β-blockers)
  - prevention, early diagnosis and treatment of anaemia
  - detection and treatment of any infection.
  - serial assessment of fetus (↑ risk IUGR with ciclosporin).
- All women will be on immunosuppressive therapy which must be continued; commonly used drugs are prednisolone, azathioprine, cyclosporin, and tacrolimus.
- Aim for vaginal delivery with continuous fetal monitoring (parenteral steroids are necessary to cover labour, due to adrenal suppression).
- Prophylactic antibiotics are recommended for obstetric procedures.
- A transplanted kidney does not obstruct labour; CS should be for obstetric reasons-the current rate is 40% (patients with pelvic osteodystrophy may need elective CS).
- Breast-feeding should be avoided with cyclosporin and tacrolimus use.

Investigations in pregnancy following renal transplantation

- At each visit:
  - FBC, U&E, urate
  - MSU
  - 24 hour urine for creatinine clearance and protein.
- Every 2–4 weeks:
  - USS for fetal growth and Doppler studies.
- Every 6 weeks:
  - calcium, phosphate, albumin and LFTs.
- Every 12 weeks:
  - CMV titres if CMV negative at the beginning of pregnancy
  - drug levels of ciclosporin and tacrolimus.

Graft rejection

- Consider the diagnosis if there is deteriorating renal function with:
- Fever.
- Oliguria.
- Renal enlargement and tenderness.

It can be difficult to diagnose and a renal biopsy may be required.

Pregnancy on dialysis

- Pregnancy is unusual because of impaired fertility.
- Manage in a tertiary referral centre with a multidisciplinary team.
- Live birth rate (excluding termination): 40–50%.
- Preterm delivery should be anticipated, may be extreme.
- Increased risk of false positive serum screening for Down's syndrome secondary to elevated levels of hCG as it is renally cleared.
- Fetal risks: miscarriage, IUGR, polyhydramnios, preterm delivery, preterm rupture of membranes, in-utero death.
- Maternal risks: placental abruption, hypertension, pre-eclampsia.
- Continue current replacement therapy, haemo- or peritoneal dialysis.
- Dialysis strategy: increase length and frequency of dialysis, aiming for urea<20 mmol/L. Avoid hypotension and minimize heparin use. Consider fetal monitoring during dialysis after 28 weeks.
- Management should also address:
  - control of blood pressure
  - ensure good nutrition
  - fluid balance
  - correction of anaemia (↑ erythropoietin ± blood transfusion)
  - avoid hypercalcaemia
  - fetal growth and well-being.

Acute renal failure

- This is characterized by oliguria (<400 mL/day), ↑ urea and creatinine, hyperkalaemia, and metabolic acidosis. It is rare in pregnancy, typically complicating the postpartum period. There are three phases:
- **Oliguria:** few days to several weeks
- **Polyuria:** 2 days to 2 weeks, dilute urine is produced, and as waste products are still not excreted, renal function still deteriorates.
- **Recovery:** urine volume returns to normal with a gradual improvement in renal function.

Causes of renal failure in pregnancy

- Haemorrhage: postpartum, abruption or placenta praevia.
- Pre-eclampsia or HELLP syndrome.
- Infection: puerperal sepsis, septic miscarriage, chorioamnionitis, pyelonephritis.
- Obstruction: ureteric damage, pelvic or broad ligament haematoma.
- Drug reaction.
- Hyperemesis.
- Adrenal insufficiency due to lack of steroid cover in woman on long-term treatment.
- Acute fatty liver of pregnancy.
- Amniotic fluid embolus.
- Haemolytic-uraemic syndrome.

⚠ Non-pregnancy-related problems may also be the cause.

Management of acute renal failure

- Seek advice from a physician or nephrologist.
- Most cases are reversible with appropriate management (permanent problems more likely with pre-existing renal disease).
- Assessment should include the following investigations:
  - FBC, coagulation, U&E, plasma osmolality, glucose, albumin.
  - Blood cultures, MSU, HVS.
  - Urinalysis and urine osmolality and electrolytes.
  - ECG (looking for changes due to ↑K^+) and arterial blood gases.
  - Fetal assessment with CTG and USS.
  - Renal USS if obstruction suspected.
- Interventions should include catheterization, central venous line, and renal biopsy if improvement is delayed; only a minority require dialysis.
- Replace fluid/blood loss but avoid fluid overload as there is a significant risk of pulmonary oedema (accurate documentation of input/output, daily weight and central venous pressure monitoring).
- Maintain blood pressure at levels that allow adequate renal perfusion.
- Review medication and stop nephrotoxic drugs.
- Correct hyperkalaemia, coagulopathy and give antibiotics if infection suspected.
- Dialysis is required for persistent hyperkalaemia, acidosis, pulmonary oedema or uraemia.

Treatment of hyperkalaemia

- 10 mL calcium gluconate (10%) IV slowly, for cardioprotection.
- 15 units soluble insulin with 50 g of glucose 50% IV over 20 minutes
- Consider use of calcium resonium.

● These are only temporary measures; dialysis may be required.

Systemic lupus erythematosus (SLE)

More common in women than men (9:1) with a higher prevalence in the Afro-Caribbean population than in whites (5:1). The incidence is 1:1000 and onset during the reproductive age is common. It is a connective tissue disease of relapses (flares) and remissions. Diagnosis is based on the 4 features from the American Rheumatism Society Criteria present either consecutively or concurrently.

Monitoring disease severity in pregnancy

- Flare-ups can be difficult to diagnose as similar symptoms occur in normal pregnancy, e.g. fatigue, hair loss, joint aches, anaemia.
  - ESR is raised in normal pregnancy and CRP is not a marker of disease activity
  - C3($\downarrow$) or anti-DNA levels ($\uparrow$) are objective index of disease activity.
- Renal disease can also be difficult to distinguish from pre-eclampsia as hypertension, proteinuria, and thrombocytopaenia are common to both conditions.
  - raised urate and liver transaminases are not features of SLE
  - falling C3 and rising anti-DNA levels suggest lupus nephritis
  - renal biopsy is diagnostic but rarely performed in pregnancy.

Maternal risks

- Long-term prognosis is not affected by pregnancy.
- There is increased risk of flare-up, especially in the puerperium.
- Hypertension, pre-eclampsia, and placental abruption are more common.

$\triangle$ Do not stop hydroxychloroquine—this may precipitate a flare.

Fetal risks

- Increased risk of miscarriage, preterm delivery, preterm rupture of membranes, IUGR, and in-utero fetal death.
- These risks are due to anticardiolipin antibodies, lupus anticoagulant, renal impairment, or hypertension. Risk are low if all these are absent.
- Congenital heart block may occur in women with anti-Ro (or La) antibodies which cross the placenta (risk of occurrence if anti-Ro +ve is 2–3%, increasing to 25% if previously affected child).
- Transient skin lesions similar to cutaneous lupus can occur in neonates (usually in first 2 weeks of life).

Management

- Multidisciplinary team management.
- Pre-pregnancy counselling of maternal and fetal risks based on blood pressure, renal function, anti-Ro, and anti-phospholipid antibody status.
- Treat hypertension and modify medication if necessary (see 📖 p. 61).
- Advise conception during periods of disease remission: less risk of flare.
- Obtain objective evidence of flare-up.
- Flare-ups should be treated by starting, or increasing dose, or steroids.
- Assess fetal growth and well-being (uterine artery Doppler at 24 weeks is a useful screening test).

Diagnosis of SLE: American Rheumatism Association criteria

Diagnosis requires 4 of the following features, either simultaneously or following each other:
- Facial butterfly rash.
- Discoid lupus.
- Photosensitivity of skin rash.
- Oral or nasopharyngeal ulceration.
- Arthritis: non-erosive, migratory of 2 or more peripheral joints.
- Serositis: pleurisy or pericarditis.
- Renal problems: proteinuria >500 mg/day or cellular casts.
- Neurological problem: psychosis or convulsions.
- Haemotological problem: haemolytic anaemia, leucopenia ($<4 \times 10^9$/L), lymphopaenia ($<1.5 \times 10^9$/L) or thrombocytopenia ($<100 \times 10^9$/L).
- Anti-DNA, anti-nuclear antibodies, chronic false-positive syphilis serology for >6 months, or positive LE cell preparation.

Anti-phospholipid antibody syndrome

This condition is diagnosed on the basis of the presence of one or more clinical features and one or more positive laboratory findings. The condition may be complicated by hypertension, pulmonary hypertension, epilepsy, thrombocytopenia, leg ulcers, and valvular problems. It is called primary if features of connective tissue disease are absent or it can occur secondary to established connective tissue disease. Lupus anticoagulant is an inhibitor of the coagulation pathway, and anti-cardiolipins are antibodies against the phospholipid components of cell walls.

Anti-phospholipid antibody syndrome: diagnostic criteria

- Clinical criteria:
  - vascular thrombosis—arterial or venous
  - 3 or more consecutive miscarriages (<10 weeks)
  - one or more fetal death >10 weeks
  - one or more preterm delivery (<34 weeks) due to pre-eclampsia or placental insufficiency.
- Laboratory criteria:
  - anti-cardiolipin antibody (IgG or IgM) in medium or high titre on at least two occasions >6 weeks apart
  - lupus anticoagulant present on at least two occasions >6 weeks apart.

Maternal risks
- These include placental abruption, pre-eclampsia.
- Previous poor obstetric history is an important predictor of outcome (the risk is less with just recurrent miscarriages).

Fetal risks
- Risks include early and late miscarriage, in-utero death, IUGR.
- Fetal outcome may be improved by multidisciplinary management, fetal monitoring (including growth, umbilical and uterine artery Dopplers), appropriate drug therapy and timely delivery.
- Anti-cardiolipin antibody is the best predictor of fetal outcome: the higher the titre the greater the fetal risk, but quantifying the risk is difficult.
- Possible mechanisms of fetal injury are recurrent placental infarction and direct cellular injury.
- Liaise with anaesthetist if the woman is on LMWH (regional anaesthesia is contra-indicated within 12 hours of a prophylactic dose of heparin and 24 hours of a therapeutic dose).

Anti-phospholipid antibody syndrome: recommendations

- **No thrombosis or pregnancy loss:**
  - no treatment or aspirin 75 mg.
- **Previous thrombosis:**
  - aspirin +LMWH.
- **Previous recurrent 1st-trimester miscarriages**:
  - aspirin ± LMWH.
- **Previous IUD or IUGR or severe pre-eclampsia:**
  - aspirin + LMWH.

Start aspirin when pregnancy confirmed; LMWH when fetal heart seen.

☙ Take home baby rate: 40% aspirin alone; 70% aspirin and LMWH.

☙ Some studies have disputed improved pregnancy outcomes with LMWH compared with aspirin alone.

Consider stopping heparin if 24 week uterine artery Dopplers normal.
- The improved live birth rate is due to ↓ miscarriages.

⚠ Steroids are not recommended → less success and more side effects.

Rheumatoid arthritis

This is more common in women than men, with an incidence of 1:1000–2000 pregnancies. It is characterized by symmetrical chronic inflammation and destruction of synovial joints. Autoantibodies are formed to immunoglobulins which are deposited as immune complexes in the synovial fluid and elsewhere. 80–90% have rheumatoid factor and 20–30% are ANA positive. It is a multisystem disorder with extra-articular features including anaemia, nodules, carpal tunnel syndrome, eye and lung involvement.

Maternal risks

- The condition improves in pregnancy in 75% of cases but flare-up is common in the puerperium.
- At this age atlantoaxial subluxation rarely causes problems during intubation.

Fetal risks

- There is usually no adverse effect on pregnancy unless the woman is anti-Ro positive or has anti-phosphlipid antibodies (5–10%).

Drugs used in the treatment of autoimmune diseases

- **Safe to continue in pregnancy:**
  - paracetamol
  - steroids
  - hydroxychloroquine
  - sulfasalazine (in conjunction with 5 mg folic acid)
  - azathioprine.
- **Discontinue/avoid in pregnancy:**
  - NSAIDs—oligohydramnios, premature closure of ductus arteriosus and neonatal haemorrhage especially with 3rd-trimester use
  - gold—teratogenic effect seen in animals only
  - penicillamine—connective tissue abnormalities only in high doses
  - cyclofosphamide (alkylating agent)—risk of leukaemia
  - methotrexate (folate antagonist)—causes miscarriage and congenital anomalies.

Myasthenia gravis

An uncommon condition but has the highest incidence in women of childbearing age. It is caused by autoimmune disruption of nicotinic acetylcholine receptors at the skeletal muscle motor end plate, leading to muscle weakness and fatigue. 90% have acetylcholine receptor antibodies. Muscles affected include eyes (ptosis, diplopia), face, neck, limbs, and trunk. Diagnosis is confirmed by prompt but transient improvement in muscle strength with the Tensilon test. The condition can be worsened by infection, hypokalaemia, exercise, emotion, and drugs (aminoglycosides, $MgSO_4$, local anaesthetic, β-blockers, β-agonists, narcotics, and neuromuscular blocking drugs.

Effect of pregnancy on myasthenia

- No change 60%, improvement 20%, deterioration 20%.
- There is no consistent effect between pregnancies.
- Symptoms commonly worsen postpartum.
- Previous thymectomy iis associated with fewer exacerbations in pregnancy.
- Hyperemesis, delayed gastric emptying, increased volume of distribution of drugs, and increased renal clearance can lead to subtherapeutic drug levels in pregnancy.
- Increased doses of anticholinesterases may be required as pregnancy advances; this is best achieved by decreasing dose intervals.
- Parenteral anticholinesterases should be given in labour to avoid absorption problems.

Effect of myasthenia on pregnancy

- Preterm delivery, polyhydramnios, and IUGR are all increased.
- The 1st stage of labour is not prolonged (the smooth muscle of the myometrium is not affected by the condition).
- In the 2nd stage there can be skeletal muscle fatigue; instrumental delivery may be required to prevent maternal exhaustion.
- Neonatal myasthenia can occur following delivery in 20% of babies:
  - it results from transplacental passage of maternal antibodies
  - there is poor correlation between the condition and maternal disease activity or antibody levels
  - presentation is with generalized hypotonia, poor sucking/feeding, and a weak cry
  - onset is within 24 hours and the condition resolves by 2 months
  - treatment is with anticholinesterases.

⚠ $MgSO_4$ contra-indicated for the treatment of eclampsia in myasthenia.

Management

- Inform neurologist, paediatrician, and anaesthetist of pregnancy.
- The usual treatment options have all been used in pregnancy:
  - Long-acting anticholinesterases(e.g. pyridostigmine)
  - immunosuppression: steroids, azathioprine
  - plasmapharesis
  - thymectomy.

Diabetes: established disease in pregnancy

Established diabetes affects 1–2% of pregnancies. It includes type 1 and type 2 diabetes mellitus. Without good glycaemic control there is increased fetal and neonatal morbidity and mortality. Management is best undertaken by a multidisciplinary team including an obstetrician, physician/diabetologist, diabetic specialist nurse, specialist midwife, and dietitian.

Glucose metabolism is altered by pregnancy. Insulin requirements increase throughout pregnancy and are maximal at term. A normal woman can increase the amount of insulin she produces to counteract diabetogenic hormones (human placental lactogen, cortisol, glucagon, oestrogen and progesterone). She maintains her blood sugars at 4–4.5 mmol/L. Diabetic women are unable to do this and need close monitoring of their blood sugars for good control.

Effect of diabetes on pregnancy

Maternal hyperglycaemia leads to fetal hyperglycaemia which is potentially harmful to the fetus. It leads to hyperinsulinaemia through β-cell hyperplasia in fetal pancreatic cells. Insulin in the fetus acts as a growth promoter. The net effect is therefore macrosomia, organomegaly, and increased erythropoiesis. Fetal polyuria occurs, especially in the presence of poor diabetic control, and this manifests as polyhydramnios.

The high levels of insulin in fetal life, coupled with the removal of its glucose supply from the mother at birth, leads to neonatal hypoglycaemia. Early feeding and regular blood glucose monitoring should be performed to minimize the risk of this problem, as it can lead to cerebral damage untreated.

Surfactant deficiency occurs through reduced production of pulmonary phospholipids. This clinically manifests as respiratory distress syndrome, which is more common in babies born to diabetic mothers.

Effect of pregnancy on diabetes

- **Ketoacidosis**: rare, but may be associated with hyperemesis, infection, tocolysis (β-sympathomimetics), or steroid therapy.
- **Retinopathy**: there is a 2 fold increased risk of development or progression of existing disease. Rapid improvement in glycaemic control leads to increased retinal blood flow which can cause retinopathy. All diabetic women should have assessment for retinopathy in pregnancy, proliferative retinopathy requires treatment. Early changes usually revert after delivery.
- **Nephropathy** affects 5–10% of women. Renal function and proteinuria may worsen during pregnancy. This is usually temporary. There is increased maternal risk of pre-eclampsia and fetal risk of IUGR in this population and increased surveillance is required.
- **Ischaemic heart disease**: pregnancy increases cardiac workload. Women with a previous myocardial infarction should avoid pregnancy (mortality 50%). Women with symptoms should be assessed by a cardiologist before conception.

Complications of diabetes in pregnancy

Maternal
- UTI
- Recurrent vulvovaginal candidiasis.
- Pregnancy-induced hypertension/pre-eclampsia.
- Obstructed labour.
- Operative deliveries: CS and assisted vaginal deliveries.
- ↑ retinopathy (15%).
- ↑ nephropathy.
- Cardiac disease.

Fetal
- Miscarriage*
- Congenital abnormalities:*
  - neural tube defects
  - microcephaly
  - cardiac abnormalities
  - sacral agenesis
  - renal abnormalities
- Preterm labour.
- Polyhydramnios (25%).
- Macrosomia (25–40%).
- IUGR.
- Unexplained IUD.

Neonatal
- Polycythaemia.
- Jaundice.
- Hypoglycaemia.
- Hypocalcaemia.
- Hypomagnesaemia.
- Hypothermia.
- Cardiomegaly.
- Birth trauma: shoulder dystocia, fractures, Erb's palsy, asphyxia.
- Respiratory distress syndrome.

* In diabetics with poor control.

Diabetes: antenatal management

Pre-pregnancy counselling
Counselling should be offered to all diabetic women of reproductive age. This should include:
- **Achievement of optimal control**: aim for normoglycaemia—pre-meal glucose <5.5 or 2-hour glucose<7.0, HbA1c<6.5% (there is increased risk of miscarriage and congenital abnormalities with poor control).
- **Assessment of severity of diabetes**: check for hypertension, retinopathy (fundoscopy, ophthalmology assessment), nephropathy (U&E, urinalysis, urinary protein: creatinine ratio, 24 hour urine for protein, creatinine clearance), neuropathy(clinical assessment), and cardiac disease.
- **Education**: ensure understanding of effects of hyperglycaemia on fetus and the need for tight control; instruct to inform doctor as soon as pregnancy confirmed, some drugs may need stopping (ACE inhibitors).
- **General health**: stop smoking, optimize weight (aim for a normal BMI), minimize alcohol (max 1–2 units twice/week).
- **Folic acid**: ↑ risk of neural tube defects, so start on 5 mg folic acid.
- **Rubella status**: offer vaccination if not rubella immune.
- **Contraception**: ensure effective contraception until good control achieved and pregnancy desired.

Antenatal care
Manage by a multidisciplinary team with a diabetologist.
- **Control**: as for pre-pregnancy, aim for normoglycaemia. Monitor glucose at least 4 times per day, usually before meals but post-meal glucose may give tighter control. Women can alter their own insulin based on their glucose. Insulin can be given as subcutaneous injections 2 or 4 times per day or as a continuous infusion. The latter is no better than injections.
- **HbA1c every month**: this gives an objective measurement of control over the preceding 2 months.
- **Dietitian review**: low sugar, low fat, high fibre diet—low glycaemic index.
- **Dating ultrasound:** to confirm viability and gestation.

- ☛ **Down's syndrome screening**: consider nuchal translucency or invasive testing. Serum screening is affected by diabetes (↓ αFP) therefore less accurate unless appropriate normograms used.
- **Anomaly scan**: 5–10 fold ↑ risk of congenital anomalies. Risk depends on glycaemic control prior to conception and early pregnancy.
- **Fetal echocardiography**: at 20–24 weeks
- **Antenatal surveillance**: individualize care. Serial USS every 2–4 weeks to detect polyhydramnios, macrosomia or IUGR. Increased surveillance if problems detected. The use of umbilical artery Doppler should be restricted to cases of IUGR; it is not of value as a screening test.
- **Hypoglycaemia**: awareness of hypoglycaemia may be lost. Educate patient and family and supply with glucagon.

Diabetes: labour and postpartum care

Timing and mode of delivery should be individualized and based on estimated fetal weight (EFW) and obstetric factors (previous mode of delivery, gestation, glycaemic control, and antenatal complications).

Timing of delivery

🖝 Some obstetricians advise elective delivery by induction of labour at 38–39 weeks if there are no maternal or fetal complications and good glycaemic control. Outcomes may not be better than awaiting spontaneous labour. Delivery should be expedited if complications occur.

Mode of delivery

Vaginal delivery is preferred. Continuous electronic fetal monitoring is advised in labour. Consider elective CS if EFW is >4.5 kg. If EFW is 4–4.5 kg use obstetric factors to influence decision. CS rates are high: 50–60%. Give antibiotic and thromboprophylaxis if CS is carried out.

🖝 Shoulder dystocia is more common at all birth weights than in the non-diabetic population. Experienced obstetricians should perform instrumental deliveries because this is an independent risk factor.

Glycaemic control

- **Diet controlled**: check blood glucose hourly. If glucose >6.0 mmol/L, start sliding scale.
- **Insulin dependent:** continue subcutaneous insulin until in established labour then convert to insulin sliding scale (Table 5.1). If induction of labour or CS, continue normal insulin until day of procedure then start sliding scale in early morning.

⚠ Avoid maternal hyperglycaemia → causes fetal hypoglycaemia.

⚠ If steroids are given for threatened preterm labour monitor glucose closely as hyperglycaemia should be anticipated.

Postpartum care

Insulin requirements fall dramatically after delivery of the placenta. Halve the sliding scale initially. Change back to SC insulin when eating and drinking. Start with the prepregnancy dose of SC insulin. If this is not known, it is roughly half the last dose. The dose may need to be further reduced if breast-feeding. Stop the sliding scale 1 hour after giving the SC dose.

▶ Aim for BM 4–9 mmol/L in the postpartum period.

- Encourage breast-feeding

⚠ Avoid oral hypoglycaemic drugs if breast-feeding, insulin is safe.
- Baby needs early feeding and glucose monitoring (liaise with paediatricians).

Contraception

- Avoid the COCP if breast-feeding or vascular complications. Progesterone-based contraception is safe and there are no contra-indications to an IUCD. This should be fitted from 6 weeks post-partum onwards. Sterilisation or vasectomy should be considered if the family is complete.

Table 5.1 Insulin: IV sliding scale
Prescription: 50 units Human Actrapid in 50 ml normal saline (sodium chloride 0.9%), via a continuous infusion pump

Blood glucose(mmol/L)	Insulin rate(mL/hour)
<3.0	0
3.1–4	0.5
4.1–6	1.0
6.1–8	1.5
8.1–11	2.0
11.1–15	3.0
>15.1	Call doctor

- Review sliding scale regularly.
- Renew insulin syringe every 24 hours.
- Intravenous fluids should always be given with the sliding scale.
  - stable situations—5% dextrose
  - high blood glucose—normal saline.

Gestational diabetes

The WHO now includes gestational impaired glucose tolerance (IGT) with gestational diabetes. A proportion of women diagnosed in pregnancy will actually have previously unrecognized type 1 or 2 diabetes (20–30%). The WHO does not advocate universal screening. Selective screening should be based on risk factors.

> ## Risk factors for gestational diabetes
>
> * Family history of 1st-degree relative with diabetes.
> * Obesity (BMI>30).
> * Previous large baby (>4 kg).
> * Previous unexplained stillbirth.
> * Previous gestational diabetes.
> * Polycystic ovarian syndrome.
> * Polyhydramnios in this pregnancy.
> * Glycosuria on 2 or more occasions in this pregnancy.
> * Abnormal timed random glucose:
>   * >5.5 mmol/L fasting or >2 hours after food
>   * >7.0 mmol/L <2 hours after food.

The diagnosis is based on an oral glucose tolerance test (OGTT) (📖 p. 237), usually undertaken at 26–28 weeks gestation. A normal result in early pregnancy does not mean that gestational diabetes will not develop and an OGTT should be repeated at 34 weeks, if concerns.

Management

* Management by a multidisciplinary team.
* Measure glucose four times per day (1 hour postprandial measurements may be more effective in preventing macrosomia than pre-meal glucose).
* Diet should be first-line treatment:
  * aim for normoglycaemia and avoid ketosis.
  * weight should remain steady if diet followed.
  * compliance is often poor—dietitian input may help.
* Start insulin if:
  * Pre-meal glucose >6.0 mmol/L
  * 1 hour postprandial glucose >7.5mmol/l.
  * AC>95th centile despite apparent good control.
* There is no increased risk of miscarriage or congenital anomalies; other fetal and neonatal risks are similar to established diabetes (IUGR is less likely).
* Antenatal and intrapartum care as for established diabetes.
* Postpartum:
  * stop insulin and glucose infusions
  * check glucose prior to discharge to ensure normal (risk of previously undiagnosed type 2 diabetes)
  * arrange OGTT at 6 week postpartum
  * education—50% risk of developing type 2 diabetes mellitus over next 25 years (this risk can be reduced by maintaining physical activity and avoiding obesity).

Oral glucose tolerance test

- Overnight fasting (8 hours minimum):
  - water only may be consumed during this time
  - no smoking
- 75 g glucose load in 250–300 mL water.
- Plasma glucose measured fasting and at 2 hours.

Results

- *Diabetes*:
  - fasting glucose ≥7.0 mmol/L
  - 2 hour glucose ≥11.1 mmol/L.
- *IGT*:
  - fasting glucose <7.0 mmol/L
  - 2hour ≥7.8 <11.0 mmol/L.

Only one value needs to be abnormal to make the diagnosis.

Thyrotoxicosis

Thyrotoxicosis occurs in 1:500 pregnancies. The most common cause is Graves' disease (95%). This is an autoimmune disease characterized by the production of TSH receptor stimulating antibodies. Most women have been diagnosed before pregnancy and may be on treatment. Many symptoms and signs occur in normal pregnancy. The most discriminating features are weight loss, tremor, persistent tachycardia, eye signs. The diagnosis is made by a low TSH and high free T_4 or free T_3 levels.

▶ Use pregnancy-specific reference ranges for each trimester. See Table 5.2 p. 241.

Effect of pregnancy on thyrotoxicosis
- Usually improves in the 2nd and 3rd trimester.
- Pregnancy is a state of relative immunodeficiency but with return of normal immunity in the puerperium it is likely to deteriorate.

Effect of thyrotoxicosis on the pregnancy
- Maternal and fetal outcome is usually good if the disease is controlled.
- Untreated or poorly controlled thyrotoxicosis is associated with sub-fertility (amenorrhoea due to weight loss) ↑ risk of miscarriage, IUGR and premature delivery.

⚠ With the stress of infection, labour, or operative delivery a 'thyroid storm' can occur in poorly controlled patients. This is a medical emergency and is characterized by pyrexia, confusion, and cardiac failure.
- Neonatal/fetal thyrotoxicosis occurs in up to 10% of babies born to women with current or past history of Graves' disease (trans-placental passage of thyroid receptor stimulating antibodies).

▶ Check antibody levels in all women with a history of Graves' disease.
- If antibodies are present, monitor by fetal heart rate, and serial USS for growth and fetal goitre (treatments include antithyroid drugs titrated to fetal heart rate, or delivery).
- Antibodies have a half-life of around 3 weeks, therefore transient neonatal hyperthyroidism may occur.

Treatment options for thyrotoxicosis
- **Antithyroid drugs:** carbimazole and propylthiouracil (PTU) are the two drugs used. The aim of treatment is to achieve clinical euthyroid with T_4 at the upper limit of normal. Use the lowest dose of drug to achieve this. Both drugs cross the placenta and may cause fetal hypothyroidism in high doses. PTU is preferred for new cases as there is less transfer across the placenta and into breast milk but do not change if on carbimazole in pregnancy. β-blockers may safely be used for symptom relief in new cases for a short period of time.
- **Surgery:** Thyroidectomy can be safely done in pregnancy. Indications include dysphagia, stridor, suspected carcinoma, and allergies to both antithyroid drugs.

☞ Radioactive iodine is contraindicated in pregnancy and breast-feeding.

Causes of thyrotoxicosis

- Graves' disease.
- Toxic multinodular goitre.
- Toxic adenoma.
- Carcinoma.
- Subacute thyroiditis.
- Amiodarone.
- Lithium.

⚠ Women with hyperemesis or a molar pregnancy may mimic biochemical hyperthyroidism as hCG, at high levels, can stimulate TSH receptors. They usually have no clinical signs of thyrotoxicosis and should not be treated.

Key points for management

- Graves' disease often improves in pregnancy but relapses postpartum.
- With treatment the outlook is good for mother and baby.
- Untreated thyrotoxicosis is dangerous for mother and baby.
- Propylthiouracil and carbimazole may be used as treatment; both cross the placenta.
- Avoid radioactive iodine.
- Check for TSH receptor stimulating antibodies.
- Monitor thyroid function every 4–6 weeks in new cases, less frequently in stable cases.
- Monitor fetus by fetal heart rate and serial USS for growth and presence of goitre.
- Breast-feeding is safe with doses of PTU <150 mg/day and carbimazole <15 mg/day. Monitor TFTs in baby at higher doses.

Hypothyroidism

Hypothyroidism complicates around 1% of pregnancies. Most cases have been diagnosed previously and patients are on replacement therapy. New diagnosis in pregnancy is rare. The commonest cause is autoimmune, and may be associated with other autoimmune conditions.

- Classical symptoms and signs may be seen in normal pregnancy. The most discriminatory features are cold intolerance, bradycardia, and slow relaxation of tendon reflexes.
- The diagnosis is made by a low free T_4. TSH is also raised but in isolation is not diagnostic.

▶ Use pregnancy-specific reference ranges for each trimester (Table 5.2). Free T_4 levels are normally lower in the 2nd and 3rd trimester. TSH level most useful.

Effect of pregnancy on hypothyroidism

No effect usually. Most women do not need to alter their dose of levothyroxine. The most common reason for increasing levothyroxine is an inadequate prepregnancy dose.

Effect of hypothyroidism on pregnancy

- Untreated hypothyroidism is associated with anovulatory infertility.
- Severe or untreated hypothyroidism in pregnancy is associated with increased risk of miscarriage, fetal loss, pre-eclampsia, and low birth weight.
- The fetus requires maternal T_4 for normal brain development before 12 weeks; after this time $T_3/T_4/TSH$ do not cross the placenta (inadequate replacement may lead to reduced IQ in the offspring).

▶ Aim for optimal control before conception.

- Women on adequate replacement therapy are euthyroid at the onset of pregnancy and have good maternal and fetal outcomes.
- Neonatal/fetal hypothyroidism is very rare and caused by the transplacental transfer of TSH receptor blocking antibodies, which may be seen in atrophic thyroiditis.

Treatment

- Most women should continue their maintenance dose of thyroxine, the dose should only be increased if they are under-replaced (shown by TSH level).
- TSH levels need to be checked before conception and in each trimester, unless there has been a dose adjustment, in which case it should be repeated in 6 weeks.
- If the diagnosis is made in pregnancy, in the absence of cardiac disease, consider a starting dose of 100 micrograms daily.
- In practice, aim for a TSH level of <2.5 mu/L
- Thyroxine can be safely taken during breast-feeding.

Causes of hypothyroidism

- Hashimoto's thyroiditis.
- Atrophic thyroiditis.
- Congenital absence of thyroid.
- Iatrogenic:
  - thyroidectomy
  - radioiodine
  - drugs (amiodarone, lithium, iodine, antithyroid drugs).
- Pituitary cause (rare).

Table 5.2 Reference ranges for thyroid function tests (TFTs) by trimester

	Non-pregnant	1st trimester	2nd trimester	3rd trimester
TSH (mu/L)	0–4	0–1.6	0.1–1.8	0.7–7.3
Free T_4 (pmol/L)	11–23	11–22	11–19	7–15
Free T_3 (pmol/L)	4–9	4–8	4–7	3–5

Other thyroid diseases

Postpartum thyroiditis

This is an autoimmune condition causing destructive thyroiditis. It presents postpartum due to return to normal immunity after the relative immuno-suppression of pregnancy. Preformed T_4 is released which may cause transient hyperthyroid symptoms followed by hypothyroidism as the reserve of T_4 is used up.

It can present for up to a year after delivery but usually occurs 3–4 months postpartum. The incidence varies (5–10%) and it may manifest as transient hypothyroidism (40%), hyperthyroidism (40%), or biphasic with first hyperthyroidism then hypothyroidism (20%). There may be a family history of thyroid disease in 25% of cases. Many women are asymptomatic and often symptoms are vague and may be attributed to the postpartum state. Initiation of treatment should be based on symptoms and not biochemical results. Some women may not require any treatment. Most recover spontaneously. Risk of recurrence in future pregnancy is 70%. Risk of permanent hypothyroidism is 5% per year for antibody-positive women (90% of patients have thyroid peroxidase antibodies).

- The hyperthyroid phase should be treated with β-blockers (not antithyroid drugs).
△ Differential diagnosis: Graves' disease.

- The hypothyroid state should be treated with thyroxine; treatment should be withdrawn after 6 months to check for recovery.
△ Differential diagnosis: Hashimoto's thyroiditis or Sheehan's syndrome.

▶ Long term follow-up should be with annual TFT.

Thyroid nodules

- Thyroid nodules are common, affecting 5% of women in their reproductive years.

△ A small proportion of thyroid nodules are malignant.
- Differential diagnosis is a solitary toxic nodule, subacute (de Quervain's) thyroiditis, or a bleed into a cystic lesion.
- Investigations:
  - TFT and thyroid antibodies
  - thyroglobulin level: suggests malignancy if >100 µg/L
  - USS: cystic nodules are more likely to be benign than solid nodules
  - fine needle aspiration for cytology (cystic lesion)
  - biopsy (solid lesion).

△ Radioiodine is contraindicated in pregnancy.
- Malignant lesions can be surgically treated in the 2nd and 3rd trimesters, and postoperatively thyroxine can be safely given to completely suppress TSH in TSH-dependent tumours.

Thyroid nodules: symptoms or signs suggestive of malignancy

- Past history of radiation to neck or chest.
- Fixed lump.
- Lymphadenopathy.
- Rapid growth of painless nodule.
- Voice change.
- Neurological involvement such as Horner's syndrome.
- PCR of fetal cells in maternal blood may help determine fetal sex.

Phaeochromocytoma

This is a tumour of the adrenal medulla that causes excess secretion of catecholamines. They are bilateral in 10% of cases and malignant in 10%. In non-pregnant hypertensive patients the incidence is around 1:1000; it is exceedingly rare in pregnancy. A high index of clinical suspicion is required to make the diagnosis—the condition should be considered in hypertensive pregnant women if there are atypical features. Untreated, mortality is high: maternal mortality ~17% and fetal mortality ~26%. Maternal mortality can be reduced to ~4% with treatment.

Symptoms and signs

- Hypertension.
- Sweating.
- Palpitations.
- Anxiety.
- Headache.
- Vomiting.

⚠ Symptoms may mimic pre-eclampsia and may be paroxysmal.

Investigations

- Raised 24 hour urinary catecholamines or their metabolites such as vanillylmandelic acid (VMA) confirm the diagnosis—a level 2× normal is highly suggestive and 3× normal diagnostic (methyl-dopa and labetolol can interfere with the results).
- Imaging is required to localize the tumour (USS, CT, or MRI are all used but MRI is preferable in pregnancy).

Management

- Multidisciplinary management including endocrine physician and surgeon.
- The main risk from this condition is potentially fatal hypertensive crises that can cause strokes, congestive cardiac failure, and arrhythmias.
- Patients should be commenced on α-blockers (phenoxybenzamine) to control BP, then β-blockers (propranolol) to control tachycardia.

⚠ Do **not** start β-blockers until a few days after α-blockers or a hypertensive crisis may ensue.

- Surgery is the only cure for the condition and should only be undertaken once pharmacological blockade has been achieved (if the diagnosis is made after 24 weeks, surgery should be delayed until fetal maturity is achieved)
- CS is preferred for delivery as it minimizes potential catecholamine surges (removal of the adrenal tumour can be done at the time of CS or later)
- Anaesthetic experience is vital as the patient may have a catecholamine surge during delivery due to inadequate pharmacological blockade.

Congenital adrenal hyperplasia (CAH)

This is an autosomal recessive disorder affecting the synthesis of glucocorticoids and mineralocorticoids. In response to low levels of these hormones, the pituitary gland produces large amounts of ACTH and this results in excessive production of sex steroids. A number of enzyme deficiencies can lead to this condition: the commonest is 21-hydroxylase deficiency. Many different gene mutations exist which result in variable clinical presentations. Treatment is replacement with corticosteroid ± fludrocortisone.

Affected individuals present in several ways:
- Salt-losing crisis in neonate.
- Masculinization of female fetus (ambiguous genitalia at birth).
- Precocious puberty in boy.

▶ If a couple has an affected child, the risk in subsequent pregnancies is 1:4.

Maternal and fetal risks

Pregnancies in women with CAH, diagnosed in infancy, are uncommon. Many are subfertile due to anovulation; others have psychosexual and emotional difficulties or anatomical problems related to corrective surgery for virilization.
- ↑ risk of miscarriage, pre-eclampsia and IUGR.
- ↑ risk of CS due to android-shaped pelvis.

Management

- Maternal steroid therapy should be continued at same dose throughout pregnancy.
- Genetic counselling should be offered to all couples after the birth of an affected child; antenatal diagnosis can be untaken in subsequent pregnancies, but the female fetus is at risk of virilization before these tests can be undertaken,

▶ Start dexamethasone, 1.5 mg/day, as soon as pregnancy confirmed, and before 5 weeks gestation (dexamethasone crosses placenta and suppresses excessive fetal ACTH production, which prevents masculinization and neuroendocrine effects to female fetus)
- Usually CVS is the preferred method of antenatal diagnosis.
- If the fetus is male, or an unaffected female, stop dexamethasone.
- If the fetus is an affected female options include continuation of dexamethasone throughout pregnancy or termination of pregnancy.

⚠Mother needs to be monitored for gestational diabetes and ↑BP.
- If invasive testing is declined, dexamethasone should be given and fetal sex determined by USS.
- Suppression of virilization with dexamethasone is not always successful and parents should be appropriately counselled.
- During labour increase steroid dose—hydrocortisone 100 mg IV every 6 hours.
- Postnatally the child needs to be reviewed by a paediatrician and evidence of virilization sought; replacement glucocorticoid and mineralocorticoid therapy should be continued.

Antenatal diagnosis

- Amniocentesis (≥16 weeks):
  - fetal sex
  - 17-hydroxyprogesterone and androgen levels in amniotic fluid
  - HLA typing of amniotic cells.
- Chorionic villus sampling (≥10 weeks):
  - fetal sex
  - gene probe for specific mutations of 21-hydroxylase.
- PCR of fetal cells in maternal blood may help determine fetal sex.

Addison's, Conn's, and Cushing's syndromes

Addison's disease

Adrenocortical failure with deficiency of glucocorticoids and mineralocorticoids; may be associated with other autoimmune conditions: pernicious anaemia, diabetes, or thyroid disease. Most common cause in the UK is autoimmune destruction of the adrenals. Worldwide, TB is an important cause. It is rare to make a new diagnosis in pregnancy.

- Diagnosis is based on ↓ cortisol, ↑ ACTH, poor response to synacthen (synthetic ACTH).

▶ Cortisol measurements are normally higher in pregnancy therefore care should be taken in interpreting results.

- Pregnancy does not affect the course of Addison's disease and if the condition is treated there are no adverse fetal effects.
- Patients should continue with their usual steroid doses (hydrocortisone 20–30 mg/day and fludrocortisone 100 micrograms/day) throughout pregnancy.
- Increased or intravenous doses of steroids are required to cover periods of stress, such as infection, hyperemesis, labour, or surgery.
- In the puerperium physiological diuresis can cause profound hypotension therefore tail steroids down to maintenance over several days.
- Breast-feeding is safe.

Conn's syndrome

- This is a rare cause of hypertension in pregnancy. Primary hyperaldosteronism is caused by adrenal aldosterone-secreting adenoma or carcinoma or bilateral adrenal hyperplasia.
- Clinical features are hypokalaemia (K^+ <3.0 mmol/L) and hypertension
- Diagnosis is based on ↓ K^+, ↑ plasma aldosterone, ↓ renin.
- Treat hypertension as usual (but avoid spironolactone which is used outside pregnancy) and give potassium supplements.

Cushing's syndrome

- This is a condition of glucocorticoid excess; very rare in pregnancy as anovulation leads to infertility. Causes in pregnancy are excessive pituitary ACTH secretion (44%), adrenal adenoma (44%), or adrenal carcinoma (12%).
- Diagnosis based on ↑ cortisol, which fails to suppress with the high dose dexamethasone suppression test (ACTH levels depend on cause).
- Maternal morbidity and mortality are raised specific risks include pre-eclampsia, diabetes, and poor wound healing.
- Fetal loss, prematurity, and perinatal mortality are increased and adrenal insufficiency can occur in the neonate.
- Surgery is the treatment of choice for adrenal and pituitary causes, it may be successfully performed in pregnancy.
- There is limited knowledge of use of drugs in pregnancy. Medical treatment include drugs that suppress cortisol production (metyrapone) or ACTH activity(cyproheptadine),
- Avoid breast-feeding.

Clinical features of Addison's disease

- Weight loss.
- Vomiting.
- Postural hypotension and syncope.
- Weakness.
- Hyperpigmentation (skin folds, scars, mouth).

Clinical features of Cushing's syndrome

- Bruising.
- Myopathy.
- Hypertension.
- Excessive weight gain/oedema.
- Hirsutism.
- Excessive striae.
- Headaches.
- Acne.
- Obesity.
- Impaired glucose tolerance/diabetes.

Investigations in Cushing's syndrome

- 24 hour urinary free cortisol or plasma free cortisol.
- Dexamethasone suppression test:
    - dexamethasone 0.5 g every 6 hours for 48°hours.
    - urinary free cortisol for last 24°hours of test
    - plasma cortisol 6°hours after last dose of dexamethasone
    - cortisol level is raised and there is failure to suppress.
- Plasma ACTH levels: ↑ if pituitary cause, ↓ if adrenal cause.
- Imaging: MRI of pituitary or adrenal gland may identify a mass.
- Visual fields: if pituitary mass suspected.

🔷 Cortisol levels are markedly raised in normal pregnancy compared with the non-pregnant state but diurnal variation persists. Use pregnancy-specific reference ranges.

Hyperprolactinaemia

Prolactinomas are the commonest pituitary tumours seen in pregnancy. They can be classified according to their size into microprolactinoma (<1 cm) and macroprolactinoma (>1 cm). Outside pregnancy diagnosis is based on a raised serum prolactin level in conjunction with imaging of the pituitary fossa by CT or MRI. In pregnancy, there is a 10-fold physiological rise in prolactin levels, so prolactin level is not a useful test in diagnosis or follow-up.

Clinical features of prolactinoma

- Amenorrhoea.
- Galactorrhoea.
- Headache.
- Visual field defects (bitemporal hemianopia).
- Diabetes insipidus.

Effect of pregnancy on prolactinomas

There is a possibility that prolactinomas will increase in size in pregnancy and cause symptoms. The highest risk (15%) is in the 3rd trimester with macroprolactinomas. Pregnancy should be delayed until tumour shrinkage has occurred with drug therapy. This reduces the risk of symptomatic tumour expansion to 4%. The risk is small for microprolactinomas (1.6%).

Effect of prolactinoma on pregnancy

Untreated, high prolactin levels lead to infertility. With preconception treatment fertility can be restored. Most cases have no complications in pregnancy. Breast-feeding is not contra-indicated.

Management

- Outside pregnancy dopamine receptor agonists (cabergoline and bromocriptine) reduce prolactin levels; these should be stopped upon confirmation of pregnancy.
- The patient should report symptoms that might suggest tumour expansion—headache, visual disturbance, thirst, and polyuria; this should then be investigated by CT or, preferably, MRI of the pituitary.
- Formal visual field testing is not routinely recommended in pregnancy, but should be used for symptomatic patients and those with macroprolactinomas.
- Bromocriptine can safely be re-started if there is concern regarding tumour expansion and can be continued during breast-feeding but may suppress milk production.
- Surgery is reserved for macroprolactinomas that fail to shrink despite drug therapy but is usually delayed until after delivery.

Causes of hyperprolactinaemia

- Normal pregnancy and breast-feeding.
- Pituitary adenomas.
- Hypothalamus or pituitary stalk lesions.
- Empty sella syndrome.
- Hypothyroidism.
- Chronic renal failure.
- Drugs: phenothiazines, metoclopramide, methyldopa.

Hypopituitarism

This is anterior pituitary failure. Diagnosis is based on reduced levels of anterior pituitary and target organ hormone levels: thyroxine, TSH, cortisol, ACTH, follicle stimulating hormone, luteinizing hormone, and growth hormone. There is also a failed response to an insulin stress test with lack of increase in growth hormone, ACTH, and prolactin levels.

Causes of hypopituitarism

- Pituitary surgery.
- Radiotherapy.
- Pituitary or hypothalamic tumours.
- Postpartum pituitary infarction (Sheehan's syndrome).
- Autoimmune lymphocytic hypophysitis.

⚠ Imaging of the pituitary area, by MRI or CT, should be undertaken to exclude a space-occupying lesion.
- Pregnancy is possible but may require ovulation induction with gonadotrophins.
- Once pregnancy is achieved the feto-placental unit can sustain pregnancy by sufficient production of oestradiol and progesterone.
- Maternal and fetal outcome is normal if the condition is adequately treated.
- Inadequately treated cases are at increased risk of adverse outcomes including maternal hypotension, hypoglycaemia and mortality, miscarriage, and stillbirth.
- Treatment involves replacement therapy with levothyroxine and hydrocortisone (additional intravenous hydrocortisone is required in labour).
- Milk production may be impaired because of prolactin deficiency.

Sheehan's syndrome

- This is caused by avascular necrosis of the pituitary, as a result of hypotension usually secondary to a postpartum haemorrhage. The pituitary is particularly vulnerable in pregnancy due to its 2–3-fold increase in size. Partial or complete pituitary failure can occur. The posterior pituitary is unaffected as it has a different blood supply. Treatment is as above. Pregnancies have been reported following this diagnosis.

Clinical features of Sheehan's syndrome

- Failure of lactation.
- Persistent amenorrhoea.
- Loss of pubic and axillary hair.
- Hypothyroidism.
- Adrenal insufficiency (vomiting, hypotension, hypoglycaemia).

Diabetes insipidus

- Incidence 1:15 000 pregnancies.
- Caused by a lack of antidiuretic hormone (ADH).
- Four types:
  - **central**: lack of ADH production by the posterior pituitary caused by expanding tumours
  - **nephrogenic**: ADH resistance in the kidney
  - **transient**: production of an enzyme by the placenta that results in increased breakdown of ADH, occurs in association with pre-eclampsia or acute fatty liver of pregnancy.
  - **psychogenic**: compulsive water drinking.
- Clinical features: excessive thirst and polyuria.
- Pregnancy may unmask the condition or make it worse (60%).
- Treatment is with desmopressin intranasally.

Obesity in pregnancy: maternal risks

- Obesity is an increasing problem in the developed world.
- The WHO definition of normal weight is a BMI between 18.5 and 24.9:
  - overweight is BMI between 25.0 and 29.9
  - obese is BMI ≥30.
- 1 in 5 pregnant women in the UK are now obese.
- The 2003–5 CEMACH report identified that obesity carries a greater risk of maternal death.

Maternal risks associated with obesity

Hypertension and pre-eclampsia

- Over twice as likely to develop gestational hypertension.
- Women with a BMI >30 have a significantly ↑ risk of pre-eclampsia.
- Excessive weight gain in pregnancy is associated with higher rates of pre-eclampsia in already overweight women.

Gestational diabetes

- Over 3 times more likely to develop gestational diabetes compared with women with a normal BMI.

Thromboembolism

- The incidence of thromboembolic disease in pregnancy is doubled in obese women.

Antenatal care in obese women

It may be difficult to palpate the uterus in obese women, leading to:
- missed diagnosis of breech presentation
- missed diagnosis of IUGR or macrosomia
- unsuccessful ECV attempts.
△ USS is also technically difficult and may be inaccurate

Postnatal complications associated with obesity

- Increased rates of postoperative complications also occur, including:
  - wound infection and endometritis
  - lower respiratory tract infection
  - PPH.
- Also associated with a reduction in breast-feeding frequency.

Peripartum risks of obesity

- Difficulty in siting regional anaesthesia due to body habitus.
- If a GA is needed:
  - intubation is technically more difficult
  - ↑ risk of aspiration.
- Difficulty monitoring both the fetus and uterine contractions.
- Higher rate of:
  - induction of labour
  - failed induction
  - CS.
- If vaginal delivery, there is an ↑ rate of:
  - instrumental deliveries
  - shoulder dystocia
  - 3rd and 4th degree perineal tears.
- High pre-pregnancy BMI and weight gain in the interpregnancy interval has been shown to ↓ the success of VBAC by 50%.

Strategies for managing pregnancy in obese women

- Counselling regarding weight loss and lifestyle changes pre-pregnancy would be ideal.
- Increased vigilance for pre-eclampsia:
  - regular antenatal checks with urine dipstick analysis (low threshold for quantifying proteinuria with a 24 hour collection)
  - measure arm circumference to ensure the correct size BP cuff.
- Increased vigilance for diabetes:
  - consider random blood sugar at booking
  - urine dipstick analysis at each visit for glycosuria
  - consider GTT in the 2nd trimester.
- Increased vigilance for both macrosomia and IUGR:
  - may need serial USS to monitor growth as symphysis–fundal height measurement may not be accurate.
- May require USS at 36 weeks gestation for presentation (to prevent an undiagnosed breech) if unable to palpate the fetus accurately.
- Further weight gain during the pregnancy should be discouraged.

Obesity in pregnancy: fetal risks

Miscarriage
- Overweight women have a significantly ↑ rate of early miscarriage (both spontaneous and IVF pregnancies):
  - thought to be related to ↓ insulin sensitivity.

Congenital abnormalities
- ☙ Conflicting evidence regarding obesity and congenital abnormalities.
- Some groups have reported an ↑ rate of neural tube defects, heart and intestinal abnormalities:
  - increased serum insulin, triglycerides, uric acid, and oestrogens in addition to increased insulin resistance, hypoxia and hypercapnia have been proposed as mechanisms for these effects

Stillbirth
- Significant risk factor for antepartum stillbirth:
  - the risk of stillbirth ↑ consistently with ↑ prepregnancy BMI
  - morbidly obese women are three times more likely to have a stillbirth than women with a normal BMI.

Macrosomia
- Well-recognized risk factor for fetal macrosomia (independent of maternal diabetes) which carries ↑ risk of:
  - instrumental delivery
  - CS
  - 3rd degree perineal tears
  - PPH.

Long-term risks for fetus

- Maternal weight is an independent determinant of childhood obesity.
- Macrosomic fetuses have an ↑ risk of adolescent and adult obesity related to an ↑ incidence of the metabolic syndrome.

Summary of risks relating to obesity in pregnancy

For the mother

- Maternal death or severe morbidity.
- Cardiac disease.
- Spontaneous 1st trimester or recurrent miscarriage.
- Pre-eclampsia.
- Gestational diabetes.
- Thromboembolism.
- Post-CS wound infection.
- Infection from other causes.
- Postpartum haemorrhage (PPH).
- Low breast-feeding rates.

For the baby

- Still birth and neonatal death.
- Congenital abnormalities.
- Prematurity.

📖 Saving mothers' lives. The 7th report on Confidential enquiries into maternal deaths in the UK; CEMACH 2007. www.cemach.org.uk

Drugs in pregnancy

Drugs in general should be avoided in pregnancy. However, even in pregnancy medication is sometimes necessary, especially where the benefits outweigh the risks. Most drugs cross the placenta to a certain extent and therefore are potentially teratogenic. The exception is very large molecules such as heparin and insulin. As women delay becoming pregnant until later life, more and more women will become pregnant whilst taking medication for common conditions such as essential hypertension. Similarly, some women with conditions that were once thought incompatible with pregnancy are now becoming pregnant due to improved medication (e.g. cystic fibrosis or transplant patients).

Timing of exposure

Drugs can cause teratogenesis in the fetus. This is defined as dysgenesis of fetal organs in terms of either structure or function. Other manifestations include IUGR or fetal death.

The timing of exposure is critical. There are three main phases of human development:

- **Pre-embryonic:**
  - conception to 17 days after conception (implantation and blastocyst formation)
  - adverse effects usually result in miscarriage.
- **Embryonic:**
  - day 17 to day 55 after conception (organogenesis)
  - congenital malformations are likely due to the sensitivity of the rapidly dividing tissues
  - the earlier the timing of the insult, the greater the damage.
- **Fetal phase:**
  - from 8 weeks after conception to term.
  - any effects of drugs impact on fetal growth and function of organs.

General principles

Your hospital pharmacy and the British National Formulary (BNF) Appendices 4 and 5 are useful sources of information regarding prescribing in pregnancy.

• Only prescribe drugs if the benefit outweighs the risks

⚠ Always think: is this drug really necessary?
• In general, try to avoid all drugs especially in the 1st trimester.
• Try to give the smallest effective dose for the shortest period of time.
• Avoid polypharmacy (multiple drugs may increase in the chance of congenital malformations, e.g. antiepileptics).
• Prescribe drugs that have been widely used before and are considered safe in pregnancy.
• Very few drugs have been proved to be teratogenic.

Help and advice can be obtained from the UK National Teratology Information Service (NTIS). This is funded by the Health Protection Agency to provide a 24-hour service on all aspects of toxicity of drugs and chemicals in pregnancy throughout the United Kingdom.

For Common drugs, and their Safety and usage in pregnancy and breast-feeding, please see Table on inside back cover.

📖 www.nyrdtc.nhs.uk/Services/teratology/teratology.html

Labour and delivery

Labour: overview

Labour is the process by which the fetus is delivered after the 24th week of gestation. Although it may be difficult to time the onset of labour, it can be defined as the point when uterine contractions become regular and cervical effacement and dilatation becomes progressive. Labour is characterized by:

- Onset of uterine contractions which ↑ in frequency, duration, and strength over time.
- Cervical effacement and dilatation.
- Rupture of membranes with leakage of amniotic fluid.
- Descent of the presenting part through the birth canal.
- Birth of the baby.
- Delivery of the placenta and membranes.

The mechanism of labour

The head usually engages in the transverse position and the passage of the head and body follows a well-defined pattern through the pelvis (Fig. 6.1). Not all the diameters of the fetal head can pass through a normal pelvis (see Chapter 1). The process of labour therefore involves the adaptation of the fetal head to the various segments of the pelvis.

Sequence for the passage through the pelvis for a normal vertex delivery

- **Engagement and descent:** the head enters the pelvis in the ocipitotransverse positon with flexion ↑ as it descends.
- **Internal rotation to occipitoanterior:** occurs at the level of the ischial spines due to the forward and downward sloping of the levator ani muscles.
- **Crowning:** the head extends, distending the perineum until it is delivered.
- **Restitution:** the head rotates so that the occiput is in line with the fetal spine.
- **External rotation:** the shoulders rotate when they reach the levator muscles until the biacromial diameter is anteroposterior (the head externally rotates by the same amount).
- **Delivery of the anterior shoulder:** occurs by lateral flexion of the trunk posteriorly.
- **Delivery of the posterior shoulder:** occurs by lateral flexion of the trunk anteriorly and the rest of the body follows.

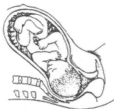

(1)
1st stage of labour. The cervix dilates. After full dilation the head flexes further and descends further into the pelvis.

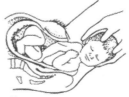

(4)
Birth of the anterior shoulder. The shoulders rotate to lie in the anteroposterior diameter of the pelvic outlet. The head rotates externally, 'restitutes', to its direction at onset of labour. Downward and backward traction of the head by the birth attendant aids delivery of the anterior shoulder.

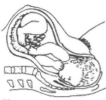

(2)
During the early second stage the head rotates at the levels of the ischial spine so the occiput lies in the anterior part of pelvis.
In late second stage the head broaches the vulval ring (crowning) and the perineum stretches over the head.

(5)
Birth of the posterior shoulder is aided by lifting the head upwards whilst maintaing traction.

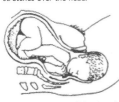

(3)
The head is born. The shoulders still lie transversely in the midpelvis.

Fig. 6.1 Mechanism of labour and delivery. Reproduced from Collier J, Longmore M, Brinsden M. *Oxford handbook of clinical specialties*, 6th edn, OUP, 2003. By permission of Oxford University Press.

Labour: 1st stage

The 1st stage is divided into two phases:
- **Latent phase:** the period taken for the cervix to completely efface and dilatate up to 3 cm.
- **Active phase:** from 3 cm to full dilatation (10 cm).

Braxton–Hicks contractions are mild, often irregular, non-progressive contractions that may occur from 30 weeks gestation (more common after 36 weeks) and may often be confused with labour. However, contractions in labour are painful, with a gradual increase in frequency, amplitude, and duration.

Failure to progress

Slow progress in the latent phase is managed conservatively. Delay in the active phase is identified when progress on the partogram falls to the right of the **alert line** drawn at 1 cm/hour. When to intervene is contentious, the NICE guidelines recommend that if an **action line** is used it should be a 4-hour action line (Fig. 6.2). Delay is suspected if there is <2 cm dilatation in 4 hours or a slowing in progress in parous women.

If the labour was slow from the early active phase, it is termed **primary dysfunctional labour**. If the rate of progress was slow after previous adequate progress then it is termed **secondary arrest**.

Some causes of poor progress in the 1st stage:
- Inefficient uterine activity (power).
- Malpositions, malpresentation, or large baby (passenger).
- Inadequate pelvis (passage).
- A combination of two of the above or all three.

Poor progress in the 1st stage

Assessment
- Review the history.
- Abdominal palpation; fetal size, frequency, and duration of contractions.
- Review fetal condition; CTG and colour of amniotic fluid.
- Review maternal condition including hydration and analgesia.
- Vaginal assessment; caput, moulding, position, and station of the head.

Management
- Amniotomy (ARM) and reassess in 2 hours.
- Amniotomy + oxytocin infusion and reassess in 2 hours:
  - this should always be considered in nulliparous women.
- Lower segment CS (if there is fetal distress).

⚠ For multiparous women and those with a previous CS an experienced obstetrician should review before starting oxytocin.

📖 NICE guideline: Intrapartum care; September 2007. www.nice.org.uk

Monitoring in labour (recorded on the partogram)

- The fetal heart rate (FHR) should be monitored every 15 minutes (or continuously with a CTG).
- The contractions should be assessed every 30 minutes.
- Maternal pulse should be checked hourly.
- BP and temperature should be checked 4 hourly.
- VE should be offered every 4 hours to assess progress.
- Maternal urine is tested 4 hourly or when passed for ketones and protein.

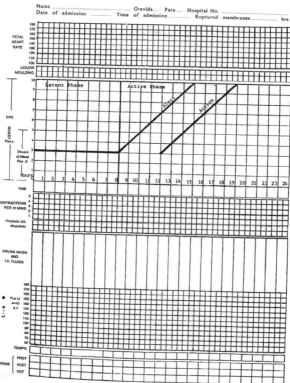

Fig. 6.2 Partogram.

Labour: 2nd stage

The 2nd stage is the time from full cervical dilatation until the baby is born.

Description of a normal 2nd stage

- The active 2nd stage commences when the mother starts expulsive efforts using her abdominal muscles with the Valsalva manoeuvre to 'bear down'.
- Women may choose many different positions to deliver in: squatting, standing, on all fours, or supine:
  - lithotomy is required for instrumental deliveries.
- As the head comes down, it distends the perineum and anus:
  - a pad may be used to support the perineum and cover the anus, while the other hand is used to maintain flexion and prevent sudden deflexion and to control the rate of delivery of the head (this attempts to slow perineal distension, minimizing tears by preventing rapid delivery).
- An episiotomy may be performed if there is concern that the perineum is tearing towards the anal sphincter:
  - episiotomy should not be used routinely.
- With the next contraction gentle traction guides the head towards the perineum until the anterior shoulder is delivered under the subpubic arch.
- Gentle traction upwards and anteriorly helps to deliver the posterior shoulder and the remainder of the trunk.
- The cord is double-clamped and cut:
  - delaying clamping for 2–3 minutes results in higher haematocrit levels in the neonate.
- The condition of the baby is assessed at 1, 5, and 10 minutes using the Apgar scoring system, and if all is well baby is handed to the mother as soon as possible.

▶ If the woman has an epidural *in situ* and the CTG is reassuring, 1 hour is usually allowed for passive descent before active pushing is commenced. During this hour it is important to ensure that good contractions are maintained and oxytocin may be commenced.

▶ Birth should take place within 3 hours of the start of 2nd stage for nulliparous women and within 2 hours for multiparous women.

Delay in the 2nd stage of labour

Nulliparous women

- Suspected if delivery is not imminent after 1 hour of active pushing
  - VE should be offered and amniotomy recommended
- If not delivered in 2 hours
  - Requires review by obstetrician to consider instrumental delivery or CS

Multiparous women

- Diagnosed if delivery is not imminent after 1 hour of active pushing
  - Requires review by obstetrician to consider instrumental delivery or CS

⚠ Delay in the 2nd stage in a multiparous woman must always raise suspicions of malposition or disproportion

Labour: 3rd stage

The 3rd stage is the duration from delivery of the baby to delivery of the placenta and membranes.

Active management of the 3rd stage

This consists of:
- Use of uterotonics.
- Early clamping and cutting of the cord.
- Controlled cord traction.

This has been shown to:
- ↓ rates of PPH >1000 mL.
- ↓ mean blood loss and postnatal anaemia.
- ↓ length of the 3rd stage.
- ↓ the need for blood transfusions.

The side effects may be:
- Nausea and vomiting.
- Headache.

Physiological management of the 3rd stage

- May be used if requested by low risk women.
- No Syntometrine® or oxytocin is given.
- Cord is allowed to stop pulsating before it is clamped and cut.
- The placenta is delivered by maternal effort alone.

⚠ The cord must not be pulled and the uterus not pushed upwards or held.

A planned physiological 3rd stage should be changed to active management in the event of:
- Haemorrhage.
- Failure to deliver the placenta within 1 hour.
- Maternal desire to shorten the 3rd stage.

Care immediately after delivery

Most complications of the 3rd stage, such as PPH, uterine inversion, or haematoma formation, occur in the first 2 hours after delivery. Usually the women are kept in the delivery unit during this time to observe their pulse, BP, temperature, uterine size and contractions, fresh bleeding per vaginum, or painful swelling of the vulva or perineum. Where there is an increased risk of PPH, an oxytocin infusion (40 units in 500 mL saline) should be given prophylactically for 3–4 hours.

Encouragement should be given for skin-to-skin contact as soon as possible and the mother and baby should not be separated for the 1st hour. Support should be provided for breast-feeding, which should be initiated in the 1st hour.

If there are no complications during these 2 hours, the mother may then be transferred to the postnatal ward. Some women wish to go home after a further 3–4 hours of observation.

Description of an actively managed 3rd stage

- Syntometrine® IM (ergometrine 0.5 mg + oxytocin 5 IU) or oxytocin 10 IUIM is given as the anterior shoulder of the baby is born.
- A dish is placed at the introitus to collect the placenta and any blood loss, and the left hand is placed on the abdomen over the uterine fundus.
- As the uterus contracts to 20-week size, the placenta separates from the uterus through the spongy layer of the decidua basalis.
- The uterus will then feel firmer, the cord will lengthen and there is often a trickle of fresh blood (separation bleeding).
- Controlled cord traction (CCT) is applied with the right hand, whilst supporting the fundus with the left hand (Brandt–Andrew's technique).

⚠ Multiple pregnancy must be excluded before uterotonics are given.

▶ NICE recommends the use of oxytocin 10 IU rather than Syntometrine® as it appears to have similar efficacy but with fewer side effects.

Induction of labour: indications

Approximately 10–15% of all pregnancies are induced and the overall success rate is about 60–80% at term. The chance of achieving a vaginal birth after attempting induction of labour (IOL) before 34 weeks is estimated to be <35%. It should be considered whenever the overall benefit of achieving a vaginal birth outweighs the risks of continuing pregnancy. The indication may be obstetric or medical. Induction of labour on maternal request or for physician's convenience should be avoided as it is an intervention and hence is associated with risks to the mother and the fetus.

Obstetric indications for induction of labour

- Uteroplacental insufficiency(one of the most common indications).
- Prolonged pregnancy (41–42 weeks).
- Intrauterine growth restriction (IUGR).
- Oligo- or anhydramnios.
- Abnormal uterine or umbilical artery Dopplers.
- Non-reassuring cardiotocograph (CTG).
- Prelabour rupture of membranes (PROM).
- Severe pre-eclampsia or eclampsia after maternal stabilization.
- Intrauterine death of the fetus (IUD).
- Unexplained antepartum haemorrhage at term.
- Chorioamnionitis.

There is inadequate evidence for induction for suspected fetal macrosomia. Some advocate induction of labour around 40–41 weeks with an aim of preventing further intrauterine growth and associated risks like shoulder dystocia and birth trauma.

Medical indications

With underlying maternal medical conditions, planned early induction of labour may potentially limit the maternal risks associated with pregnancy. Careful timing is required to balance the best interests of the mother with any potential risks of prematurity. Such situations may include:

- Severe hypertension.
- Uncontrolled diabetes mellitus.
- Renal disease with deteriorating renal function.
- Malignancies (to facilitate definitive therapy).

Cervical ripening

Predictors for successful induction of labour

Strong predictors for a successful induction (i.e. that results in a vaginal birth) are:
- Gestational age at induction.
- Parity.
- Modified Bishop's score of the cervix (Table 6.1):
  - gives an overview of the 'ripeness' of the cervix and higher the score, greater is the chance of a successful vaginal birth.

Mechanical methods of cervical ripening

- Separation of the membranes from the cervix leads to the local release of prostaglandins.
- The most commonly used method is artificial separation of membranes ('stretch and sweep').
- This can be performed if the cervical os admits a finger, and involves digitally separating the membranes from the cervix.
- This may be uncomfortable for the woman.

Pharmacological methods

Prostaglandins (PGE2)
- The preferred agents for cervical ripening.
- Usually given intravaginally into the posterior fornix.
- Although the gel form is absorbed well, tablets are being increasingly used as they are easier to remove if uterine hyperstimulation occurs (5–7%).
- Vaginal prostaglandins (3 mg tablets, 2 mg gel) increases vaginal delivery rates within 24 hours with no increase in operative delivery rates.

Oxytocin infusion
- Has been shown to increase cervical prostaglandin levels.
- As most receptors are located in the myometrium, it is more suitable for initiating uterine contractions.
- Best used where membranes have ruptured, whether spontaneously or after amniotomy

▶ Other agents have been tried but there is limited evidence for their safety and efficacy.

Other methods

There is no evidence to suggest that the following are effective in cervical ripening or induction of labour:
- Sexual intercourse.
- Herbal remedies (raspberry leaf tea).
- Nipple stimulation.
- Acupuncture.
- Castor oil.

Table 6.1 Modified Bishop's score: to assess the favourability for induction of labour (data from Calder et al, 1974) A score >8 indicates a favourable cervix

Score	0	1	2
Position of cervix	Posterior	Axial	Anterior
Length of cervix	2 cm	1 cm	<0.5 cm
Consistency of cervix	Firm	Soft	Soft and stretchy
Dilatation of cervix	0	1 cm	> 2cm
Station of the presenting part (distance in cm in relation to the ischial spines)	−2	−1	0

Induction of labour: methods

Amniotomy

Artificial rupture of membranes (ARM or amniotomy) releases local prostaglandins causing cervical ripening and myometrial contractions. If regular, painful uterine contractions are not initiated or there are no cervical changes after 2 hours, then oxytocin infusion should be commenced. Starting oxytocin at the time of amniotomy has been shown to decrease the induction–delivery interval, thereby decreasing both the fetal and maternal risk of sepsis. However, it can be viewed as 'medicalization' as it has been reported that about 88% of patients will go into established labour within 24 hours of ARM alone.

It is essential to understand that by performing an ARM, a commitment has been made to deliver the fetus. A prolonged induction process with repeated vaginal examinations increases the risk of chorioamnionitis.

Prostaglandins for induction of labour

- A CTG should be performed 30 minutes before as well as after insertion of prostaglandins to confirm fetal well-being.
- VE after 6 hours; if the cervix is not favourable, another dose may be administered (>2 doses need to be reviewed by a consultant; Multips seldom require more than 1 dose.)
- Oxytocin should not be started for 6 hours to avoid the risk of uterine hyperstimulation.

Synthetic oxytocin for induction or augmentation of labour

- It should be started on a low dose (1–4 mU/min).
- It is increased (usually doubled) every 30 minutes to achieve optimal contractions (3–4 every 10 minutes, each lasting 40–60 seconds).
- Continuous CTG monitoring should be used:
  - the sensitivity of the myometrium to oxytocin ↑ during labour and it may be necessary to ↓ the rate of infusion as labour advances
  - infusion pumps should be used to carefully control the amount given and avoid the risk of uterine hyperstimulation.

☛ Women should be advised that the use of oxytocin will bring forward the time of birth but will not influence the mode of birth or other outcomes (NICE guidelines).

Risks and complications of induction of labour

- Prematurity:
  - may be iatrogenic (severe pre-eclampsia)
  - unintentional (failure to correctly assess the gestational age).
- Cord prolapse with rupture of membranes if the presenting part is not engaged.
- Side effects of pharmacological agents used:
  - pain or discomfort
  - uterine hyperstimulation
  - fetal distress
  - uterine rupture (rare but ↑ in grand multipara or a scarred uterus).
- Prostaglandins rarely cause non-selective stimulation of other smooth muscle leading to:
  - nausea and vomiting
  - diarrhoea
  - bronchoconstriction (caution in asthmatics)
  - maternal pyrexia may result due to the effect on thermoregulation in the hypothalamus.
- Caesarean section (CS) due to failed induction
- Atonic postpartum haemorrhage.
- Intrauterine infection with prolonged induction.

⚠ Oxytocin has the properties of antidiuretic hormone (ADH), U+Es should be checked if it has been used for >12 hours as it may very rarely cause dilutional hyponatraemia.

Induction of labour: special circumstances

Prelabour rupture of membranes
NICE recommends the use of prostaglandins before starting syntocinon for IOL if the cervix is unfavourable.

> **IOL with previous CS**
>
> ⚠The risk of scar dehiscence with previous uterine surgery is:
> - 5:1000 with spontaneous labour
> - 8:1000 with use of oxytocin
> - 24:1000 with prostaglandins.
>
> ▶ Women should be counselled regarding theses risks and have continous CTG monitoring throughout the whole of the induction process when contractions are present.

Stabilizing induction
This is carried out when the presenting part is not engaged or when there is an unstable lie, to avoid the risk of cord prolapse. The head is 'stabilized' by an assistant holding it suprapubically, while amniotomy is performed. Cord prolapse is excluded and oxytocin infusion started.

▶This is preferably performed in theatre with an epidural which is topped up sufficiently to allow an emergency CS in the event of cord prolapse.

Grand multipara (≥para 5)
⚠ The risk of uterine rupture is higher and hence caution should be exercised.

- ☞ Prostaglandin gel should only be used in exceptional circumstances.
- Onset of labour is awaited for 4–6 hours after ARM.
- In the absence of contractions oxytocin infusion can be started and titrated to get 3–4 every 10 minutes, each lasting >40 seconds.
- Once contractions are established it should be possible to stop the oxytocin as most will continue to labour and deliver normally.

⚠ Malpresentation (obstructed labour) must be excluded before starting oxytocin.

📖 National Institute of Clinical Excellence. Guidelines for Induction of Labour. www.nice.org.uk

Fetal surveillance in labour: overview

- It is estimated that 10% of cerebral palsy (CP) is due to intrapartum hypoxia (the rest may be attributed to antenatal events).
- The blood supply to the placental pool is restricted with contractions (especially in the 2nd stage) placing a physiological strain on the fetus.
- Ability to withstand the stress of labour is dependant on fetal physiological reserve.
- A fetus that was coping in the antenatal period but has no extra reserve may decompensate in labour.

Intrapartum surveillance

- The options for intrapartum surveillance are:
  - intermittent auscultation
  - continuous EFM (CTG).
- On admission in labour, an assessment should be made to identify fetal or maternal risk factors (see 📖 p. 279).
- If the woman has no risk factors she should be offered intermittent auscultation performed for a full minute after a contraction:
  - at least every 15 minutes in the 1st stage
  - every 5 minutes or after every other contraction in the 2nd stage.

Electronic fetal monitoring (EFM)

- Has resulted in:
  - ↑ intervention and operative delivery rates
  - without marked ↓ in CP.
- Most likely because:
  - CTG is not specific enough in detecting fetal hypoxia
  - and it is frequently poorly interpreted
  - and intrapartum hypoxia as a cause of CP is rare.
- Additional tests such as fetal scalp blood sampling in labour are required to ↑ specificity.

▶ Interest is growing in the use of fetal electrocardiographic (ECG) ST waveform analysis (STAN) to improve the positive predictive value of the CTG. So far the results look promising for successfully predicting acidosis and avoiding unnecessary interventions.

📖 RCOG National evidence based guideline 8: The use of electronic fetal monitoring http://www.rcog.org.uk

Antenatal risk factors which should prompt recommendation of EFM in labour include:

Maternal
- Previous CS.
- Cardiac problems.
- Pre-eclampsia.
- Post-term pregnancy (>42 weeks).
- Prolonged rupture of membranes (>24 hours).
- Induction of labour.
- Diabetes.
- Antepartum haemorrhage.
- Other significant maternal medical conditions.

Fetal
- IUGR.
- Prematurity.
- Oligohydramnios.
- Abnormal Doppler velocimetry.
- Multiple pregnancy.
- Meconium-stained liquor.
- Breech presentation.

Intrapartum risks requiring EFM

- Oxytocin augmentation.
- Epidural analgesia.
- Intrapartum vaginal bleeding.
- Pyrexia >37.5 °C.
- Fresh meconium staining of liquor.
- Abnormal FHR on intermittent auscultation.
- Prolonged labour.

Fetal surveillance: CTG

Definitions of terms used in EFM

- **Baseline rate** is the mean level of the FHR when this is stable and after exclusion of accelerations and decelerations.
- **Baseline variability** is the degree to which the baseline varies, i.e. the bandwidth of the baseline after exclusion of accelerations and decelerations. A variability of 5–25 beats/min is defined as normal, 0–5 beats/min as reduced, and greater than 25 beats/min as saltatory.
- An **acceleration** is a transient rise in FHR by at least 15 beats over the baseline lasting for 15 seconds or more (Fig. 6.3).
- A **deceleration** is a reduction in the baseline of 15 beats or more for more than 15 seconds.

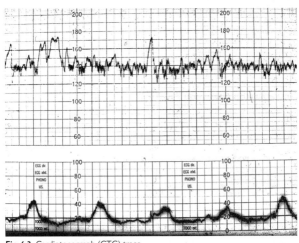

Fig. 6.3 Cardiotocograph (CTG) trace.

▶ The most useful features in assessing fetal well-being are normal variability and presence of accelerations.

⚠ Always be concerned about a CTG if you cannot identify the baseline rate.

Causes of decreased baseline variability include:

- Fetal hypoxia.
- Fetal sleep cycle (should be for <40 minutes).
- Administration of drugs including:
  - methyldopa
  - magnesium sulphate
  - narcotic analgesics
  - tranquillizers
  - barbiturates
  - general anaesthesia.
- Severe prematurity.
- Fetal heart block.
- Fetal anomalies.

Fetal surveillance: CTG abnormalities

Abnormalities in baseline rate

A **bradycardia** is a baseline FHR of less than 110 beats/min.

- 100–110 beats/minute is termed moderate baseline bradycardia and provided other parameters are normal, it is considered not to be associated with fetal compromise.
- A baseline below 100 beats/minute should raise the possibility of hypoxia or other pathology.

⚠ Beware of maternal heart rate being recorded as the FHR.

A **tachycardia** is a baseline FHR of more than 160 beats/minute and is associated with maternal pyrexia and tachycardia, prematurity and fetal acidosis.

- A baseline of 160–180 beats/minute is termed moderate baseline tachycardia and provided other features are normal, is probably not indicative of hypoxia
- A baseline >180 beats/minute should always raise suspicion of underlying pathology

Decelerations

- **Early decelerations:** uniform in appearance and timing and are defined as early when the peak of the deceleration coincides with the peak of the contraction (Fig. 6.4).
- **Late decelerations:** have at least a 15 second time lag between the peak of the contraction and the nadir of the deceleration (Fig. 6.5).

⚠ They may be suggestive of acidosis. Shallow, decelerations in the presence of reduced baseline variability on a non-reactive trace should be of particularly concern.

- **Variable decelerations:** have an irregular pattern and may be associated with cord compression (Fig. 6.6):
  - **typical** variable decelerations are U or V shaped, quick to recover, and often have 'shouldering' (they are not usually associated with fetal hypoxia)
  - **atypical** variable decelerations are those with a duration of greater than 60 seconds, a loss of more than 60 beats from the baseline, slow recovery, a combined variable, and a late deceleration component and a rising baseline rate (these are more likely to indicate fetal compromise).

Other abnormalities

- **Sinusoidal pattern:** this is rare and is seen as an undulating pattern (like a sine wave) with little, or no, variability. This can indicate significant fetal anaemia but in short spells (<10 minutes) may be a result of fetal physiological behaviour (thumb-sucking).

⚠ A sinusoidal pattern should always be taken seriously.

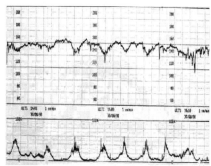

Fig. 6.4 Cardiotocograph trace with early decelerations.

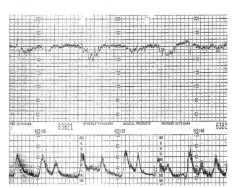

Fig. 6.5 Cardiotocograph trace with late decelerations.

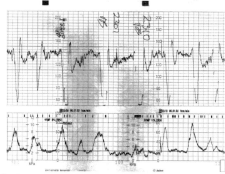

Fig. 6.6 Cardiotocograph trace with variable decelerations.

Fetal surveillance: CTG classification

In order to help with the difficulties encountered when assessing a CTG a classification scheme was introduced which can be used to define a CTG as normal, suspicious, or pathological.

Table 6.2 Fetal heart-rate feature classification

	Baseline (bpm)	Variability (bpm)	Decelerations	Accelerations
Reassuring	110–160	≥5	None	Present
Non-reassuring	100–109 161–180	<5 for ≥40 but <90 minutes	Early decelerations Variable decelerations being present for 50% of contractions for ≥ 90 minutes Single prolonged deceleration up to 3 minutes	The absence of accelerations in an otherwise normal CTG is of uncertain significance
Abnormal	<100 >180 Sinusoidal pattern for ≥ 10mins	<5 for ≥90 minutes	Atypical variable decelerations Late decelerations being present for >50% of contractions for ≥ 30 minutes Single prolonged deceleration >3 minutes	

📖 NICE Intrapartum Care Guidelines www.nice.org.uk

CTG classification using Table 6.2

- **Normal:** all four features are in the reassuring category.
- **Suspicious:** no more than one non-reassuring feature when analysing the CTG.
- **Pathological:** two or more non-reassuring features or one or more abnormal features.

Maternal factors that may contribute to an abnormal CTG

- The woman's position:
  - advise her to adopt left lateral.
- Hypotension.
- Vaginal examination.
- Emptying bladder or bowels.
- Vomiting.
- Vasovagal episodes.
- Siting and topping-up of regional anaesthesia.

Fetal blood sampling

- This is used to improve the specificity of CTG in the detection of fetal hypoxia.
- It should be obtained if the trace is pathological, unless obvious immediate delivery is required (e.g. bradycardia of >3 minutes).
- The woman should be in left lateral.

Interpretation of the FBS results

- **Normal** (pH≥ 7.25):
  - repeat FBS within 1 hour if CTG remains pathological.
- **Borderline** (pH 7.21–7.24):
  - repeat FBS within 30 minutes if CTG remains pathological.
- **Abnormal** (pH≤ 7.20):
  - immediate delivery.

Meconium-stained liquor

Meconium is primarily made up of water, bile pigment, mucus, and amniotic fluid debris. Its detection in amniotic fluid causes anxiety as it is associated with increased perinatal morbidity and mortality and may be aspirated by the fetus.

- Meconium-stained amniotic fluid (MSAF) is rare in pre-term infants(<5%) and is associated with infection and chorioamnionitis.
- Incidence of MSAF gradually increases from 36–42 weeks.
- Passage of meconium signifies the maturation of the central nervous and the gastrointestinal systems. In some cases it is thought to be due to hypoxia that causes peristalsis of the bowel and relaxation of anal sphincters.

Classification of MSAF

- **Grade 1 (light):** meconium lightly stains the amniotic fluid which is usually copious.
- **Grade 2 (moderate):** dark green staining of amniotic fluid which appears opalescent.
- **Grade 3 (thick):** thick, opaque meconium in scanty amniotic fluid.

Meconium aspiration syndrome

Meconium aspiration syndrome (MAS) occurs in 1 in 1000 births in Europe. It may happen in utero when fetal breathing movements draws amniotic fluid into the airway. The likelihood of fetal gasping is increased by fetal distress but 50% of MAS occurs in fetuses which were not acidotic in labour.

Meconium causes mechanical blockage of the airway and acts as a chemical irritant causing pneumonitis, and alveolar collapse. It also predisposes to secondary bacterial infection.

Suction of the mouth and upper airway immediately after delivery may help to clear any meconium contamination from birth. However, it will not help with pre-existing in utero aspiration.

Management of meconium-stained liquor

- Recommend immediate induction of labour if pre-labour rupture of membranes.
- Advise continuous fetal monitoring.
- Advise delivery in a unit able to provide fetal blood sampling and advanced neonatal life support at birth:
  - if baby is born with depressed vital signs it will require laryngoscopy and suction by a health-care professional trained in advanced neonatal life support
  - if baby is born in good condition it will still require close monitoring for 12 hours.

Operative vaginal delivery: overview

Caesarean section in the 2nd stage of labour is associated with increased morbidity to the mother. Instrumental vaginal delivery helps to avoid maternal and perinatal morbidity and mortality and avoid an emergency CS.

In the UK the operative vaginal delivery rate is stable at between 10% and 15%. It is important to appreciate that forceps and ventouse are complementary to each other and that the operator's skill and experience, as well as the clinical findings, should decide which one should be used.

▶ If in doubt, senior help must be called.

Indications for instrumental delivery

Maternal
- Exhaustion.
- Prolonged 2nd stage.
  - >1 hour of active pushing in multiparaous women
  - >2 hours of in primiparaous women.
- Medical indications for avoiding Valsalva manouevre such as:
  - severe cardiac disease
  - hypertensive crisis
  - uncorrected cerebral vascular malformations.
- Pushing is not possible (paraplegia or tetraplegia).

Fetal
- Fetal compromise.
- To control the after coming head of breech (forceps).

▶ It is important to discuss with the women why an operative delivery is indicated, the instrument chosen, the likelihood of success, and the alternatives available (emergency CS). Consent (verbal or written) must be obtained.

Ways to avoid operative delivery

- Encourage continuous support in labour.
- Appropriate use of the partogram.
- Use of upright or lateral positions.
- Avoid epidural anaesthesia/use low-dose epidural.
- Appropriate use of oxytocin and delayed pushing in primiparous women with epidurals.
- Delayed pushing with an epidural when the head is in the perinial phase.

Complications of operative vaginal delivery

- Forceps are associated with increased maternal trauma (including anal sphincter trauma).
- Rotational forceps may cause spiral tears of the vagina.
- Fetal injuries with forceps are rare but may occur (mostly due to incorrect application of the blades) including:
  - facial nerve palsy
  - skull fractures
  - orbital injury
  - intracranial haemorrhage
- Ventouse is associated with fetal injuries including:
  - scalp lacerations and avulsions (rarely, alopecia in the long term)
  - cephalhaematoma
  - retinal haemorrhage
  - rarely, subgaleal haemorrhage and/or intracranial haemorrhage.

⚠ The use of sequential instruments (usually forceps after a failed ventouse) is associated with an increased risk of fetal trauma.

Operative vaginal delivery: instruments

Forceps

These consist of curved blades which sit around the fetal head and allow traction to be applied. This is usually to speed up the delivery but may be used to slow the rate of the head in a breech delivery. See Fig. 6.7.

Low cavity forceps (Wrigley's)
- Short and light.
- These are also the forceps used at CS.

Midcavity non-rotational forceps (Neville Barnes, Haig Ferguson, Simpson's)
- Used when the saggital suture is in the direct anteroposterior position (usually direct occipitoanterior—DOA).
- Malpresentation can be corrected manually between contractions and the blades applied once the head is in the DOA position.

Midcavity rotational forceps (Keilland's)
- Reduced pelvic curve on the blades of the forceps allows rotation about the axis of the handle.
- Corrects asynclitism and malposition.
- Must only be attempted by a senior operator (or under the close supervision of one).

Vacuum extraction (ventouse)

Vacuum extractor works on the principle of creating 'negative pressure' to allow fetal scalp tissues to be sucked into the vacuum cup. This creates artificial caput called a 'chignon'. The cup is held in place by the atmospheric pressure on the cup against the negative pressure created. It should not be used at <34 weeks gestation. See Fig. 6.7.

Metal cup
- Available with 60, 50, or 40 mm, standard or posterior cup.
- Pressure is created by a suction pump.
- Excessive traction is likely to cause fetal trauma.

Soft cup
- Soft and easier to apply (important in women without epidural) for occipitoanterior positions.
- Moulds around the fetal head covering a greater surface area.
- Causes fewer scalp abrasions.

Kiwi Omni Cup
- Single-use cup
- Pressure created with hand pump (quick in an emergency).
- Allows application to flexion joint in occipitolateral and posterior position.

Comparison of forceps and vacuum extractor (ventouse)

- Ventouse is more likely to fail.
- Ventouse is more likely to cause fetal trauma such as:
  - cephalohaematoma
  - retinal haemorrhage.
- Ventouse is more likely to be associated with maternal concerns about the baby.
- Forceps are more likely to cause significant maternal genital tract trauma.
- There is no difference between them for:
  - risk of delivery by CS
  - low 5 minute Apgar scores
  - need for neonatal phototherapy.

▶ Bottom line—ventouse appears safer for mother but forceps may be safer for baby.

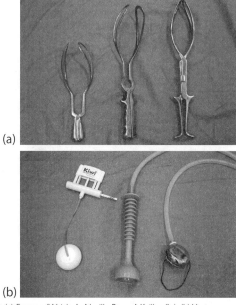

(a)

(b)

Fig. 6.7 (a) Forceps (Wrigley's, Neville-Barnes', Keilland's,). (b) Ventouse cups (Kiwi™ Omni Cup, Silc cup, Bird's cup); With permission of Clinical innovations turope Ltd, 2008 & Menox AB, Goteborg, Sweden 2008.

Operative vaginal delivery: criteria

▶ The techniques involved with both ventouse and forceps can only be learned under direct supervision from an experienced operator and are therefore not described in the book.

The following criteria should be satisfied before attempting an operative vaginal delivery. This may be best remembered as 'FORCEPS'

- **F** **F**ully dilated cervix (i.e. confirm 2nd stage).
- **O** **O**bstruction should be excluded (head ≤1/5 palpable abdominally).
- **R** **R**uptured membranes.
  Review the procedure (if forceps blades don't lock, lack of rotation or descent despite 3 attempts at traction).
- **C** **C**onsent.
  Catheterize bladder ('in and out' technique, indwelling catheters must be removed).
  Check instrument prior to application.
- **E** **E**xplain the procedure to the patient.
  Epidural (or pudendal) analgesia.
  Examine the genital tract to **E**xclude genital tract trauma.
- **P** Check **P**resentation and **P**osition of the head (must be sure before applying any instrument).
  Power: are the contractions effective? correct with syntocinon— (propulsion is better than extraction).
  Correct **P**lacement of forceps blades or ventouse cup (ensure no maternal tissues are caught).
- **S** **S**tation of the presenting part (not above ischial spines).
  Senior help should be called if needed.

See Fig. 6.8.

When to abandon and deliver by emergency Caesarean

- No evidence of progressive descent with each pull (care must be taken with the ventouse to not interpret increasing caput as descent of the head)
- Where delivery is not imminent following 3 pulls of a correctly applied instrument by an experienced operator.

📖 RCOG Guideline 26: Operative vaginal delivery. http://www.rcog.org.uk

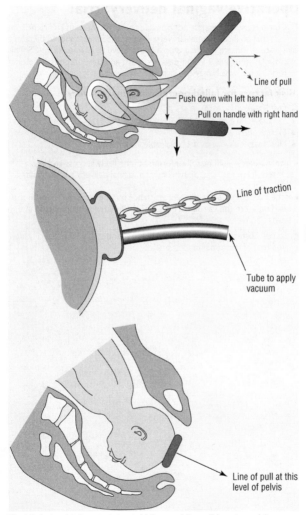

Fig. 6.8 Assisted delivery techniques: (a) forceps delivery; (b) ventouse delivery. Reproduced from Chamberlain, G. *et al.* ABC of labour care: operative delivery. BMJ 1999;318:1260–1264. with permission. © BMJ Publishing Group Ltd 1999.

Operative vaginal delivery: trial

This term is used when it is not possible to determine with sufficient confidence that an instrumental delivery will be successful. It should therefore take place in theatre where it is possible to move to an immediate CS. This avoids a failed delivery in the delivery room and the subsequent delay in performing CS, which may compromise fetal well-being.

Risk factors for failed operative vaginal delivery

- BMI >30.
- EFW > 4000 g or clinically big baby.
- Occipitoposterior position.
- Mid-cavity delivery or if 1/5 palpable abdominally.

- The woman should be fully informed of the likely success and sign a consent form for 'Trial of instrumental vaginal delivery ± emergency CS'.
- If the procedure is abandoned, assistance may be required to 'push the head up' from the vagina during CS as the head may be impacted in the pelvis.

⚠ Senior obstetric input is recommended in 2nd stage CS, especially after a failed trial of instrumental delivery.

Episiotomy

More than 85% of women delivering vaginally in the UK will sustain some degree of perineal trauma. Episiotomy is a surgical incision to enlarge the vaginal introitus and facilitate childbirth. The decision to perform an episiotomy is made by the birth attendant. The worldwide rates of episiotomy vary dramatically (14% in England, 8% in the Netherlands, 50% in the USA). This highlights that the indications are not absolute and the practice not always justified. However, there is clear evidence to recommend a *restricted* use of episiotomy.

> **WHO recommends that episiotomy should be considered in the following circumstances:**
>
> * Complicated vaginal delivery:
>   * breech
>   * shoulder dystocia
>   * forceps
>   * ventouse.
> * If there is extensive lower genital tract scarring:
>   * female genital mutilation
>   * poorly healed 3rd or 4th degree tears.
> * When there is fetal distress.
>
> ▶ It is also often recommended if there is an indication that there may be extensive perineal trauma such as the appearance of perineal button-holing.

Types of episiotomy

* Mediolateral episiotomy extends from the fourchette laterally (thus reducing the risk of anal sphincter injury).
* Midline episiotomy extends from the fourchette towards the anus (common in the USA but not recommended in the UK).

> **How to perform an episiotomy**
>
> * If the woman does not have a working regional block (epidural) then the perineum should be infiltrated with lidocaine (lignocaine).
> * Two fingers should be placed between the baby's head and the perineum (to protect the baby).
> * Sharp scissors are used to make a single cut in the perineum about 3–4 cm long (ideally this should be at the height of the contraction when the perineum is at its thinnest).
>
> See Fig. 6.9.

▶ Every effort should be made to anaesthetize the perineum early to provide sufficient time for effect.

▶ It will cause bleeding so must not be done too early and should be repaired as soon as possible.

⚠ Always check for any extension or other tears (including a PR examination to ensure no trauma to the anal sphincter).

General complications of perineal trauma including episiotomy

- Bleeding.
- Haematoma.
- Pain.
- Infection.
- Scarring, with potential disruption to the anatomy.
- Dyspareunia.
- Very rarely, fistula formation.

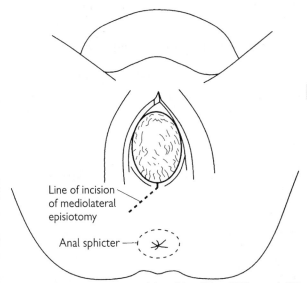

Line of incision of mediolateral episiotomy

Anal sphicter

Fig. 6.9 Performing an episiotomy. Adapted from Wyatt JP, Illingworth RN, Graham CA et al (eds) *Oxford handbook of emergency medicine.* OUP, 2006. By permission of Oxford University Press.

Perineal tears

Classification of perineal tears

- **1st degree:** injury to the skin only.
- **2nd-degree:** injury to the perineum involving perineal muscles (includes episiotomy).
- **3rd-degree:** injury to the perineum involving the anal sphincter complex:
  - 3a: <50% of the external anal sphincter (EAS) thickness torn
  - 3b: >50% of the EAS thickness torn
  - 3c: internal anal sphincter (IAS) torn.
- **4th-degree:** injury to perineum involving the anal sphincter complex (EAS and IAS) and the anal/rectal epithelium.

Principles of basic perineal repair (Fig. 6.10)

- Suture as soon as possible to reduce bleeding and infection risk.
- A rectal examination is recommended before starting to ensure there is no trauma to the anal sphincter complex.
- The attendant should have adequate training for the type of tear:
  - difficult trauma should be repaired in theatre under regional or general anaesthesia by an experienced operator.
- The woman should preferably be in lithotomy position.
- There should be a good light source and adequate analgesia.
- Use of rapid-absorption polyglactin suture material is associated with a significant reduction in pain.
- Apex of the cut should be identified and the suturing started from just above this point.
- A loose, continuous non-locking suturing technique used to appose each layer is associated with less short-term pain than the traditional interupted method.
- Perineal skin should be sutured with a subcuticular suture as this is associated with less pain.
- Anatomical apposition should be as accurate as possible and consideration given to cosmetic results.
- Rectal examination after completion ensures that no suture has accidentally passed into the rectum or anal canal.

△ Needle and swabs must be counted afterwards (lost swabs are a recurring cause of litigation in obstetrics).

📖 RCOG guideline 23: Perineal repair. http://www.rcog.org.uk

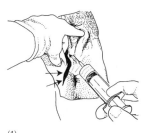

(1)
Swab the vulva towards the perineum. Infiltrate with 1% lignocaine → (arrows).

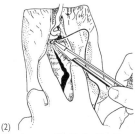

(2)
Place tampon with attached tape in upper vagina. Insert 1st suture above apex of vaginal cut (not too deep as underlying rectal mucosa nearby).

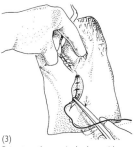

(3)
Bring together vaginal edges with continuous stitches placed 1cm apart. Knot at introitus under the skin. Appose divided levator ani muscles with 2 or 3 interrrupted sutures.

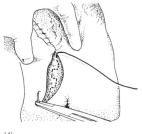

(4)
Close perineal skin (subcuticular continuous stitch is shown here).

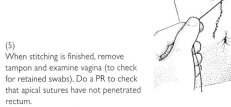

(5)
When stitching is finished, remove tampon and examine vagina (to check for retained swabs). Do a PR to check that apical sutures have not penetrated rectum.

Fig. 6.10 Episiotomy repair. Reproduced from Collier J, Longmore M, Brinsden M. *Oxford handbook of clinical specialties*, 7th edn,. OUP, 2006. By permission of Oxford University Press.

Third- and fourth-degree tears

Approximately 1% of vaginal deliveries will result in injury to the anal sphincter. Predicition and prevention are both difficult.

Factors associated with increased risk of anal sphincter trauma

- Forceps delivery.
- Nulliparity.
- Shoulder dystocia.
- 2nd stage >1 hour.
- Persistent OP position.
- Midline episiotomy.
- Birth weight >4 kg.
- Epidural anaesthesia.
- Induction of labour.

Management of 3rd- and 4th-degree tears

- All women sustaining genital tract injury should be carefully examined before suturing is started (including a rectal examination).
- Repair must be carried out by a trained senior clinician in theatre with adequate analgesia.
- The technique used can be end to end or overlapping for the EAS using either PDS or Vicryl suture material.
- The IAS should be repaired with vicryl using interupted sutures.
- Women must receive broad-spectrum antibiotics and stool softners.
- They should recieve physiotherapy input.
- Ideally they should be reviewed 6 weeks later by an obstetrician or gynaecologist.
- Women must be warned of the risk of incontinence of faeces, fluid, and flatus:
  - those experiencing symptoms at 6 weeks should be referred to a specialist gynaecologist or colorectal surgeon for investigation with endoanal ultrsonography.
- Around 60–80% will have a good result and be asymptomatic at 12 months.
- For future deliveries they should be advised that the result may not be so good from a 2nd repair:
  - if symptomatic they should be given the option of delivery by CS.

📖 RCOG guideline 29: 3rd and fourth degree tears—management. http://www.rcog.org.uk

Caesarean section: overview

Background

- CS involves delivery of the fetus through a direct incision in the abdominal wall and the uterus.
- The rates vary in different countries and populations:
  - the overall CS rate for nulliparous women in the UK has increased to about 24%
  - for multiparous women who have not previously had a CS, the rate is <5%
  - for women who have had at least one previous CS the rate is increased to about 67%. Most are elective.

Caesarean section is associated with a higher incidence of:

- Abdominal pain.
- Venous thromboembolism.
- Bladder or ureteric injury.
- Hysterectomy.
- Very rarely maternal death.

and with a lower incidence of:

- Perineal pain.
- Urinary incontinence.
- Uterovaginal prolapse.

Some interventions to decrease morbidity from CS

- Preoperative haemoglobin check and correction of anaemia.
- Intraoperative antibiotics.
- Risk assessment and appropriate thromboprophylaxis (graduated stockings, hydration, early mobilization and low molecular weight heparin).
- Indwelling bladder catheterization during the procedure.
- Antacids and H_2 receptor analogues before surgery.
- Antiemetics as appropriate.
- Regional rather than general anaesthesia.
- The risk of hypotension can be reduced using:
  - intravenous ephedrine or phenylephrine infusion
  - volume preloading with crystalloid or colloid
  - lateral tilt of 15°.
- General anaesthesia for emergency CS should include preoxygenation and rapid sequence induction to reduce the risk of aspiration.

Vaginal birth after CS (VBAC)
- Uterine rupture is very rare but is increased with VBAC:
  - 50:10 000 with VBAC and spontaneous onset of labour
  - 1:10 000 with repeat CS
- Intrapartum infant death is rare:
  - 1:1000—the same as for primiparous women
- Electronic fetal monitoring is recommended during labour as FHR changes may be the earliest signs of scar rupture.
- Women should deliver in a unit where there is immediate access to CS and on-site blood transfusion.
- With induction of labour, there is increased risk of uterine rupture:
  - 8:1000 if oxytocin infusion is used
  - 24:1000 if prostaglandins are used.
- Women with both previous CS and a previous vaginal birth are more likely to give birth vaginally.

Caesarean section: indications

The main indications for CS are:
- Repeat CS.
- Fetal compromise.
- 'Failure to progress' in labour.
- Breech presentation.

☛ Maternal request accounts for 7% of CS, but is not, on its own, an indication for CS.

Categories to determine the timing of CS

1. Immediate threat to the life of the woman or fetus (immediate, 'crash CS').
2. Maternal or fetal compromise which is not immediately life-threatening (urgent).
3. No maternal or fetal compromise but needs early delivery (scheduled).
4. Delivery timed to suit woman and staff (elective).

⚠ In cases of suspected or confirmed acute fetal compromise, delivery should be as soon as possible. The accepted standard for category 1 (immediate) CS is within 30 minutes.

Indications for a category 1 CS include:
- Placental abruption with abnormal FHR or uterine irritability.
- Cord prolapse.
- Scar rupture.
- Prolonged bradycardia.
- Scalp pH <7.20.

Indications for a category 2 CS include:
- Failure to progress with pathological CTG.

Indications for category 3 (scheduled) CS include:
- Severe pre-eclampsia.
- IUGR with poor fetal function tests.
- Failed induction of labour.

Indications for category 4 (elective) CS include:
- Term singleton breech (if ECV is contraindicated or has failed).
- Twin pregnancy with non-cephalic 1st twin.
- Maternal HIV.
- Primary genital herpes in the 3rd trimester.
- Placenta praevia.
- Previous hysterotomy or classical CS.

▶ Elective CS is usually carried out at 39 weeks, as the risk of respiratory morbidity (transient tachyopnoea of the newborn) is increased at lower gestational ages.

Caesarean section: types

Lower uterine segment incision

The two main types of skin incision are:
- **Pfannenstiel incision:** a straight horizontal incision 2 cm above the symphysis pubis—superior cosmetic result.
- **Joel–Cohen incision:** also a straight horizontal incision, but higher, about 3 cm below the level of the ASIS—allows quicker entry to the abdomen.

A transverse incision in the uterine lower segment is used in >90% of CS as it is associated with:
- Reduced adhesion formation
- Decreased blood loss
- Lower incidence of scar dehiscence in subsequent pregnancies.

However, if the lower segment is poorly developed, a low transverse incision carries a risk of lateral extension into the uterine vessels and haemorrhage. In these women, a lower segment vertical incision may be used, as it has a lower risk of lateral extension and a lower probability of dehiscence in a subsequent pregnancy compared with a classical incision.

Following delivery of the fetus and completion of the 3rd stage, the lower uterine segment is closed in one or two layers.

☞ Double-layer closure is usually practised; however, research comparing single- vs double-layer closure is ongoing.

Classical CS

This involves a vertical incision into the upper uterine segment. It is rarely performed, but indications may include:
- Structural abnormality of the uterus.
- Difficult access to the lower uterine segment due to fibroids or severe adhesions over the lower segment.
- Postmortem caesarean delivery (if the fetus is viable).
- Anterior placenta praevia with abnormally vascular lower uterine segment.
- Contraction ring.
- Very preterm fetus (especially breech presentation) where the lower segment is poorly formed.
- Elective Caesarean hysterectomy.
- Transverse lie of the fetus with ruptured membranes.

This incision allows rapid delivery and has a lower risk of bladder injury. However, the closure is more complicated and time-consuming and there is a higher incidence of infection and adhesion formation.

⚠ There is a greater risk of uterine rupture in subsequent pregnancies with a greater risk of the fetus being expelled into the peritoneal cavity. For these reasons, a classical incision is an absolute contraindication to a trial of a vaginal delivery (VBAC).

Caesarean section: complications

Intraoperative complications

Major complications are most common with an emergency CS and 82% of anaesthesia-related maternal deaths occurred in women undergoing CS, most frequently with general anaesthesia.

▶ Intraoperative complications occur in 12–15% of women and include:
- Uterine or uterocervical lacerations (5–10%).
- Blood loss >1L (7–9%).
- Bladder laceration (0.5–0.8%).
- Blood transfusion (2–3%).
- Hysterectomy (0.2%).
- Bowel lacerations (0.05%).
- Ureteral injury (0.03–0.09%.).

Risk factors predisposing to uterocervical lacerations include:
- Low station of the presenting part and full dilatation.
- Birth weight >4000 g.
- ↑ maternal age.
- Category 1 CS.

Risk factors predisposing to intraoperative haemorrhage include:
- Placenta praevia or abruption.
- Extremes of fetal birth weight.
- BMI >25.

Postoperative complications

▶ Postoperative complications occur in up to 1/3 of women and include:
- Endometritis (5%).
- Wound infections (3–27%).
- Pulmonary atelectasis.
- Venous thromboembolism.
- Urinary tract infections.

Risk factors independently associated with infection are:
- Preoperative remote infection.
- Chorioamnionitis.
- Maternal severe systemic disease.
- Pre-eclampsia.
- High BMI.
- Nulliparity.
- ↑ surgical blood loss.

Long-term effects of CS

In subsequent pregnancies there is a higher risk of:
- Uterine rupture (1:200 with spontaneous labour).
- Placenta praevia (47% ↑ of background risk).
- Placenta accreta.
- Antepartum stillbirth:
  - risk doubles with a previous CS.

Women undergoing multiple CS (≥3) are at higher risk of:
- Excessive blood loss (8%).
- Difficult delivery of the neonate (5%).
- Dense adhesions (46%).
- The risk of any major complication is higher (9%).
- Complications are ↑ with ↑ number of CS:
  - 4% for 2nd
  - 8% for 3rd
  - 13% for 4th.

Prelabour rupture of membranes (PROM) at term

Definition
Prelabour rupture of membranes (PROM) is defined as leakage of amniotic fluid in the absence of uterine activity after 37 completed weeks of gestation.

Incidence
- 8% of term pregnancies (2–3% before 37 weeks).

Aetiology
- Unknown.
- Clinical or subclinical infection.
- Polyhydramnios.
- Multiple pregnancy.
- Malpresentations.

Clinical assessment
It is important to establish a correct diagnosis to plan further management. If unnecessary interventions are undertaken there is a risk of increased maternal and fetal morbidity.

History
Women give a history of a sudden gush of fluid leaking from the vagina, recurrent dampness, or constant leaking.

Examination
- There is no need to carry out a speculum examination with certain history of ruptured membranes at term.
- If the history is uncertain, a speculum examination should be offered (liquor should be seen pooling in the upper vagina or trickling through the cervical os):
  - coughing or straining (Valsalva manoeuvre) may help to demonstrate leaking fluid
  - note the colour of the liquor (?blood or meconium stained).
- Temperature, pulse, and BP.
- Obstetric examination of the abdomen (including lie and presentation).
- CTG.

▶ If conservative management is planned, avoid digital examination as it increases the incidence of chorioamnionitis, postpartum endometritis, and neonatal infection.

⚠ Any concern regarding fetal well-being is an indication to deliver.

⚠ Signs of chorioamnionitis should prompt treatment with antibiotics and rapid delivery.

Clinical features of chorioamnionitis

- Fetal tachycardia.
- Maternal tachycardia.
- Maternal pyrexia.
- Rising leucocyte count.
- Rising CRP.
- Irritable or ↑ tender uterus.

Prelabour rupture of membranes (PROM): management

If there are no contraindications to waiting, women should be offered the choice between immediate induction and expectant management.

Expectant management vs immediate induction

- 60% of women will labour spontaneously within 24 hours.
- No evidence of a difference in the mode of delivery for either.
- 1% risk of serious neonatal infection (compared to 0.5% for women with intact membranes).

With expectant management:

- Women are more likely to develop chorioamnionitis and endometritis with expectant management of >24 hours.
- The baby is more likely to be admitted to SCBU:
  - no evidence of a difference in eventual neonatal outcome (morbidity/mortality) with expectant management of <24 hours.

▶ The NICE guidelines recommend induction after 24 hours.

Conservative management advice

- If the woman opts for this she should be advised to:
- Record her temperature every 4 hours (during waking hours).
- Urgently report any change in colour or offensive smell.
- Avoid sexual intercourse (showering and bathing is okay).
- Report any ↓ in fetal movements.
- Deliver in a unit with neonatal services and remain in hospital for >12 hours after delivery to allow close observation of the baby.
- Consider induction if not in labour by 24 hours.
- Seek medical advice if any concerns regarding the baby's well-being in the 1st 5 days of life (especially in the 1st 12 hours).

✒ The use of antibiotics is controversial. NICE does not recommend prophylactic antibiotics for either the woman or the baby in the absence of symptoms, even if her membranes have been ruptured for >24 hours.

▶ In labour regular maternal observations are essential to pick up signs of infection early. Fetal heart rate monitoring should be carried out as it may be tachycardic in the presence of infection.

⚠ If there is clinical evidence of infection a full course of broad spectrum IV antibiotic therapy should be started after blood cultures have been sent.

Known group B *Streptococcus* carriers (see Chapter 4)

- Immediate induction should be encouraged (↓ neonatal infection).
- Mothers should be offered benzyl penicillin in labour.
- Neonates should to be screened soon after birth.

📖 NICE guideline: Intrapartum care; September 2007. www.nice.org.uk

Abnormal lie: transverse and oblique

Transverse and oblique lie (see Chapter 2, Fig 2.4 p. 87)

These occur in 1:300 pregnancies and result in a shoulder, limb, or cord presentation. If this persists, vaginal delivery is not feasible.

Diagnosis

- The maternal abdomen is unusually wide and the fundus is lower than expected for the gestation.
- Neither fetal pole is palpable entering the pelvis.
- Fetal head is identifiable at one side.
- On vaginal examination the pelvis is empty.
- A limb or cord may prolapse through the cervix.

Management

- When this presents in labour, fetal well being should be established and an USS performed to try to identify the cause

⚠ Placenta praevia must be excluded before attempting vaginal examination

- CS is indicated in almost all cases
- An unstable lie at term due to multiparity alone may warrant a gentle attempt at external cephalic version (ECV) if the following criteria are met:
  - the membranes must be intact
  - labour not advanced
  - the fetus must have no signs of compromise.
- If the ECV is successful cord presentation or prolapse should be excluded before labour is allowed to establish.
- CS for transverse lie, especially with placenta praevia or fibroids requires an experienced obstetrician and cross-matched blood.
- A vertical uterine incision on the uterus or acute tocolysis with a transverse incision may be necessary for safe delivery of the fetus.

Malpresentations in labour: overview

- More than 95% of fetuses at term present with the vertex (an area subtended by the two parietal eminences, anterior and posterior fontanelle).
- Malpresentation describes any presentation other than a vertex lying in close proximity to the internal os of the cervix and includes:
  - breech (most common malpresentation with an incidence of 3–4% at term; see Chapter 2).
  - Brow.
  - Face.
  - Shoulder.
  - Arm.
  - Cord.

Some causes of malpresentation

Maternal
- Multiparity.
- Pelvic tumours.
- Congenital uterine anomalies.
- Contracted pelvis.

Fetal
- Prematurity.
- Multiple pregnancy.
- Intrauterine death.
- Macrosomia.
- Fetal abnormality including:
  - hydrocephalus
  - anencephaly
  - cystic hygroma.

Placental
- Placenta praevia
- Polyhydramnios
- Amniotic bands.

Malpresentations: brow and face

Brow presentation

Incidence ranges between in 1:1000 to 1:3500 deliveries. The head occupies a position midway between full flexion (vertex) and full extension (face). It can revert to a face or vertex presentation, but if it persists vaginal delivery is not usually possible. See Fig. 6.11a.

Diagnosis
- Often diagnosed in advanced labour (may be suspected on abdominal palpation when both occiput and chin are palpable).
- The head does not descend below the ischial spines.
- Vaginal examination is diagnostic as the frontal sutures, anterior fontanelle, orbital ridges, eyes, and the root of nose are palpable.

Management
- Watch and wait: may become a vertex or face presentation.
- If progress is slow or if the brow persists then CS is indicated.

Face presentation

The incidence of face presentation is between 1:600 and 1:1500 deliveries. It is due to hyperextension of the fetal neck. See Fig. 6.11b.

Diagnosis
- Face presentation is diagnosed in labour on vaginal examination.
- The orbital ridges, nose, malar eminences, mentum, gums, and mouth can be distinguished:

▶ It may be mistaken for a breech, but presence of gum margins will help to differentiate between a mouth and an anus.

Management
- 90% are mentoanterior (MA) and the head can flex to allow vaginal delivery.
- Expectant management should be considered with mentoposterior (MP) as about 20–30% will rotate on reaching the pelvic floor.
- Persistent MP face presentations cannot deliver vaginally as it would require the head to over extend.
- If there is poor progress or failure to rotate, CS is indicated.
- Fetal monitoring should be external and fetal blood sampling is contraindicated.
- The use of ventouse is absolutely contraindicated but forceps delivery is possible with a MA position well below spines.

⚠ Attempts to convert face presentations manually into vertex or use of forceps to rotate persistent MP positions can lead to complications of cord prolapse and fetal cervical cord injury.

📖 See Chapter 1, Fig. 1.6 and 1.7: Diameters and presenting parts of the fetal head

Cord presentation

This occurs when one or more loops of cord lie below the presenting part and the membranes are still intact. It is associated with malpresentation, abnormal lie and a high head. The risk is of cord prolapse when the membranes rupture. This is an obstetric emergency (see Chapter 10).

Diagnosis

- The diagnosis of cord presentation is often made on USS but may be found on VE in labour.
- It can be suspected clinically when persistent variable fetal heart decelerations occur early in labour.
- ARM is contraindicated as it will cause cord prolapse.

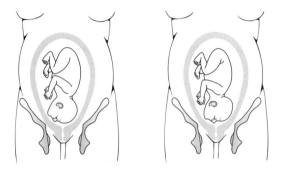

Brow presentation   Face presentation

Fig. 6.11 Malpresentations: (a) brow presentation; (b) face presentation.

Retained placenta and placenta accreta

Retained placenta should be suspected if it is not delivered within 30 minutes of the baby in an actively managed 3rd stage and 1 hour in a physiological 3rd stage.

⚠ Care must be taken as blood can gather behind the placenta leading to a significant occult blood loss—beware of the high uterus full of blood!

Management of retained placenta
- IV access, FBC and cross-match.
- If it was physiological management, revert to active management:
  - give Syntometrine® or oxytocin
  - try controlled cord traction.
- Injection of 20 IU of oxytocin in 20 mL of saline into the umbilical vein.
- If the oxytocin is not effective within 30 minutes, transfer to theatre for regional block and manual removal of the placenta.

Intraoperative prophylactic antibiotics should be given.

☝ The use of a 40 IU IV oxytocin infusion to help deliver the placenta is controversial. The NICE guidelines do not recommend using it before the placenta is delivered.

Placenta accreta, increta, and percreta

This abnormal placentation occurs in about 1:7000 pregnancies, but is much more common if there have been prior Caesarean deliveries. The placenta is normally separated from the myometrium by the decidua basalis. However, if the decidua is abnormal the villi may invade further through the uterine wall. There are three types but they are all often referred to as just accreta:
- **Placenta accreta:** placental villi are attached to the myometrium.
- **Placenta increta:** villi invade into the myometrium.
- **Placenta percreta:** villi pass through the myometrium upto the serosa, potentially involving other visera (bladder or bowel).

Risk factors for placenta accreta may include:
- Uterine surgery such as CS or myomectomy.
- Repeated surgical termination of pregnancy.

Management of placenta accreta-post delivery
- With heavy bleeding:
  - blood replacement
  - tamponade with balloon (e.g. Rusch)
  - hysterectomy.
- With minimal bleeding leaving the placenta in situ is an option with close monitoring.

How to perform a manual removal of placenta (MROP)

- One hand is placed on the abdomen to steady the uterus (reduces the risk of perforation).
- The other hand is gently inserted through the cervix into the uterus.
- The fingers are used to identify the plane between the placenta and the uterine wall, and gently separate it.
- The placenta should be removed in one piece and inspected to ensure it is complete.
- The uterine cavity is then explored again to make sure it is completely empty.
- Oxytocin infusion is continued for 4 hours prophylactically.
- Intravenous antibiotics are given.

Postpartum haemorrhage (PPH)

- **Primary PPH** is defined as a blood loss of 500 mL or more from the genital tract occurring within 24 hours of delivery.
- **Secondary PPH** is defined as 'excessive' loss occurring between 24 hours and 6 weeks after delivery.

- Major cause of maternal morbidity and mortality:
  - globally >125 000 women die of PPH each year
  - major cause of maternal deaths in the UK (often after CS).
- Incidence is 2–11% in the UK.
- With a low BMI or low Hb, <500mL loss may cause haemodynamic disturbance requiring prompt and appropriate management.

Causes of primary PPH

- Uterine atony.
- Genital tract trauma.
- Coagulation disorders.
- Large placenta.
- Abnormal placental site.
- Retained placenta.
- Uterine inversion.
- Uterine rupture.

Uterine atony (90%)
This is caused by failure of the uterus to contract after delivery. It may be due to many factors; overdistended uterus with twins or polyhydramnios, prolonged labour, infection, retained tissue, failure to actively manage 3rd stage of labour, or rarely due to placental abruption (diffuse bleeding into the uterine muscle that prevents contraction).

Genital tract trauma (7%)
Tears, episiotomy, lacerations of the cervix, and rupture of uterus.

Coagulation disorders
Severe PET, placental abruption, and sepsis may contribute to PPH. Autoimmune diseases, liver disease, inherited or acquired cogulation disorders are rare causes. Sometimes the patients may be on heparin which can lead to excessive bleeding.

Abnormal placental site
Placenta previa, placenta accreta, and percreta are associated with PPH. Appropriate preplanning is needed to avoid morbidity and mortality.

Uterine inversion and rupture are rare causes of excessive bleeding.

📖 For management see Chapter 10—massive obstetric haemorrhage, p. 380.

Antenatal risk factors for PPH

- Previous PPH.
- Previous retained placenta.
- Maternal Hb ≤8.5 g/dL at onset of labour.
- ↑ BMI.
- Para 4 or more.
- Antepartum haemorrhage.
- Overdistention of the uterus (multiple pregnancy or polyhydramnios).
- Uterine abnormalities.
- Low-lying placenta
- Maternal age >35 years.

⚠ The presence of any risk factors for PPH should lead to the woman being advised to deliver in an obstetric unit (facilities for blood transfusion and surgical management of PPH).

Intrapartum risk factors for PPH

- Induction of labour.
- Prolonged 1st, 2nd, or 3rd stage.
- Use of oxytocin.
- Precipitate labour.
- Vaginal operative delivery.
- CS.

Home birth: overview

Home birth can be safe for women screened as low risk and emotionally satisfying for the mother, her partner, and family. For women identified as having risk factors, hospital delivery is safer. Debates about the safety of home births focus on the risk of preventable perinatal morbidity and mortality, and on broader issues of appropriate screening and referral.

The numbers
- The proportion of births at home fell markedly from 80% in 1930 to 1% in 1990.
- As a result of Government committee recommendation (HMSO 1993) stating that a full choice including home births should be offered to pregnant women, the UK home birth rate is steadily increasing and is now approaching 2%.
- Some studies suggest that 10–14% of women would choose the option of home birth if given the opportunity.
- In women booked for home births:
  - change to hospital care is nearly 29%
  - transfer in labour is up to 15% in multiparae and 30% in nulliparae.
- The risk of intrapartum fetal death in appropriately selected low risk women is 1:1000.
- It is difficult to compare directly the perinatal mortality rates for home and hospital, as more complex deliveries occur in hospital.

Reasons for women to choose home birth
- Wish to be in a familiar setting in which they feel relaxed and in control.
- Fear of hospital setting.
- To have a continuing relationship with a known midwife.
- To be with more family members who provide support.
- Previous home birth.
- To avoid unnecessary intervention.

Discussion points when considering home birth
- In the presence of obvious risk factors (hypertension, diabetes, placenta praevia) the advice must be to deliver in hospital.
- If the woman is low-risk and wishes to have home birth, she should be counselled appropriately, provided with the relevant facts, reassured that adverse emergencies are rare and that hospital backup would be available if any problems arise.
- If a risk arises before birth, the booking should be changed.
- If the risk is minimal, the lead professional in charge should offer the woman and her partner the opportunity to review their choice and respect their decision.

Home birth: risks and GP involvement

The potential risks of home birth are rare, but should be discussed with the women as part of her decision. These include:

- Should a complication occur transfer to hospital may be required.
- Should there be a delay in transfer, response to acute complications such as intrapartum fetal hypoxia or postpartum haemorrhage may be delayed, potentially leading to a worse outcome.
- The facilities for neonatal resuscitation will be limited but the midwife is well trained in basic neonatal resuscitation.
- Inadequate lighting and analgesia may make diagnosis of the extent of perineal tears difficult, necessitating transfer to hospital.

Discussion of the risks and other factors, including the type of pain relief available, will help the women to make an informed choice. Clear documentation of these discussions in the antenatal period is essential for medico-legal reasons.

The GP's role

- The GP should be fully informed about the local options for place of birth, and will then be in a position to provide the options to the woman in a clear, understandable, and balanced manner.
- GPs who do not wish to provide care for home births should refer women to a community midwife, supervisor of community midwives at the district maternity unit, or a GP who provides full maternity services.
- In case of any unfortunate event occurring with the intrapartum care of a woman being looked after by her GP and if the case proceeds to a litigation, the GP would not be judged by the standards of a consultant obstetrician, but by those of a GP with similar skills and standing (the Bolam test).
- The GP does not have to attend a home birth even when the woman has been accepted by them for full maternity care, unless asked to do so by the midwife.
- The GP should provide support to women and midwife and help in identifying any deviations from normal course of labour and arrange for hospital care.
- Where the midwife feels that the GP is supportive, the likelihood of transfer to hospital is reduced.

📖 The GP's guide to home birth. http://www.jr2.ox.ac.uk/bandolier/band32/b32–8.html

Home birth: the evidence

A Cochrane review suggests no strong evidence to favour either home or hospital birth for selected, low-risk pregnant women. In places where it is possible to establish a home birth service backed up by a modern hospital system, all low-risk women should be offered the possibility of considering a planned hospital, midwifery-led unit, or home birth.

Meta-analysis of several methodologically sound observational studies comparing the outcomes of planned home births (irrespective of the eventual place of birth) with planned hospital births for women with similar characteristics showed:

- No increase in maternal mortality.
- No statistically significant differences in perinatal mortality.
- In the home births group there were significantly fewer medical interventions (including in women transferred to hospital).
- Fewer babies had low Apgar scores, neonatal respiratory problems, and instances of birth trauma with home births.

A randomized controlled trial would help to resolve the controversy over the relative safety of home and hospital birth; because maternal and perinatal mortality are so low in low-risk pregnancies if we consider these as primary outcome measures, large numbers need to be studied.

Home birth: general points

GPs and midwives have the responsibility for creating the right circumstances for safe and satisfying home births.
This means:

- Selecting women without risk factors.
- Establishing an infrastructure for safe obstetric care which should include:
  - hygiene during delivery
  - keeping the baby warm
  - care of the eyes.
- Providing support and care during labour, delivery and in the immediate postnatal period.
- Arrangements for transfer to hospital in the event of any unforeseen complication.
- Care should be provided based on a pre-arranged protocol that provides guidance as to the conduct of labour and what action needs to be taken should the woman need help.

Chapter 7

Obstetric anaesthesia

Pain relief in labour

Uterine contractions in labour are associated with pain. Professionals can help to reduce women's fears by giving precise, accurate, and relevant information antenatally including the types of analgesia available in their unit.

Ideal pain relief in labour

Should:
- Provide good analgesia.
- Be safe for the mother and baby.
- Be predictable and constant in its effects.
- Be reversible if necessary.
- Be easy to administer.
- Be under the control of the mother.

Should not:
- Interfere with uterine contractions.
- Interfere with mobility.

Non-pharmacological methods
- Education regarding what to expect is important as it may help reduce fear and the sense of loss of control.
- A trusted companion present throughout labour and birth reduces the need for pain relief.
- Warm bath, acupuncture, hypnosis, and homeopathy are also helpful.

Transcutaneous electrical nerve stimulation (TENS) is a safe form of analgesia. It may help with short labours and postpone the need for stronger analgesia but may not be adequate as labour advances.

Pharmocological methods

Nitrous oxide (Entonox)
Entonox is premixed nitrous oxide and oxygen as a 50:50 mixture. It is self-administered and has quick onset of action and a short half-life. Side effects include feeling faint, nausea and vomiting.

Narcotic agents
- **Pethidine** is administered at a dose of 50–150 mg; the onset of action is in 15–20 minutes. It lasts about 3–4 hours and can be repeated. It is usually given with an antiemetic. If given within 2 hours of delivery, it can cause neonatal respiratory depression and naloxone may be needed.
- **Diamorphine** is also used in some units at a dose of 2.5–5 mg. There is controversy about the extent and timing of neonatal respiratory depression but it may be up to 3–4 hours after the last dose.
- **Meptazinol** is an opioid which may cause less respiratory depression. The onset of action starts in 15 minutes and lasts for about 2–7 hours.

Pudendal nerve block and local perineal infiltration
- Pudendal nerve block is used for operative vaginal delivery and is performed by the obstetrician:
  - Lidocaine (lignocaine) is injected 1–2 cm medially and below the right and left ischial spines; this is done trans vaginally with a specially designed pudendal needle.
- Local anaesthetic such as lidocaine (lignocaine) is infiltrated in the perineum before performing an episiotomy at the time of delivery, or before suturing tears and episiotomies.

Epidural analgesia: overview

Safe and effective analgesia for labour is still something that is not available for the vast majority of women in the world today. Although the provision of epidural analgesia during labour has been one of the greatest advances in the care of women during this difficult and distressing time, it still carries a small but definite complication rate.

Consent for analgesia in labour

Women in labour present a particular group of patients in whom the obtaining of fully informed consent may be difficult because of a variety of factors such as pain, fatigue, or the effects of narcotic analgesia administered previously. Ideally anaesthetists should try to explain the risks and benefits of epidural analgesia to women in the antenatal period.

Anatomy

The epidural space lies between the spinal dura and the vertebral canal. The superior margin is the foramen magnum, inferiorly the sacrococcygeal membrane. Posteriorly lies the ligamentum flavum and the anterior surfaces of the laminae, anteriorly the posterior longitudinal ligament. Within the epidural space lie the spinal nerve roots as well as the spinal arteries and extradural veins. The usual distance between skin and the epidural space in the lumbar region in adults is about 4–5 cm. It is important to realize that the epidural space is continuous the whole way down the back. The lumbar region is chosen for the provision of labour analgesia as this is where the nerves roots involved in the production of pain during labour are found.

The pain of the first stage of labour is caused by uterine contractions and is referred by afferent Aδ and C fibres mainly to dermatones T10–L1 and by distension of the perineum during the second stage of labour to S2–4.

Epidural analgesia: advantages and disadvantages

Advantages of epidural analgesia include:

- It provides effective analgesia in labour.
- Reduced maternal secretion of catecholamines, which benefits the fetus.
- Can be used when topped up for an operative delivery and for any complications of the 3rd stage of labour, e.g. retained placenta or repair of perineal tears
- Can provide effective postoperative analgesia.
- Can be used as an additional method of controlling blood pressure in pre-eclampsia.

Disadvantages and complications of epidural analgesia

- Failure to site, or a patchy or incomplete block.
- Hypotension from sympathetic blockade.
- Decreased mobility.
- Tenderness over the insertion site; however, there is no association between epidural analgesia and long-term backache.
- Inadvertent dural puncture:
  - incidence <1 in 100
  - may develop a postdural puncture headache, which is characterized by ↑ on sitting up or standing and may need treatment with an epidural blood patch.
- Respiratory depression:
  - from the catheter migrating into the subarachnoid space followed by bolus of local anaesthetic (total spinal)
  - from accumulation of epidurally administered opiates.
- Extremely rare complications resulting in neurological deficits:
  - epidural abscess formation
  - epidural haematoma
  - damage to individual nerves or the spinal cord itself.
- Increased risk of operative delivery.

An alternative to epidural: Remifentanil PCA

There are a few women in whom epidural analgesia is contra-indicated and who are not able to obtain adequate analgesia from more conventional methods such as nitrous oxide. The administration of remifentanil (a powerful opiate which is rapidly metabolized and unable to cross the placenta) via a patient-controlled IV system has shown promise in providing analgesia.

Contra-indications to epidural analgesia

- Septicaemia.
- Infection at site of insertion.
- Coagulopathy/thrombocytopaenia (platelet count < 75 × 10^9).

⚠ Beware of a falling count over the past few days—always check the platelet count if this has occurred. If the platelet count is between 75 and 100 × 10^9, do clotting studies before proceeding with the epidural.
- Raised intracranial pressure.
- Haemorrhage and cardiovascular instability/hypovolaemia.

▶ There may be limited circumstances where an epidural is appropriate in these cases.
- Known allergy to amide (lidocaine-type) local anaesthetic solutions or opioids.
- Fixed cardiac output states, e.g. severe aortic stenosis, hypertrophic obstructive cardiomyopathy (HOCM).

Anaesthetic techniques for Caesarean section: spinal

Regional anaesthetic techniques are undoubtedly safer for the women and most anaesthetists would counsel women having a CS to opt for one of them. However, the choice of anaesthetic technique may be influenced by the urgency of the CS. Facilities for conversion to general anaesthesia (GA) such as drugs and endotracheal tubes must always be available as conversion to GA may be required if the block wears off during surgery, or is too high, or if the woman requests it due to pain or discomfort.

Spinal anaesthesia

- This technique accounts for the majority of CS performed in the UK.
- Fasting and antacid precautions are ideal, as GA may be required if the block is unsatisfactory.
- Good intravenous access is essential to provide fluids rapidly to counteract hypotension that may occur. Vasopressor drugs, such as phenylephrine or ephedrine, should also be available.
- Hyperbaric bupivacaine 0.5% in a dose of 12.5–15 mg is usually used, together with an opiate such as fentanyl (20 micrograms) or diamorphine (around 250 micrograms).

> ### Advantages and disadvantages of spinal anaesthesia
>
> *Advantages*
> - Technically relatively easier than epidurals to perform.
> - Enable mother to bond immediately with baby.
> - The most reliable option for establishing a dense, bilateral block.
>
> *Disadvantages*
> - May cause severe hypotension.
> - May wear off if surgery is unexpectedly prolonged.

⚠ Hypotension is common due to sympathetic blockade and inadequate tilt leading to aortocaval pressure, and must be prevented by the use of fluids, adequate left lateral tilt, and vasopressors if appropriate.

▶ Patients must be warned of the risk of intraoperative pain and the small chance of conversion to GA.

▶ The full extent of the block must be tested and recorded by the anaesthetist, prior to the commencement of surgery.

Anaesthetic techniques for Caesarean section: epidural

Conversion of a functioning epidural from analgesia to anaesthesia is the choice when a woman requires an operative or instrumental delivery, provided there is sufficient time (it takes about 20 minutes or longer).

Advantages and disadvantages of epidural anaesthesia

Advantages
- Can be topped up to prolong the anaesthesia, should the surgery be extended.
- Can be used for good postoperative analgesia.

Disadvantages
- More likely than spinal anaesthesia to produce patchy or unilateral blockade.
- Takes longer to establish an adequate block.
- Can be technically difficult to perform, with a higher incidence of headache in the event of inadvertent dural puncture.
- The catheter might migrate into the subarachnoid, intravenous or subdural space, resulting in unpredictable and possibly fatal complications when large doses of local anaesthetic agents are administered.
- Larger doses of local anaesthetic agents are required, leading to the possibility of toxicity if the catheter has migrated intravenously.

Technique for siting an epidural

- The procedure should be explained and consent sought.
- There should be no clotting abnormalities present.
- Establish wide-bore IV access.
- Position the woman, either on her side or sitting, with the back curved to open intervertebral spaces.
- Full aseptic technique should be followed while performing the epidural.
- A suitable interspace, usually L3/4, is identified and lidocaine (lignocaine)1% injected.
- The epidural space is identified by a loss of resistance technique, usually to saline 0.9%.
- Once the space is identified, a catheter is threaded into the space, the needle withdrawn and the catheter firmly fixed to the skin.
- A test dose of local anaesthetic, usually bupivacaine, can be given to check that the epidural catheter has not inadvertently entered the subarachnoid space.
- Various regimens exist for the delivery of the local anaesthetic solution to the epidural space either involving bolus administration, infusions, or patient-controlled epidural administration devices.
- Careful monitoring is mandatory following epidural top up doses including blood pressure reading every 5 minutes for 20 minutes following the administration of a top up dose.
- Block height and the degree of motor block should be recorded.
- Continuous electronic fetal monitoring is required if an epidural has been sited.

Anaesthetic techniques for Caesarean section: combined spinal epidural (CSE)

These are usually performed by inserting a spinal needle through an epidural needle, although two separate injections may be performed.

Advantages and disadvantages of the CSE

Advantages
- The epidural component can be used to top up the block.
- A smaller volume of local anaesthetic can be used intrathecally and the block extended gradually with the epidural component (this may cause less cardiovascular instability and be useful in women with cardiac disease).
- The epidural component can provide postoperative analgesia.

Disadvantages
- There is a higher risk of failure of the intrathecal component.
- Possible higher risk of meningitis than with either spinal or epidural alone.
- The epidural component of the technique is untested and any local anaesthetic agents must be given in small boluses, in case the catheter is in the subarachnoid space.

▶ CSE anaesthesia combines the advantages of spinal anaesthesia, i.e. speed of onset and dense block with the ability to prolong the period of anaesthesia and analgesia via the epidural route.

Anaesthetic techniques for Caesarean section: general anaesthesia

There has been a general trend throughout the developed world away from using GA for CS. However, it is still necessary in the presence of contra-indications to regional anaesthesia or in an emergency.

Problems with GA
- Potential airway difficulties:
  - incidence of failed intubation in pregnant women is approximately 1:300 compared with 1:3000 in the general surgical population.
- Pulmonary aspiration of gastric contents.
- Awareness:
  - rare with modern anaesthetic techniques, but may occur if inadequate levels of inhalational agents are used.

GA technique in pregnancy
- Adequate assessment of the airway is essential, as well as questioning about relevant medical, obstetric, drug treatment, and allergies.
- Antacid prophylaxis must be administered.
- Left lateral tilt maintained at all times to prevent aortocaval compression.
- Adequate pre-oxygenation must precede induction of GA, regardless of the obstetric indications for the CS.
- ECG, pulse oximetry, and capnographic monitoring must be available.
- For full discussion of GA for CS, readers are advised to consult a specialist anaesthetic text.

△ Emergency GA is associated with increased maternal morbidity and mortality

▶ There are few absolute indications for general anaesthesia for CS.

Chapter 8

Neonatal resuscitation

Overview

Most babies establish normal respiration and circulation without help after delivery. However, all babies should be assessed at delivery. Newborn infants who are born at term, have clear liquor, and are breathing and crying with good tone, will require only drying and keeping warm. Less than 1% of babies need resuscitation and anticipation of problems before delivery is the key to success.

It is necessary to call paediatricians to attend deliveries where further support may be necessary such as:

- Preterm deliveries.
- Emergency Caesarean deliveries.
- Vaginal breech birth.
- Thick meconium stained liquor.
- Major fetal abnormality.
- Other concerns (e.g. maternal drug use).

Trained personnel should be available round the clock. The environment should be warm, well lit, and draught free with a flat surface available for resuscitation. Equipment should be checked on a daily basis and before each delivery. Some of the important items are:

- Resuscitaire (radiant warmer) (see Fig. 8.1).
- Source of air/oxygen with pressure-limited gas delivery.
- Appropriate size face masks, oropharyngeal airways, endotracheal tubes.
- Suction device with different size suction catheters.
- Stethoscope.
- Laryngoscope with straight laryngeal blades (size 0, 1).
- Instruments for clamping and cutting the umbilical cord.
- Emergency resuscitation box for advanced resuscitation.

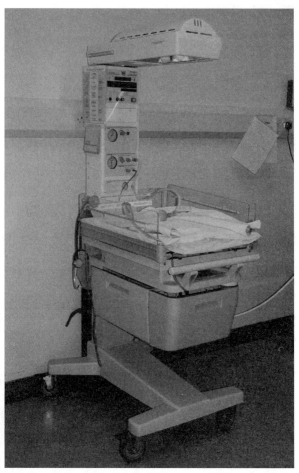

Fig. 8.1 Neonatal radiant warmer (Resuscitaire). Reproduced with permission of Dräger Medical UK, 2008

Practical aspects

Temperature control

Hypothermia can lower oxygen tension, increase metabolic acidosis, lead to hypoglycaemia, and inhibit the production of surfactant. Low temperature is associated with poor neonatal outcome.

Heat loss should be prevented by:
- Protecting the baby from draught.
- Keeping the delivery room warm.
- Drying the term baby immediately after delivery, covering the head and body with warm towel to prevent further heat loss.
- Placing baby on warm surface under radiant warmer, if resuscitation is needed.

▶ For a preterm baby born before 28 weeks of gestation (< ~1 kg birth weight), the most effective way of keeping the baby warm is not to dry and wrap it in warm towels but to cover the head and body (apart from the face) with a plastic bag before placing under a radiant heater. Plastic wrapping should therefore be available at all deliveries of extremely preterm infants.

Initial assessment at delivery

The immediate assessment includes colour, tone, breathing, and heart rate. APGAR scoring has been used for the initial assessment of the baby. However, it is a retrospective, highly subjective tool and was never intended to identify babies needing resuscitation.

- **Colour**: baby may be centrally pink, cyanosed, or pale (peripheral cyanosis is common and does not by itself indicate hypoxaemia).
- **Tone**: a very floppy baby is likely to be unconscious, and may need respiratory support.
- **Breathing**: the rate, depth, and symmetry of respiration together with any abnormal breathing pattern such as grunting and gasping should be noted.
- **Heart rate**: best evaluated by auscultating with a stethoscope (palpating the umbilical cord is often effective but can be misleading).

After the initial assessment, infants can be generally classified into one of four groups and further management can be guided by this (Table 8.1).

Table 8.1 Classification of babies at birth with appropriate action

	Assessment	Clinical condition	Action
Group1	Healthy	Vigorous baby—crying Becoming pink Good tone Heart rate >100	Dry and warm Hand to mother for skin to skin contact

Group 2	Primary Apnoea	Apnoeic or inadequate
		  breathing
		Remaining blue
		  reduced tone
		Heart rate >100
			Dry and warm
			Tactile stimulation
			Facial oxygen
			Consider mask ventilation
			  if not improving

Group 3	Terminal apnoea	Apnoeic
		Blue or pale Floppy
		Heart rate <100
			Dry and warm
			Mask ventilation—if no
			  improvement will need
			  intubation, ventilation
			  and chest compressions
			  if heart rate not
			  improving

Group 4	Fresh stillbirth	Apnoeic Pale Floppy No heart rate	Full cardiopulmonary resuscitation

ABC

⚠ Call for skilled help as soon as a problem is identified.

Airway

The head should be placed in neutral position—this is different from the head position for adult resuscitation because of the relatively large occiput of babies. Over-extension of the neck can occlude the airway. A jaw thrust may be helpful, but care must be taken not to compress the airway under the chin. Use of an appropriately sized Guedel airway can be considered, particularly in infants with micrognathia. Suction of the airway is only required if there is blood or particulate material in the oropharynx. Aggressive pharyngeal suction should be avoided and suction should always be done under direct vision with a laryngoscope.

⚠ Blind suction is not helpful; it may lead to trauma and induce bradycardia or laryngospasm.

Breathing

Mask ventilation may be necessary if the infant is apnoeic, has irregular breathing, or is bradycardic. The aim is to achieve adequate lung inflation and to deliver oxygen. In most cases mask ventilation is as effective as intubation in the initial resuscitation scenario.

It is essential to use the correct-sized mask. The mask should cover the nose and mouth but should not extend beyond the chin or over the orbits. Mask ventilation can be performed using a bag and mask, or via a constant flow T-piece system (Fig. 8.2).

The lungs of newborn infants are fluid-filled immediately after birth and the first 5 breaths given should sustain an inflation pressure of approximately 30 cm of water (for a term infant) for 2–3 seconds (inflation breaths). These long breaths aim to displace the lung fluid and expand the lungs. If effective, chest wall movement and improvement of heart rate should be seen. If the heart rate rises, but baby is still not breathing, continue to ventilate at 30–40 breaths per minute (maintain the inflation for ~1 second for each breath).

⚠ If there is no improvement, the airway should be checked again. Help should be sought early as endotracheal intubation may be necessary if there is no improvement.

Circulation

⚠ Chest compressions are effective only if the lungs have been successfully inflated.

Chest compressions aim to deliver oxygenated blood to the heart allowing the circulation to recover. Chest compressions should be commenced if the infant remains bradycardic despite adequate ventilation.

How to perform chest compressions in the neonate

- Both thumbs should be placed over the lower 1/3 of sternum, encircling the chest with both hands; other fingers lie behind the baby supporting the back.
- For effective chest compressions, the chest is compressed to a depth of 1/3 the anteroposterior diameter.
- 3:1 ratio of compression and ventilation is used, i.e. 90 compressions and 30 breaths per minute, each breath lasting for 1 second.
- The quality of compressions and ventilation are more important than the rate.

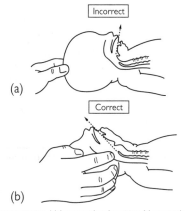

Fig. 8.2 Neonatal resuscitation (a) Incorrect head position. Neonates have a prominent occiput therefore in the prone position will naturally adopt a flexed head posture which compromises the airway. (b) Correct 'neutral' head position. The neutral position is neither extended nor flexed but opens the airway to allow effective inflation breaths.

Drugs

Drugs are rarely indicated in neonatal resuscitation. They should be considered only if adequate ventilation and effective chest compression have failed to increase the heart rate above 60/minute. In the resuscitation situation, drugs should be given via an umbilical venous catheter.

Drugs used in neonatal resuscitation

- **Adrenaline**: 1:10 000, dose 0.1–0.3mL/kg equivalent to 10–30 micrograms/kg; route through umbilical venous catheter or IV.

▶ It is no longer recommended that adrenaline is given down the endotracheal tube (ETT).

- **Sodium bicarbonate**: dose 1–2 mmol/kg (2–4 mL/kg of 4.2% NaHCO₃); route through IV or UVC. Reversing the intracardiac acidosis may help bump-start the heart.

▶ Use of repeated doses of NaHCO₃ should be avoided without proper evidence of metabolic acidosis from blood gas analysis.

- **Glucose 10%:** dose 2 mL/kg/dose (200 mg/kg/dose), route through IV or UVC. Glucose should be given if there is hypoglycaemia.
- **Volume replacement**: crystalloid (0.9% saline, 10mL/kg/dose) is the preferred fluid, if the infant appears to be in shock. Blood should be given if there is evidence of hypovolaemia and evidence of acute blood loss.
- **Naloxone** is no longer kept in the resuscitation trolley.

⚠ These are not resuscitation drugs and should only be considered after there is a secure airway, and effective aeration of the lungs and a normal heart rate.

Actions in the event of a poor response to resuscitation

Check for a technical problem
- Is the gas flow connected?
- Is there a leak in the circuit? Check the tubing.
- Is the ETT in the trachea? If in doubt remove ETT, give breaths by mask, and replace ETT if necessary.
- Is the ETT blocked? If in doubt remove ETT, give breaths by mask, and replace ETT if necessary.
- Check the blow-off valve pressure (30 cm of water for term infant).

Does the baby have other pathology?
- Pneumothorax.
- Congenital lung problem, e.g. diaphragmatic hernia.
- Lung hypoplasia.
- Hydrops fetalis.
- Perinatal asphyxia.

Recent advances

Infants with meconium-stained liquor

There is now evidence that suctioning of the meconium from the infant's airway after delivery of the head but before delivery of the shoulder is not beneficial and so it is no longer recommended.

▶ No suctioning should be performed if the infant is active, vigorous and crying.

If an infant is born through thick meconium and is floppy and depressed after birth, it is reasonable for a skilled person to inspect the larynx directly with a laryngoscope and suction the oropharynx and trachea. There is no role for bronchial lavage.

Preterm infants

It is easier to maintain the preterm infant's temperature by placing it into a plastic bag (while wet, leaving the face uncovered) and then under a radiant heater. This is more effective than drying and wrapping for infants <28 weeks gestation.

Also, preterm infants usually require less pressure to inflate their lungs and therefore the blow-off valve on the resuscitaire should be initially set at 20–25 cm of water (rather than 30 cm of water for term infants). In addition, exogenous surfactant is important in the initial stabilization of extremely preterm infants.

Use of air vs oxygen in resuscitation

There is evidence that using air for the resuscitation of near-term and term babies is as effective as using oxygen, although there is still active debate. It is therefore reasonable to resuscitate infants in air, with supplemental oxygen available if needed.

Communication with parents

Resuscitation decisions

If resuscitation is required, parents should be fully informed of the procedure undertaken and the purpose.

The decision to resuscitate an extremely preterm infant should be a combined decision of parents, paediatric, and obstetric staff. This is a difficult conversation but one that is best had early. The obstetricians caring for any women who has a strong probability of delivering very prematurely must raise the issue early and actively involve their paediatric colleagues. The decision taken about resuscitation should also influence the level of fetal monitoring in labour.

The decision to discontinue resuscitation should involve senior paediatric staff. Proper birth plans should be in place in cases of severe congenital malformations. All communication with parents should be documented in the mother's notes and later in the baby's notes after delivery.

Stopping resuscitation

If there are no signs of life after 10 minutes of continuous and effective resuscitation, stopping must be considered as the outcome is universally poor. The decision should be made by the resuscitation team and the most senior paediatrician available. Local and national guidelines are very helpful in making such decisions.

📖 Biarent D, Binghma R, Richmond S et al. European Resuscitation Council Guidelines for resuscitation. *Resuscitation* 2005; 67(S1):S97–S133.

📖 Resuscitation Council (UK). Resuscitation at birth. Newborn life support course provider manual, 2nd edn. London, Resuscitation Council (UK) 2006.

Postnatal care

Normal changes in the puerperium

The puerperium begins after the delivery of the placenta and lasts until the reproductive organs have retuned to their pre-pregnant state (about 6 weeks).

Hormones
- **Human placental lactogen and βhCG:** levels fall rapidly; by 10 days neither should be detectable.
- **Oestrogen and progesterone:** non-pregnant levels are achieved by 7 days postpartum.

Genital tract
- **Uterus:** This should undergo rapid involution. The weight of the uterus falls from 1000 g post-delivery to about 500 g at the end of a week. By 2 weeks, it returns to pelvis and is no longer palpable abdominally.
- **Vagina:** Initially vaginal wall is swollen, but rapidly regains its tone although remaining fragile for 1–2 weeks. Gradually the vascularity and oedema decrease, and by 4 weeks rugae reappear, but are less prominent than in a nullipara.
- **Cervix:** The cervical os gradually closes after delivery. It admits 2–3 fingers for the first 4–6 days and by the end of 10–14 days is dilated to barely more than 1 cm.

Perineum
Perineal oedema may persist for some days. It may take longer in women who had perineal tears that needed repair.

Lochia
Lochia constitutes of sloughed-off necrotic decidual layer mixed with blood. It is initially red (lochia rubra), becomes paler as the bleeding is reduced (lochia serosa), and finally becomes a yellowish white (lochia alba). The flow of lochia may last for 3–6 weeks.

Breast
Between the 2nd and 4th days the breasts become engorged, the vascularity is increased, and areolar pigmentation increases. There is enlargement of the lobules resulting from an increase in the number and size of the alveoli.

Cardiovascular system
After the 3rd stage of labour, the cardiac output initially increases due to an expansion in plasma volume then rapidly decreases to about 40% of the pre-labour levels as a result of diuresis. It returns to normal by 2–3 weeks postpartum. Heart rate also decreases and is partly responsible for the reduced cardiac output. Blood loss at delivery and excretion of extracellular fluid are responsible for alterations in the blood volume.

Major postnatal problems

The three major causes of morbidity in the postnatal period are:
- Secondary postpartum haemorrhage (PPH) (see text box 🕮 below and Chapters 6 and 10).
- Venous thromboembolism (VTE) (see text box 🕮 p. 351 and Chapter 10).
- Puerpural pyrexia.

Puerperal pyrexia

Puerperal pyrexia is defined as the presence of fever in a mother ≥38°C in the first 14 days after giving birth.

- Puerperal sepsis was the most common cause of maternal mortality before the mid-1930s, accounting for >40% of all maternal deaths.
- The control and cure of puerperal infection began in 1935 with the introduction of the first sulphonamides.
- The incidence of puerperal pyrexia has fallen to 1–3% of all births, miscarriages, and terminations.
- The CEMACH report 2003–5 (see 🕮 Chapter 11, p. 410) has highlighted the increasing number of maternal deaths due to genital tract sepsis (18 over the 3 year period) so vigilance remains vitally important.

Factors predisposing to puerperal pyrexia

Antepartum
- Anaemia.
- Duration of membrane rupture.

Intrapartum
- Duration of labour.
- Bacterial contamination during vaginal examination.
- Instrumentation.
- Trauma, e.g. episiotomy, vaginal tears, Caesarean section (CS).
- Haematoma.

Secondary PPH (see Chapters 6 and 10)
- Defined as any 'abnormal' bleeding occurring between 24 hours and 6 weeks postnatally.
- In developed countries, 2% of postnatal women are admitted to hospital with this:
  - 50% undergo surgical evacuation.
- In developing countries it is a major cause of maternal death.
- Caused by retained products, endometritis, or a tear.
- Management depends on the cause (see Chapters 6 and 10).

VTE (see Chapter 10)

⚠ Venous thromboembolism (VTE) remains the main cause of maternal death in the UK.

It may be asymptomatic until it presents with a PE but some of the signs and symptoms may include:

Deep vein thrombosis (DVT):
- leg pain or discomfort (especially in the left leg)
- swelling
- Tenderness
- Erythema, increased skin temperature and oedema
- Lower abdominal pain (high DVT)
- Elevated white cell count

Pulmonary thromboembolism (PE):
- Dyspnoea
- Collapse
- chest pain
- haemoptysis
- faintness
- raised JVP
- focal signs in chest
- symptoms and signs associated with DVT.

⚠ In the postnatal period there should be high level of suspicion for women presenting with any symptoms and urgent investigation is warranted.

Puerperal pyrexia: genital causes

Uterine infection (endometritis)

Predisposing factors

- Caesarean section.
- Intrapartum chorioamnionitis.
- Prolonged labour.
- Multiple pelvic examinations.
- Internal fetal monitoring.
- Other risk factors, e.g. anaemia, low socio-economic status.

Symptoms

- Fever usually in proportion to the extent of infection.
- Foul, profuse and bloody discharge.
- Subinvolution of uterus.
- Tender bulky uterus on abdominal examination.

Perineal wound infection

- Includes infection of episiotomy wounds and repaired lacerations.
- Perineum becomes painful.
- May cause breakdown of wound.

Complications of pelvic infection

- Wound dehiscence.
- Adnexal infections.
- Pelvic abscess.
- Septic thrombophlebitis.
- Septicaemia.
- Subsequent subfertility.

Puerperal pyrexia: non-genital causes

Breast causes (mastitis, breast abscess)
- About 15% of women develop fever from breast engorgement.
- Fever may be high as 39° C.
- Is associated with painful and hard breast.
- May need antibiotics in presence of infection.
- Breast-feeding should be continued.
- Abscess may need surgical drainage.

Urinary tract infection (UTI)
- About 2–4% women develop UTI postpartum.
- Hypotonic bladder may result in stasis and reflux of urine.
- Catheterization, birth trauma, and pelvic examinations during labour.
- Presenting symptoms include increased frequency of micturition, dysuria, or urgency.
- Rigors may be present in pyelonephritis.
- Most common organisms involved are *E. coli*, *Proteus*, and *Klebsiella*.

Thrombophlebitis
- Superficial or deep venous thrombosis of legs may cause pyrexia.
- Caused by venous stasis.
- Diagnosis is made by the observation of a painful, swollen leg, usually accompanied by calf tenderness.

⚠ High risk of postpartum DVT and PE—be vigilant and get appropriate investigations urgently.

Respiratory complications
- Usually seen within the first 24 hours after delivery.
- Almost invariably in women delivered by CS.
- Complications due to atelectesis, aspiration, and/or bacterial pneumonia.

Abdominal wound infection
- Incidence following CS is about 6%.
- With prophylactic antibiotics, the rate of infection could be <2%.
- Risk factors include:
  - obesity
  - diabetes
  - corticosteroid therapy
  - poor haemostasis at surgery with subsequent haematoma.

⚠ VTE can also cause low-grade pyrexia and must always be considered in the differential diagnosis.

Puerperal pyrexia: management

Investigations

Investigations should be aimed at identifying the most likely source of infection, the causative organism and antibiotic sensitivity. These may include:

- FBC.
- Blood cultures.
- MSU.
- Swabs from cervix and lochia for *Chlamydia* and bacterial culture.
- Wound swabs.
- Throat swabs.
- Sputum culture and chest radiograph.

Management of puerperal pyrexia

Supportive

- Analgesics and anti-inflammatory drugs (NSAIDs).
- Wound care in cases of wound infection.
- Ice packs for pain from perineum or mastitis.

Antibiotics

- A regimen with activity against the *Bacteroides fragilis* group and other penicillin-resistant anaerobic bacteria is better than one without.
- There is no evidence that any one regimen is associated with fewer side effects, except that cephalosporins are associated with less diarrhoea.
- No specific recommendations can be made for the treatment of women who develop endometritis after receiving antibiotic prophylaxis for CS.
- Combination of clindamycin and an aminoglycoside (such as gentamicin) is appropriate for the treatment of endometritis.
- Tetracyclines should be avoided in breast-feeding women.
- Involvement of microbiologists is indicated in women who fail to respond to antibiotics.

Surgical

- Incision and drainage of breast abscess.
- Secondary repair of wound dehiscence.
- Drainage of pelvic haematomas and abscesses.

📖 French LM, Smaill FM. Antibiotic regimens for endometritis after delivery. *Cochrane Database of Systematic Reviews* 2004.

Prevention of puerperal pyrexia

- Women suspected to have a UTI during antenatal period should be investigated and any infection treated vigorously.
- Advice should be offered with regard to breast-feeding and care of breasts during the antenatal period.
- Prevention and treatment of pre-existing anaemia (especially important in women from developing countries).
- Rigid antiseptic measures taken during labour and delivery also help to eliminate infection, including:
  - hand washing and use of alcohol hand gel by midwives and doctor before examining the patient
  - examining in a sterile environment and using sterile instruments
  - use of antiseptic creams and lotions
  - catheterizing only when it is indicated and using all sterile precautions while introducing the catheter
- Prophylactic antibiotic administration at CS.
- Treatment with broad-spectrum antibiotics while waiting for the culture results.

Features of septicaemic shock

- Tachycardia (>90 bpm).
- Tachyopnoea (>20 breaths per minute).
- Pyrexia (>38° C).
- Hypothermia (<35° C).
- Hypotension (systolic BP <90 mm/Hg in the absence of other causes such as bleeding).
- Hypoxaemia.
- Poor peripheral perfusion (mottled skin).
- Oliguria.
- Metabolic acidosis.
- Elevated lactate.
- Positive blood cultures.
- Abnormal coagulation and bleeding.
- Abnormal liver and renal function.

Other postnatal problems

Pain

- Common in postpartum period.
- 'After-pains' due to uterine contractions cause lower central abdominal pain mainly in first 4 days.
- Perineal pain could be severe, especially after instrumental delivery, episiotomy, or vaginal tears:
  - increasing pain may be a sign of infection
  - if infected, antibiotics are prescribed depending on the local policy.

▶ Randomized controlled trials of oral analgesia for perineal pain show that paracetamol and NSAIDs are as effective as oral narcotic medications. Some may find topical application of local anaesthetic helpful.

Bladder problems

- **Urinary retention:** following instrumental delivery or extensive tears (especially periurethral), pain and oedema can cause voiding difficulties and retention. Reassurance along with analgesics is helpful in most situations. Occasionally, catheterization is required to protect the bladder from over distention. Urinary retention can also occur with an epidural as bladder sensation and the desire to void is masked.
- **UTI:** Low threshold for suspicion of UTI as catheterization during labour may predispose. Confirm with MSU and treat with appropriate antibiotics and plenty of oral fluids.

⚠ An indwelling catheter should be used after a dense regional block, such as a spinal, until full sensation returns to the lower body to protect the bladder from damage by over-distension.

Bowel problems

Constipation may continue into the puerperium. Pain and fear of wound disruption following perineal tears could further exacerbate the problem, as can opiate analgesia. Advice should be offered to increase the intake of fibre and fluids. Osmotic stool softeners such as lactulose may be helpful. Women with 3rd or 4th degree tears should be prescribed stool softeners and laxatives (see Chapter 6, 📖 p. 300).

Symphisis pubis discomfort

Symptoms include severe pubic and groin pain exacerbated by weight bearing. Most cases resolve by 6–8 weeks. Conservative approach includes rest, a belt that wraps around the femoral trochanters to discourage separation, weight-bearing assistance, and analgesics.

Maternal obstetric paralysis

This is very rare but manifests as intrapartum foot drop due to lumbosacral trunk compression by the fetal head at the pelvic brim. The primary pathology is predominantly demyelination, and recovery is usually complete in up to 5 months. Referral for neurological assessment and input is recommended.

Identifying mental health problems (see 📖 Chapter 12)

- Lack of social and psychological support during puerperium is a common problem and may occur in 7–30% of women in developed countries.
- Psychological well-being of women should be carefully and continually assessed in the postnatal period.

⚠ Mental illness is one of the leading causes of maternal death in the UK. The majority of these deaths are the result of suicide, which is itself most strongly associated with perinatal depression. Over half of suicides occur between 6 weeks prenatally and 12 weeks postnatally (see Chapter 12).

Other postnatal care issues

Lifestyle

Both care and information provided should be culturally appropriate. The cultural practices of women from ethnic minority groups should be incorporated into their postnatal care. Advice should be given regarding diet, exercise, breast-feeding, weight and shape, rest, and support for coping with changes.

Postpartum contraception

- Discussion of contraception should be a routine part of postpartum care.
- Contraception is not needed in first 3 weeks.
- Breast-feeding (lactational amenorrhoea) may be used as contraception (see Breast-feeding, 📖 p. 360).
- Breast-feeding women can start POP without the need for additional contraceptive protection.
- The combined oral contraceptive pill (COCP) should be avoided in lactating women as it can affect milk composition and increase the incidence of breast-feeding failure.
- Bottle-feeding women can start COCP 21 days postpartum.

▶ There may be an increased risk of VTE with earlier commencement of COCP.

Maternal immunization

Rubella

Women found to be seronegative on antenatal screening for rubella should receive rubella vaccination after delivery, before discharge from the maternity unit. Breast-feeding is not a contraindication for rubella immunization but women should be warned to avoid conceiving in the following 3 months although the risk is only theoretical.

Anti-D

The RCOG recommend the administration of anti-D 500iu to every non-sensitized RhD-negative woman within 72 hours after the delivery of an RhD-positive infant (see Chapter 3, 📖 p. 133).

Hepatitis B

There are no specific recommendations for postpartum vaccination of Hep B. However, it could be offered to individuals who are at increased risk because of their lifestyle or occupation. Neither pregnancy nor lactation should be considered a contraindication for Hep B vaccination of susceptible women. Neonatal vaccination is recommended for the babies of women at risk or who already have the virus.

Breastfeeding: overview

Breast-feeding is strongly supported by several international organizations and health-care institutions. WHO and UNICEF launched the Baby-friendly Hospital Initiative (BFHI) in 1992, to strengthen maternity practices to support breast-feeding. The foundation for the BFHI is the ten steps to successful breast-feeding described in *Protecting, Promoting and Supporting Breast-feeding*: a Joint WHO/UNICEF Statement. Breast milk provides enormous medical and physical benefits to the infant.

Breast-feeding rates in England and Wales at 1 week postpartum were only 57% among the 71% of women who initially breast-fed. These rates further decline to 43% at 6 weeks and only 22% of women were still giving breast milk at 6 months.

📖 WHO. *Evidence for the ten steps to successful breast-feeding*. www.who.int/child-adolescent-health/

Colostrum

- Thick yellow fluid produced from around 20 weeks gestation.
- It has a high concentration of secretory IgA.
- It is rich in proteins which play an important part in gut maturation and immunity for the infant.
- It is produced in small quantities following the birth of the baby.

Human milk

- The amount of milk produced rapidly ↑ to ~500 mL at 5 days postpartum
- It has 57–65 kcal/dL (2.4–2.7MJ/L) and is more energy efficient than formula milk.

Initiation and frequency

Initiation
- Skin-to-skin contact should start as soon as possible after delivery.
- Early contact ↑ breast-feeding both after delivery and 2–3 months later.
- Feeding within the first 2 hours after birth increases the duration of breast-feeding when compared to a delay of 4 hours or more.

Frequency
- Varies widely.
- Demand feeding should be encouraged because of its benefits of less weight loss in the immediate postpartum period and increased duration of breast-feeding subsequently.
- Frequent feeding is associated with less hyperbilirubinemia during the early neonatal period.
- For mothers, demand feeding helps to prevent engorgement, and breastfeeding is established more easily.

Demand feeding: facts and figures

- Exclusively breast-fed term infants feed a median of 8 times/day:
  - 6 times during the day, and twice in the night.
- Feeds tend to be infrequent in the first 24–48 hours and could be as few as 3 feeds in the first 24 hours (this should not cause concern in an otherwise well baby).
- The frequency increases gradually and reaches peak around 5th day of life.
- WHO recommends exclusive breast-feeding for 4–6 months, with introduction of appropriate complementary foods after this period.

Breastfeeding: benefits

Human breast milk contains numerous protective factors against infectious disease and may influence immune system development. These include the effect of colostrum on immunity, fewer diarrhoeal diseases, the benefits of omega-3 fatty acids on visual developments in small infants, as well as improved bonding and less breast disease for the mother later.

For the infant

Gastrointestinal illness

Infants who are exclusively breast-fed for 6 months experience less morbidity from gastrointestinal infection than those who are mixed breast-fed at 3–4 months.

UTIs

Breast milk is a part of the natural defence against UTIs.

Respiratory infection

Exclusive breast-feeding protects against chest infections.

Atopic illness

Breast-fed babies are less likely to have atopic illnesses such as eczema and asthma

Leukemias

Breast-feeding is associated with a reduced risk of childhood acute leukaemia, acute lymphoblastic leukaemia, Hodgkin's disease and neuroblastoma in childhood.

Giardiasis

Children born to non-immune mothers are at significantly higher risk of acquiring *Giardia* infection and developing giardiasis with more severe symptoms compared with children of immune mothers.

Intelligence

It remains unclear whether the child's intelligence is affected by breast-feeding, although it remains an unequalled way of providing ideal nutrition.

For the mother

Uterine involution

Breast-feeding helps in uterine involution and reduces the risk of post-partum haemorrhage.

Amenorrhoea and contraception

- Lactational amenorrhoea and full or nearly full breast-feeding for up to 6 months is nearly 99% effective as contraception.
- At 12 months the effectiveness during amenorrhoea dropped to 97%.
- Amenorrhoea can be helpful for anaemia in developing countries.

Other benefits

Breastfeeding protects the mother against premenopausal breast cancer, ovarian cancer, and osteoporosis.

Breastfeeding: potential problems

Inadequate milk supply

Inadequate milk supply
- <1% of women are physiologically incapable of producing an adequate milk supply.
- Treatment for insufficient milk includes: adequate fluids, nutrition, secure and private environment, dopamine antagonists, thyrotropin-releasing hormone, and oxytocin.

Problems with milk flow

Breast engorgement, mastitis, and breast abscess (see 📖 p. 365)
- Limitations on feeding frequency and duration.
- Problems with positioning the baby at the breast.
- Allowing baby unrestricted access to the breast is the most effective method of treating.

Sore or cracked nipples
- It could be because of incorrect attachment of the baby to the breast.
- It may be necessary to rest the breast and express the breast milk manually until the crack has healed.

Lactation after breast cancer

- There will be little or no enlargement of the treated breast during pregnancy.
- The ability to lactate and breastfeed from untreated breast remains normal.
- Tamoxifen inhibits milk production.

Drugs that may reduce milk production

- Progestins.
- Oestrogens.
- Ethanol.
- Bromocriptine.
- Ergotamine.
- Cabergoline.
- Pseudoephedrine.

Breast problems

Mastitis (non-infective)

- Results from obstruction of milk drainage from one section of the breast, which may be due to:
  - restriction of feeding
  - a badly positioned baby
  - blocked ducts
  - compression from fingers holding the breast or from wearing too small a bra.
- Is characterized by swollen, red and painful area on breast, tachycardia, pyrexia, and an aching, flu-like feeling, often accompanied by shivering and rigors.
- Resolves with relieving the obstruction by continuing to breast-feed with correct positioning of the baby.
- *Mastitis (infective)*
- If non-infective mastitis is not managed appropriately, it may become infected.
- *Staphylococcus aureus* is the most common organism involved.
- The antibiotics that should be used include penicillinase-resistant penicillins (e.g. cloxacillin, flucloxacillin, amoxicillin + clavulanate) or cefalosporins (cefalexin, cefadrine, cefaclor).
- Breast-feeding should be continued.

Breast abscess

- Possible complication of inappropriately managed infective mastitis.
- It may need surgical drainage under anaesthetic.
- In severe cases breastfeeding may have to cease on the affected side.

Drugs and breastfeeding

Almost all drugs pass to some extent in breast milk, but the significance of this depends on factors such as the degree of passage into milk, the amount of milk ingested by the infant, if the infant absorbs the drug, and if the drug affects the infant. There are limited human studies to advise on which drugs are contraindicated in pregnancy.

▶ Prescribe medication only when absolutely indicated. Choose ones with shorter half-lives, less toxicity, those commonly used in infants, and those with reduced bioavailability. Only a few medications are unsafe.

Medications with poor oral bioavailability and low risk

- Heparin.
- Insulin.
- Aminoglycoside antibiotics.
- Third generation cephalosporins.
- Omeprazole and lansoprazole.
- Inhaled steroids and beta agonists.

Drugs generally contraindicated in breastfeeding mothers

- Amiodarone.
- Antineoplastic.
- Chloramphenicol.
- Ergotamine.
- Cabergoline.
- Ergot alkaloids.
- Iodides.
- Methotrexate.
- Lithium.
- Tetracycline.
- Pseudoephedrine.

Drugs to avoid in breastfeeding mothers

- Acebutolol.
- ACE inhibitors (except captopril).
- Alcohol.
- Caffeine.
- Cocaine.
- Marijuana.
- Fluoxetine.
- Iodine.
- Sulphonamides.

Viruses and breastfeeding

Human immunodeficiency virus (HIV)
HIV can be transmitted through breast milk. The risk factors are:
- Maternal viral load.
- Duration of breastfeeding.
- Oral lesions in infant and maternal breast lesions.

⚠ In developed countries, breastfeeding by HIV-infected mother should be avoided.

Human lymphotropic virus (HTLV-1)
Breast-fed babies of HTLV-1 infected mothers are likely to become infected, especially with prolonged breast-feeding.

⚠ HTLV-1 seropositive women are advised not to breastfeed.

Hepatitis B virus (HBV)
Infants born to HBV-positive mothers, already exposed to maternal blood, amniotic fluid, and vaginal secretions during delivery, may breast-feed. Babies of all mothers positive for HBV surface antigen should be immunized at birth. Babies of mothers positive for HBVe antigen are also given immunoglobulins as additional protection.

▶ Breast-feeding does not appear to increase the rate of infection among infants.

Herpes simplex virus (HSV)
If there are no breast lesions, breastfeeding should be encouraged.

Chickenpox/varicella
If the mother contracts chickenpox while breastfeeding, she should continue to breastfeed, because the antibodies in her milk confer immunity against chickenpox to her baby. This passive immunization may even spare the baby from symptoms of chickenpox.

Cytomegalovirus (CMV)
CMV is possibly the most commonly detectable virus in human milk. No serious illness or clinical symptoms in neonates secondary to breast-feeding has been reported.

Rubella
Can be passed on to the infant if mother has active infection. However, the baby does not become ill as transmission of maternal antibodies serves as natural vaccine. If the mother is immunized to rubella postpartum, the breast-feeding infant will not show symptoms of the illness.

Obstetric emergencies

Sudden maternal collapse

⚠ **Immediate maternal resuscitation is vital**

A Airway: open airway with head tilt and chin lift; a jaw thrust may be required (care must be taken if a cervical spine injury is suspected).

B Breathing: Assess for chest movements and breath sounds and feel for breathing. If no breathing, put out cardiac arrest call and give 2 rescue breaths.

C Circulation: carotid pulse should be checked and circulation optimized by aggressive intravenous fluids and blood transfusion if indicated.
► CPR should be initiated as necessary.
⚠ In a pregnant patient, a lateral tilt to relieve aortocaval compression is essential.

D Drugs: to maintain circulation, combat infection, antidotes if drug overdose, anticoagulants in cases of massive embolism.

E Environment: avoid injury (eclampsia), ensure safety of the patient and staff.

F Fetus: once maternal condition is stable, assess fetal well-being and plan delivery as appropriate.

General investigations

- **History:** from the patient or her relatives.
- **Observations:** BP, pulse, respiration, oxygen saturation, temperature, and urine output every 15 minutes.
- **Bloods:** FBC, coagulation profile, U+Es, LFTs, uric acid, group and save or cross-match, and blood glucose.

Specific investigations

- If a cardiorespiratory cause is suspected:
  - ECG, chest radiograph, arterial blood gases.
- If pulmonary embolism is suspected:
  - Doppler ultrasound of calf veins, ventilation (Q) scan or ventilation/perfusion (V/Q) scan.
- If intracranial pathology is suspected:
  - cerebral imaging (CT/MRI).

Treatment

Specific treatment depends on the cause. It is important to ensure multi-disciplinary input early to optimize outcome. If bleeding, the woman may require immediate laparotomy to control it and anaesthetic and ITU assistance are urgently required. If focal neurological signs are present, early neurosurgical input may save lives.

Some causes of sudden maternal collapse

Obstetric
- Massive obstetric haemorrhage (⚠ may be concealed):
  - placenta praevia
  - placental abruption
  - postpartum haemorrhage (PPH)
  - uterine rupture
  - supralevator haematoma following genital tract trauma.
- Severe pre-eclampsia with intracranial bleeding.
- Eclampsia.
- Amniotic fluid embolism.
- Neurogenic shock due to uterine inversion.
- Surgical complications:
  - bleeding after Caesarean section (CS)
  - broad ligament haematoma.
- Severe sepsis due to chorioamnionitis.
- Cardiac failure due to peripartum cardiomyopathy.

Medical/surgical causes
- Massive pulmonary embolism.
- Cardiac failure:
  - structural or functional cardiac disorders
  - myocardial infarction.
- Shock:
  - anaphylactic
  - septic.
- Intra-abdominal bleeding:
  - hepatic
  - splenic
  - aortic rupture.
- Intracerebral haemorrhage.
- Overdosage or substance abuse.
- Metabolic/endocrine:
  - diabetic coma.
- Cerebral infection:
  - encephalitis
  - cerebral malaria.

Cord prolapse

In cord prolapse the umbilical cord protrudes below the presenting part after the rupture of membranes. This may cause compression of the umbilical vessels by the presenting part and vasospasm from exposure of the cord. These acutely compromise fetal circulation and if delivery is not immediate may lead to neurological sequelae or fetal death.

> **Predisposing factors for cord prolapse**
>
> - Abnormal lie or presentation (transverse lie, breech).
> - Multiple pregnancy.
> - Acute polyhydramnios.
> - Prematurity.
> - High head.
> - Unusually long umbilical cord.

Prevention

When the presenting part is high or if there is polyhydramnios, a stabilizing induction (see 📖 Chapter 6, p. 270) may be performed. During artificial rupture of membranes (ARM), if cord presentation is detected (i.e. presence of cord below the presenting part with intact membranes), the procedure should be abandoned and senior help should be summoned.

> **Management of cord prolapse**
>
> - ⚠The fetus should be delivered as rapidly as possible; this may be by instrumental delivery or category 1 CS.
> - Prevent further cord compression during transfer for CS:
>   - knee-to-chest position
>   - fill the bladder with about 500 mL of warm normal saline to displace the presenting part upwards (remember to unclamp the catheter before entering the peritoneal cavity at CS)
>   - a hand in the vagina to push up the presenting part (may not always be practical).
> - Prevent spasm by avoiding exposure of the cord:
>   - reduce the cord into the vagina to maintain body temperature and insert a warm saline swab to prevent the cord coming back out.
>   ⚠ It is important to avoid handling the cord as much as possible, as this provokes further spasms.
> - Tocolytics (terbutaline 250 micrograms SC) may be administered to abolish uterine contractions and improve oxygenation to the fetus:
>   - may cause PPH at CS due to uterine atony; tackle with oxytocics but propranolol 1 mg intravenously may be given if needed.
> - Neonatal team must be present at delivery.

Shoulder dystocia: overview

Shoulder dystocia is defined as any delivery that requires additional obstetric manoeuvres after the gentle downward traction on the head has failed to deliver the shoulders. It complicates about 1:200 deliveries, and has the potential for serious fetal complications.

Complications of shoulder dystocia

Fetal

- Hypoxia and neurological injury (cerebral palsy).
- Brachial plexus palsy.
- Fracture of clavicle or humerus.
- Intracranial haemorrhage.
- Cervical spine injury.
- Rarely, fetal death.

Maternal

- PPH.
- Genital tract trauma including 3rd and 4th degree perineal tears.

Mechanism

- Usually the anterior shoulder is impacted against the symphysis pubis often due to the failure of internal rotation of the shoulders.
- Rarely, the posterior shoulder may be impacted against the sacral promontory resulting in bilateral impaction, this causes greater problems at delivery.

Risk factors

Prediction of shoulder dystocia by the use of risk factors has a poor predictive value. It is estimated that only 50% of shoulder dystocia is associated with a birth weight of >4 kg. However, it is important to be aware of the antepartum and intrapartum risk factors, so that shoulder dystocia may be anticipated. This will allow senior input being made available.

Risk factors for shoulder dystocia

Antenatal

- Previous history of shoulder dystocia.
- Fetal macrosomia.
- BMI >30 and excessive weight gain in pregnancy.
- Diabetes mellitus.
- Post-term pregnancy.

Intrapartum

- Lack of progress in late first stage of labour.
- Induction of labour.
- Prolonged 2nd stage.
- Instrumental vaginal delivery (especially rotational deliveries).
- Oxytocin augmentation of labour.

Shoulder dystocia: management

Prompt, skilful, and well-rehearsed manoeuvres may improve outcome. An mnemonic '**HELPERR**' (ALSO course) has been suggested to aid in remembering the sequence. The main objectives are to facilitate the entry of the anterior (or posterior) shoulder into the pelvis and to ensure rotation of the shoulders to the larger oblique or transverse diameter of the pelvis.

H Call for help (including additional midwife, senior obstetrician, neonatologist, anaesthetist).

E Episiotomy—remember shoulder dystocia is a bony problem but an episiotomy may help with internal manoeuvres.

L Legs into Mc Roberts' (hyperflexed at the hips with thighs abducted and externally rotated).

P Suprapubic pressure applied to the posterior aspect of the anterior shoulder (must know which side the fetal back is on) to dislodge it from under the symphysis pubis; if continuous pressure fails, a rocking movement may be tried.

E Enter pelvis for internal manoeuvres, which include:
- pressure exerted on the posterior aspect of anterior shoulder to adduct and rotate the shoulders to the larger oblique diameter (Rubin II)
- if this fails combine it with pressure on the anterior aspect of the posterior shoulder (Woods' screw)
- if this fails, reversing the manoeuvre may be tried with pressure on anterior aspect of anterior shoulder and posterior aspect of posterior shoulder in the opposite direction (reverse Woods' screw)

R Release of posterior arm by flexing the elbow, getting hold of the fetal hand, and sweeping the fetal arm across the chest and face to release the posterior shoulder.

R Roll over to 'all fours' may help aid delivery by the changes brought about in the pelvic dimensions (Gaskin manoeuvre).

Other manoeuvres

- **Zanvanelli:** replacement of the head into the vagina by reversing the mechanism of labour (i.e. flexion and 'de-restitution') and performing a CS may be used as a last resort. Tocolysis may be required to facilitate this procedure.
- **Symphysiotomy:** may be performed to 'open up' the pelvic girdle. This can result in severe maternal morbidity (urethral injury, incontinence, altered gait, and chronic pelvic pain). Urethral injury should be avoided by displacing the urethra with a metal catheter at the time of symphysiotomy.

📖 Advanced Life Support in Obstetrics (ALSO) course. www.also.org.uk

Other considerations in the event of a shoulder dystocia

⚠ It is essential not to exert traction on the head without dis-impaction of the shoulders as this increases the risk of brachial plexus injury.

- Time-keeping is essential and it is good practice to allocate a member of the team to document the timeline of events.
- The paediatric team must be called urgently as a need for neonatal resuscitation should be anticipated.
- PPH should also be anticipated and prophylactic measures considered, such as a 40 IU oxytocin infusion.
- The genital tract should be carefully examined for trauma.
- Carefully document the timing and sequence of events, who was involved and what each person did, as soon as possible afterwards.
- It is important to explain the delivery and discuss the outcome with the parents after the event.
- An incident report form should be filled for risk management.
- If an injury has occurred, it may become a medico-legal issue, making documentation even more important.

Fetal distress of second twin

See 📖 Chapter 2 (Multiple pregnancy: labour, p. 79).

Common causes of distress in the 2nd twin include:

- Placental abruption (indicated by profuse bleeding).
- Cord prolapse.
- Tetanic uterine contraction.

▶ The 2nd twin must be delivered by the fastest, safe route.
- If it is **cephalic** and if the presenting part is at or below the ischial spines, an instrumental vaginal delivery may be attempted. In preterm twins (before 34 weeks), a ventouse delivery should be avoided.
- With a **breech** presentation, a 'breech extraction' may be attempted by an experienced clinician. This involves grasping the feet of the fetus and gently pulling it through the vagina. In modern obstetric practice, 2nd twin with fetal distress is the only acceptable indication for this procedure.
- With a **transverse** lie, internal podalic version with breech extraction may be attempted.

If vaginal delivery is not possible, immediate CS (category 1) should be performed.

Massive obstetric haemorrhage: causes

This is an important cause of maternal morbidity and mortality. Identification of risk factors, institution of preventive measures, and prompt and appropriate management of blood loss is likely to improve outcome. It is also important to remember that all bleeding can be concealed.

▶ Massive obstetric haemorrhage refers to the loss of 30–40% (generally about 2 L) of the patient's blood volume. This may be caused by an insult leading to hypovolaemia (then coagulopathy) or from direct coagulation failure (leading to hypovolaemia).

Consequences of massive obstetric haemorrhage include:

- Acute hypovolemia.
- Sudden and rapid cardiovascular decompensation.
- Disseminated intravascular coagulation (DIC).
- Iatrogenic complications associated with fluid replacement and multiple blood transfusions.
- Pulmonary oedema.
- Transfusion reactions.
- Adult respiratory distress syndrome (ARDS).
- Sheehan's syndrome (hypopituitarism).

Causes of massive obstetric haemorrhage

Antepartum
- Placental abruption.
- Placenta praevia.
- Severe chorioamnionitis or septicaemia.
- Severe pre-eclampsia (hepatic rupture).
- Retained dead fetus.
- Associated with ectopic pregnancy.

Intrapartum
- Intrapartum abruption.
- Uterine rupture.
- Amniotic fluid embolism.
- Complications of CS; angular or broad ligament tears.
- Morbidly adherent placenta (accreta).

Postpartum
- Primary PPH is usually due to:
  - atonic uterus ('tone')
  - genital tract trauma ('trauma')
  - coagulopathy ('thrombin')
  - retained products of conception ('tissue').
- Secondary PPH is due to:
  - infection (often associated with retained products of conception)
  - rarely, gestational trophoblastic disease
  - very rarely, uterine arteriovenonous malformation including a pseudo-aneurysm.

Massive obstetric haemorrhage: pathophysiology

Pregnancy is associated with an increase in blood volume (see 📖 Chapter 1, Physiology of pregnancy: haemodynamics, p. 000). The blood flow to the pregnant uterus at term is about 500–800 mL/min with the placental circulation accounting for about 400 mL/min. It is therefore quite easy for a large proportion of the circulating volume to be lost in a short time.

A loss of about 500–1000 mL (10–15% of blood volume) is usually well tolerated by a fit, healthy young woman, as she is able to maintain her cardiovascular parameters by effective compensatory mechanisms until about 30–40% of the blood volume is lost.

Blood loss >1000 mL may result in:

- Acute hypovolaemia.
- Shock with sudden reduction in perfusion to vital organs.
- Loss of clotting factors ('washout phenomenon').
- DIC.
- Hypoxia leading to anaerobic metabolism, accumulation of lactic acid, and metabolic acidosis.
- Multi-organ dysfunction/failure.

Pulse rate rather than blood pressure is more useful in assessing the degree of blood loss, especially with occult loss such as concealed abruption or scar rupture. In these situations, the degree of haemodynamic instability may be out of proportion to the visually estimated blood loss. Table 10.1 shows cardiovascular responses to blood loss.

Disseminated intravascular coagulopathy (DIC)

The main cause of DIC is massive blood loss but it can occur with other conditions such as amniotic fluid embolism. It occurs due to the depletion of fibrinogen, platelets, and coagulation factors that are consumed or lost with the blood. Infusions of replacement fluids further dilute the remaining coagulation factors and combined with hypotension-mediated endothelial injury may trigger DIC.

The most useful tests to diagnose DIC are fibrin degradation products (FDPs), fibrinogen, PTT, and APTT. Early involvement of a senior haematologist is vital to advise on appropriate replacement of blood products.

- **Fresh frozen plasma (FFP):** contains all the clotting factors required. Ideally, 4 units of FFP should be given with each 6 units of rapidly transfused blood.
- **Cryoprecipitate:** contains more fibrinogen but lacks antithrombin III which is often depleted in massive obstetric haemorrhages.
- **Platelet concentrate:** rarely indicated, but may be required if surgical intervention is planned.
- **Recombinant activated factor VII:** used successfully in severe coagulopathy but is expensive and not always readily available.

Table 10.1 Blood loss and cardiovascular parameters

Blood loss	Heart rate	Systolic BP	Tissue perfusion
10–15%	Increased	Normal	Postural hypotension
15–30%	Increased +	Normal	Peripheral vasoconstriction
30–40%	Increased ++	70–80 mmHg	Pallor, oliguria, confusion, restlessness
40%+	Increased+++	<60 mmHg	Collapse, anuria, dyspnoea

Massive obstetric haemorrhage: resuscitation

Massive obstetric haemorrhage is a life-threatening emergency requiring swift and appropriate treatment. Most units will have a local guideline for its management which will take into account such things as local hospital geography and staff availability. It should include such details as who to contact and agreed timescales for laboratory results.

Management should consist of immediate resuscitation with restoration of the circulating volume and rapid treatment of the underlying cause in order to stop ongoing blood loss.

Initial measures for resuscitation

- Call for help, which should include alerting the senior obstetrician, anaesthetists, haematologist, hospital porter, blood bank, and theatres.
- Left lateral tilt if antepartum, to relieve venocaval compression and improve venous return.
- High-flow facial oxygen (regardless of oxygen saturation).
- Assess airway and respiratory effort—intubation may be indicated to protect the airway if there is a decreased level of consciousness due to hypotension.
- Two large-bore IV cannulae (14 gauge):
  - take blood whilst cannulating for FBC, cross-match, U+Es, LFTs, coagulopathy screen
  - start intravenous crystalloids to correct hypovolemia.
- Catheterize and measure hourly urine output.
- Blood transfusion;
  - O Rhesus –ve blood can be used immediately until cross-matched blood is available.
- Replace clotting factors:
  - FFP (4 units for every 6 units of blood)
  - cryoprecipitate
  - recombinant activated factor VII if indicated.
- As soon as appropriate in the resuscitation process, transfer the woman to a place where there is adequate space, lighting, and equipment to continue treatment (usually theatre).
- Assess need for central venous pressure (CVP) line.

⚠ One member of the team should be assigned to record the vital signs, urinary output, type and quantity of fluid replacement, drugs given, and timeline of events.

▶ Once the bleeding has been stopped and the woman stabilized, she should be managed in a high dependency unit (HDU) or intensive care unit (ICU).

Massive obstetric haemorrhage: medical management

The exact management plan will depend on the cause of the bleeding. The most common cause is uterine atony, often secondary to retained tissue, but genital tract trauma and underlying coagulation disorders must also be considered.

Principles for stopping the bleeding

- Empty uterus (fetus or tissue).
- Treat uterine atony (physically, medically, surgically).
- Repair genital tract trauma.

Medical management of uterine atony

⚠ Should be accompanied by physical attempts to contract the uterus such as rubbing up contractions and bimanual compression if necessary.

- 500 micrograms of ergometrine is given IV (may be given IM if difficulties with IV access).
- Start oxytocin infusion (40 IU).
- If the bleeding does not stop, 10 units of oxytocin may be given IV.
- If the atony continues, carboprost 250 micrograms IM is given in the thigh or directly into the myometrium and repeated at 15 minute intervals up to a total of 4 doses.
- If the bleeding still persists (or ergometrine is contraindicated) then 800 micrograms of misoprostol (tablets) is given rectally.

▶ If all these measures fail, retained tissue must be considered and examination under anaesthesia with possible further surgical management is indicated without delay.

General interventions in the management of massive obstetric haemorrhage

- Empty uterus
  - deliver fetus
  - remove placenta or retained tissue.
- Massage uterus (to 'rub up' a contraction).
- Give drugs to ↑ uterine contraction:
  - oxytocin 40 IU infusion
  - ergometrine 500 micrograms IV or IM
  - misoprostol 800–1000 micrograms
  - carboprost 250 micrograms
- Apply bimanual compression if necessary.
- Repair any genital tract injuries (including cervical tears).
- Uterine tamponade with a Rusch balloon.
- Laparotomy:
  - if bleeding from placental bed, may need over-sewing and insertion of a Rusch balloon
  - if uterus is atonic, not responding to drug treatment but the bleeding is ↓ with compression, a B-Lynch or vertical compression suture should be placed
  - internal iliac or uterine artery ligation (proceeds to hysterectomy in 50% of cases)
  - uterine artery embolization may be helpful but is not always an option in emergency situations
  - total or subtotal hysterectomy.

▶ Compression of the aorta may be used to gain temporary control while a definitive treatment gets under way.

Massive obstetric haemorrhage: surgical management

Tamponade test

A Rusch ballon catheter, Sengstaken–Blakemore tube, or Cooke's balloon is inserted into the uterine cavity and filled with 100–500 mL of warm saline (warm saline accelerates the clotting process). If the bleeding is controlled then the balloon is left in situ for 12–24 hours and removed. This test is therapeutic as it stops bleeding in 80% of cases, and prognostic in revealing within 15 minutes whether further surgical intervention is needed.

Interventions after laparotomy

- ⚠ Ensure that the uterine cavity is definitely empty as even very small pieces of retained tissue can cause atony.
- If the bleeding is from large placental sinuses following CS then under-sewing the placental bed ± insertion of a Rusch balloon may control the bleeding.
- If the bleeding is from uterine atony unresponsive to drug treatment but which ↓ with manual compression, a B-Lynch or vertical compression suture should be attempted (this provides continuous compression and reduces the blood flow into the uterus)
- Systematic pelvic devascularization by ligation of uterine, tubal branch of the ovarian or anterior division of internal iliac arteries:
  - ligation of uterine artery and utero-ovarian artery anastomosis will not control the bleeding from the vaginal branch of the internal iliac artery which supplies the lower segment of the uterus
  - internal iliac artery ligation will help in controlling both the uterine artery and the vaginal branch bleeding (bilateral ligation results in 85% reduction in the pulse pressure and 50% reduction in blood flow and bleeding is reduced by 50%).
- Hysterectomy is the last option:
  - sub-total hysterectomy is safer and quicker to perform
  - if the bleeding is from the lower segment (placenta previa, accreta or tears) then total hysterectomy is carried out.

⚠ The decision to carry out hysterectomy should not be unduly delayed as this can result in the death of the mother

Arterial embolization for massive obstetric haemorrhage

Advantages
- Less invasive than laparotomy.
- Helps to preserve fertility.
- Quicker recovery than laparotomy.

Disadvantages
- Only available in a few centres.
- It may not be possible to get the required equipment to the obstetric theatres or to transfer a woman to the radiology department.
- Appropriately trained interventional radiologists must be available.

Method
- A catheter is inserted through the femoral artery and advanced above the bifurcation of the aorta and a contrast dye is injected to identify the bleeding vessels.
- The catheter is then directed to the bleeding vessel and embolized with gelatin sponge, which is usually reabsorbed in about 10 days.

▶ If excessive bleeding is anticipated (e.g. major placenta previa with accreta), prophylactic interventional radiology can be a planned procedure where balloons are placed in the internal iliac or uterine vessels in advance if embolization is required.

Venous thromboembolism: overview

Background

Venous thromboembolism (VTE) is a leading cause of maternal morbidity and mortality in developed countries. In the UK, VTE accounted for 41 maternal deaths in 2003–2005. Thromboembolic events include venous thrombosis (DVT) of the leg, calf, or pelvis, and pulmonary embolism (PE).

- Incidence of pregnancy-associated VTE is 1–2:1000 pregnancies.
- Incidence of DVT is 3 times higher than that of PE.
- Emergency CS is associated with a higher incidence of DVT than elective CS or vaginal delivery.
- Thromboembolic disease can occur at any point in pregnancy:
  - antenatal DVT is more common than postpartum DVT
  - the event rate of VTE is higher in the puerperium.
- DVT leads to PE in approximately 16% of untreated patients.

Women with past history of VTE

The risk of VTE in pregnancy is ↑ in women with past history of VTE.
- For a single previous thrombosis with no known thrombophilia, the risk of VTE in pregnancy is increased from about 0.1% to 3%.
- The risk is higher if the woman has thrombophilia or if the previous VTE was in an unusual site or unprovoked.
- Women with previous VTE should be screened for thrombophilia before pregnancy.

Inherent pregnancy associated risk factors for VTE

Pregnancy itself is a risk factor for VTE, due to:
- Venous stasis in the lower limbs
- Possible trauma to the pelvic veins at the time of delivery
- Changes in the coagulation system including:
  - ↑ in procoagulant factors (factors X, VIII, and fibrinogen)
  - ↓ in endogenous anticoagulant activity
  - suppression of fibrinolysis
  - significant ↓ in protein S activity.

▶ All pregnant women are at risk of thrombosis from early in the first trimester until at least 6 weeks postpartum. Some women are at even higher risk during pregnancy because they have one or more additional risk factors.

📖 Saving mothers' lives. The 7th report on confidential enquiries into maternal deaths in the UK; CEMACH 2007. www.cemach.org.uk.

📖 RCOG guideline 28: Thromboembolic disease in pregnancy and the puerperium. http://www.rcog.org.uk

Other risk factors for VTE

Pre-existing risk factors
- Previous VTE.
- Congenital thrombophilia:
  - antithrombin deficiency
  - protein C deficiency
  - protein S deficiency
  - factor V Leiden
  - prothrombin gene variant.
- Acquired thrombophilia (antiphospholipid syndrome):
  - lupus anticoagulant
  - anticardiolipin antibodies.
- Age >35 years.
- Obesity (BMI > 30) either before pregnancy or in early pregnancy.
- Parity > 4.
- Gross varicose veins.
- Paraplegia.
- Sickle cell disease.
- Inflammatory disorders, e.g. inflammatory bowel disease.
- Medical disorders, e.g. nephrotic syndrome, cardiac diseases.
- Myeloproliferative disorders, e.g. essential thrombocythaemia, polycythaemia vera.

New onset or transient risk factors
- Ovarian hyperstimulation syndrome.
- Hyperemesis.
- Dehydration.
- Long-haul travel.
- Severe infection, e.g. pyelonephritis.
- Immobility (> 4 days bed rest).
- Pre-eclampsia.
- Prolonged labour.
- Midcavity instrumental delivery.
- Excessive blood loss.
- Surgical procedure in pregnancy or puerperium, e.g. evacuation of retained products of conception, postpartum sterilization.
- Immobility after delivery.

Venous thromboembolism: prevention

- LMWHs are the agents of choice for antenatal thromboprophylaxis.
- They are as effective as UFH in pregnancy, and safer.
- Monitoring anti-Xa levels is not usually required when using LMWH for thromboprophylaxis.
- In antithrombin deficiency, anti-Xa monitoring is critical, as higher doses of LMWH may be necessary.

Indications and duration of thromboprophylaxis

- **Previous VTE:** LMWH for 6 weeks postpartum.
- **Previous recurrent VTE or previous VTE and family history (1st-degree) of VTE:** LMWH antenatally, and for ≥ 6 weeks postpartum
- **Previous VTE and thrombophilia:** LMWH antenatally and for ≥6 weeks postpartum
- **Asymptomatic inherited or acquired thrombophilia:** thromboprophylaxis depends on the specific thrombophilia and the presence of other risk factors
- **Antithrombin III deficiency:** merits higher doses of LMWH as it associated with a 30% risk of VTE in pregnancy
- **≥3 persisting 'moderate' risk factors:** LMWH for 5 days postpartum.

▶ Women should be reassessed before or during labour for risk factors for VTE. Age >35 years and BMI >30 or body weight >90 kg are important independent risk factors for postpartum VTE. The combination of these risk factors with any other risk factor for VTE or the presence of two other persisting risk factors indicate the use of LMWH for 3–5 days postpartum.

Thromboprophylaxis; other considerations

- All women should undergo an assessment of risk factors for VTE in early pregnancy.
- This should be repeated if they develop any other problems.
- Women with previous VTE should be screened for inherited and acquired thrombophilia, ideally before pregnancy.
- Immobilization and dehydration should be avoided.
- Antenatal thromboprophylaxis should begin as early as practical.
- Postpartum prophylaxis should begin as soon as possible after delivery (with precautions after use of regional anaesthesia).
- Excess blood loss and blood transfusion are risk factors for VTE, so thromboprophylaxis should be commenced or re-instituted as soon as the immediate risk of haemorrhage is reduced.

📖 RCOG guideline 37: Thromboprophylaxis during pregnancy, labour and after vaginal delivery. http://www.rcog.org.uk

Risk assessment profile for VTE after CS

Low risk—early mobilization and hydration
- Elective CS, uncomplicated pregnancy and no other risk factors:

Moderate risk—consider one of a variety of prophylactic measures
- Age >35 years.
- Obesity (>80 kg).
- Parity 4 or more.
- Labour >12 hours.
- Gross varicose veins.
- Current infection.
- Pre-eclampsia.
- Immobility prior to surgery (>4 days).
- Major current illness (such as heart or lung disease, cancer, inflammatory bowel disease, nephritic syndrome).
- Emergency CS in labour.

High risk—Heparin prophylaxis ± leg stockings
- Three or more moderate risk factors.
- Extended major pelvic or abdominal surgery (such as Caesarean hysterectomy).
- Personal or family history of DVT, PE, or thrombophilia.
- Paralysis of the lower limbs.
- Antiphospholipid antibody syndrome (cardiolipin antibody or lupus anticoagulant).

📖 RCOG guideline 37: Thromboprophylaxis during pregnancy, labour and after vaginal delivery. http://www.rcog.org.uk

Venous thromboembolism: diagnosis

Symptoms and signs of VTE

Deep vein thrombosis
- Leg pain or discomfort (especially in the left leg).
- Swelling.
- Tenderness.
- Pyrexia.
- Erythema, increased skin temperature and oedema.
- lower abdominal pain (high DVT).
- Elevated WBC.

Pulmonary embolism
- Dyspnoea.
- Collapse.
- chest pain.
- Haemoptysis.
- Faintness.
- Raised JVP.
- Focal signs in chest.
- Symptoms and signs associated with DVT.

⚠ In pregnancy there should be high level of suspicion for women presenting with any symptoms and urgent investigation undertaken. If VTE is suspected, treatment should be commenced while diagnostic tests are awaited.

Investigations
- Thrombophilia screen.
- FBC, U+E, LFTs.
- Coagulation screen.

Diagnostic imaging
- Ultrasound (compression or duplex)
- Contrast venography with shielding of the uterus
- MRI.

If PE suspected:
- ECG
- CXR
- Arterial blood gases (ABG)
- Ventilation/perfusion lung scanning (V/Q or Q scan)
- spiral CT/MRI scan
- bilateral duplex ultrasound leg examinations.

If diagnostic imaging reports a low risk of VTE, yet there is high clinical suspicion, anticoagulant treatment should be continued, with repeat testing in 1 week. Among women with clinically suspected VTE, <50% have the diagnosis confirmed as some of the symptoms and signs are commonly found in normal pregnancy.

D-dimers and pregnancy

- D-dimer is now used as a screening test for VTE in the non-pregnant where it has a high negative predictive value.
- D-dimer can be elevated due to the physiological changes in the coagulation system and particularly if there is a concomitant problem such as pre-eclampsia.
- Thus a 'positive' D-dimer test in pregnancy is not necessarily consistent with VTE.
- However, a low level of D-dimer is likely to suggest that there is no VTE.

Venous thromboembolism: treatment

Anticoagulation

Unfractionated heparin (UFH)

- Has been the standard treatment in the initial management of VTE including massive PE. The regimen is:
- Loading dose of 5000 IU, followed by continuous IV infusion of 1000–2000 IU/h with an initial infusion concentration of 1000 IU/mL.
- Measure APTT level 6 hours after the loading dose, then at least daily.
- The therapeutic target APTT ratio is usually 1.5–2.5× the average laboratory control value.
- Prolonged UFH use during pregnancy, may result in osteoporosis, fractures, and allergic skin reactions.

Low molecular weight heparins (LMWHs)

- More effective than UFH, with lower mortality and fewer haemorrhagic complications in non-pregnant subjects.
- LMWHs are as effective as UFH for treatment of PE.
- A twice-daily dosage regimen for LMWHs is recommended in the treatment of VTE in pregnancy, (enoxaparin 1 mg/kg twice daily; dalteparin 100 units/kg twice daily up to a maximum of 18 000 units/24 hours).
- Long-term users of LMWHs have a lower risk of osteoporosis and bone fractures than UFH users.
- The peak anti-Xa activity (3 hours post-injection) should be measured to ensure the woman is appropriately anticoagulated.
- The target range for the anti-Xa level is 0.35–0.70 IU/mL.

VTE: other considerations

- Therapeutic anticoagulation should be continued for at least 6 months.
- After delivery, treatment should continue for at least 6 weeks.
- Warfarin can be used postnatally and it is safe for breastfeeding.
- The leg should be elevated and a graduated elastic compression stocking applied to reduce oedema; mobilization is recommended.
- An inferior vena caval filter may be considered for recurrent PEs despite adequate anticoagulation or if anticoagulation is contraindicated
- In life-threatening massive PE thrombolytic therapy, percutaneous catheter thrombus fragmentation or surgical embolectomy may be required.
- Where DVT threatens leg viability, surgical embolectomy or thrombolytic therapy may be considered.

Anticoagulation during labour and delivery

- The women should be advised that once she thinks that she is in labour, she should not inject any further heparin.
- To avoid the risk of epidural haematoma:
  - regional anaesthesia should be avoided until at least 12 hours after the last dose of LMWH (24 hours if she is on a therapeutic dose)
  - LMWH should not be given for at least 4 hours after the epidural catheter has been removed
  - the epidural catheter should not be removed within 10–12 hours of a LMWH injection.
- There is an increased risk of wound haematoma following CS of around 2%.
- Wound drains should be considered.
- The skin incision should be closed with staples or interrupted sutures.
- Women on anticoagulant therapy at high risk of haemorrhage should be managed with UFH, as it has a shorter half-life and is more completely reversed with protamine sulphate.

Amniotic fluid embolism: overview

Amniotic fluid embolism (AFE) is a rare and often fatal maternal complication. It is not predictable or preventable and is usually rapidly progressive. It accounts for 8% of the direct maternal deaths in the UK and 10% of all maternal deaths in the USA.

- Incidence 1:8000–30 000 births.
- Reported mortality ranges from 13% to 80%.
- The interval from onset of symptoms to death varies from 10 minutes to 32 hours.
- Can cause permanent neurological sequelae in up to 85% of survivors.
- Tends to occur:
  - with spontaneous or artificial rupture of membranes (70%)
  - at CS (19%)
  - during delivery or within 48 hours (11%)
  - rarely during or after termination of pregnancy, manual removal of placenta, or amniocentesis.

Causes

Presumed causal roles have been attributed to strong uterine contractions, excess amniotic fluid, and disruption of the uterine vasculature.

AFE is characterized by the acute onset of:

- Hypoxia and respiratory arrest (27–51%).
- Hypotension (13–27%).
- Fetal distress (17%).
- Convulsions (10–30%).
- Shock.
- Altered mental status.
- Cardiac arrest.

⚠ Although only 12% will present with DIC, virtually all cases will go on to develop it within 4 hours

---

Risk factors for AFE

- Multiple pregnancy.
- Older maternal age.
- Caesarean or instrumental vaginal delivery.
- Eclampsia.
- Polyhydramnios.
- Placenta praevia.
- Placental abruption.
- Cervical laceration.
- Uterine rupture.
- Medical induction of labour.

Amniotic fluid embolism: diagnosis and management

Diagnosis

The diagnosis is clinical and essentially a diagnosis of exclusion. The differential diagnosis should include:

- Pulmonary embolism.
- Anaphylaxis.
- Sepsis.
- Eclampsia.
- Myocardial infarction.

△ In some patients severe haemorrhage with DIC may be the first sign.

The clinical diagnosis is supported by the retrieval of fetal elements in pulmonary artery aspirate and maternal sputum. However, the diagnosis is only definitively confirmed by the presence of fetal squamous cells and debris in the pulmonary vasculature at a postmortem examination.

Investigations

- ABG.
- Electrolytes including calcium and magnesium levels.
- FBC(↑ WBC).
- Coagulation profile.
- CXR (pulmonary oedema).
- ECG (ischaemia and infarction).

Management of AFE

- Rapid maternal cardiopulmonary resuscitation and admission to ICU under multidisciplinary senior input from obstetrics, anaesthetics, and haematology.
- Pulmonary artery wedge pressure monitoring will assist in the haemodynamic management and blood aspirated via the catheter can be examined to aid with the diagnosis.
- Oxygen to maintain saturation close to 100% (helps to prevent neurological impairment from hypoxia).
- Fluid resuscitation is imperative to counteract hypotension and haemodynamic instability.
- For refractory hypotension, direct-acting vasopressors such as phenylephrine are required to optimize perfusion pressure.
- Inotropic support may be needed.
- DIC should be managed with the help of a haematologist (see massive obstetric haemorrhage, 📖 p. 000).
- Plasma exchange techniques may be helpful in clearing fibrin degradation products from the circulation.
- If not yet delivered, continuous fetal monitoring is indicated:
  - delivery by CS within 5 minutes of cardiac arrest is recommended to facilitate cardiopulmonary resuscitation of the mother.

Uterine inversion

Uterine inversion can cause serious maternal morbidity or death. The incidence is about 1:2000–3000 deliveries. Maternal mortality can be as high as 15%.

Risk factors for uterine inversion

- Strong traction on umbilical cord with excessive fundal pressure.
- Abnormal adherence of the placenta.
- Uterine anomalies.
- Fundal implantation of the placenta.
- Short cord.
- Previous uterine inversion.

Signs and symptoms

- Haemorrhage (present in 94% of cases).
- Severe lower abdominal pain in the 3rd stage.
- Shock out of proportion to the blood loss (neurogenic, due to increased vagal tone).
- Uterine fundus not palpable abdominally (or inversion may be just felt as a dimple at the fundus).
- Mass in the vagina on VE.

Management of uterine inversion

- Call for help (including a senior obstetrician and anaesthetist).
- Immediate replacement by pushing up the fundus through the cervix with the palm of the hand (the Johnson manoeuvre).
- IV access with 2 large bore cannulae.
- Bloods for FBC, coagulation studies, and cross-match 4–6 units.
- Immediate fluid replacement.
- Continuous monitoring of vital signs.
- Transfer to theatre and arrange appropriate analgesia.
- If the placenta is still attached to the uterus it is left in situ to minimize the bleeding and removal attempted only after replacement.
- Tocolytic drugs, such as terbutaline, or volatile anaesthetic agents may be tried to make replacement easier.
- If manual reduction fails then hydrostatic repositioning (O'Sullivan's technique) may be tried:
  - warm saline is rapidly infused into the vagina with one hand sealing the labia (a silicone ventouse cup may be used to improve the seal)
  - uterine rupture should be excluded first.
- Sometimes both manual and hydrostatic methods fail and a laporotomy is needed for correction (Haultain's or Huntingdon's procedure)

Miscellaneous obstetric issues

Fibroids in pregnancy

- Incidence in pregnancy varies from 0.1% to 3.9%.
- May be higher in women over 35, primigravida, and those of Afro-Caribbean origin.
- USS is usually used to make the diagnosis but fibroids can be confused with solid ovarian or other tumours.
- Only 42% of fibroids in pregnancy are detected clinically.

Effects of pregnancy on fibroids

Fibroids commonly but not invariably enlarge in pregnancy. There is initial myometrial hyperplasia followed by hypertrophy. Whether fibroids increase, decrease, or stay the same after pregnancy remains controversial.

Effects of fibroids on pregnancy

Pain due to:
- Red degeneration (necrobiosis).
- Torsion of a pedunculated fibroid.
- Fibroid impaction.
- ⚠ Pain may be severe enough to require morphine via PCA.

1st and 2nd trimesters
- The risk of spontaneous miscarriage may be ↑:
  - preconception myomectomy seems to improve the likelihood of a successful pregnancy with recurrent pregnancy loss, especially when no other cause can be found.
- May ↑ the risk of 2nd-trimester miscarriages.
- Invasive procedures, such as amniocentesis and CVS, may be technically difficult.

3rd trimester
- ↑ risk of threatened preterm labour (reported rate up to 22%).
- Placentation over a fibroid is a strong risk factor for abruption.
- It is unclear whether fibroids are associated with IUGR.
- Large fibroids may exert pressure on the fetus, causing limb reduction defects, congenital torticollis, and head deformities (fetal compression syndrome).
- Very rare complications include disseminated intravascular coagulation, spontaneous haemoperitoneum, uterine inversion, uterine incarceration, acute renal failure, and urinary retention.

Delivery
- The incidence of Caesarean section (CS) is doubled, as malpresentations, dysfunctional labour, and obstructed labour are more common, especially when the fibroids are in the lower uterine segment.
- ↑ risk of postpartum haemorrhage (PPH).
- A higher incidence of retained placenta (may be due to lower-segment fibroids obstructing delivery of the placenta).

Management of fibroids in pregnancy

- Conservative management:
  - symptomatic treatment of pain
  - monitoring of the fetus.
- Surgical procedures for fibroids during pregnancy carries a risk of significant haemorrhage, therefore myomectomy is not performed in pregnancy.
- A myomectomy during CS is also avoided as it carries a high morbidity from haemorrhage:
  - rarely, it may be necessary to remove a fibroid to gain access to the fetus or to facilitate uterine repair.

Ovarian cysts in pregnancy

- Incidence of 1–2%.
- The majority are small (3–4 cm), persistent follicular cysts.
- Cysts ≥6 cm occur in 0.5–2:1000 pregnancies.
- Most common ovarian cysts seen in pregnancy include:
  - functional ovarian cysts (follicular, corpus luteum, and theca-lutein)
  - benign cystic teratomas
  - serous cystadenomas
  - mucinous cystadenomas
  - endometriomas
  - malignant tumours (2–3%).

Effects of ovarian cysts on pregnancy

- Impaction of the cyst may lead to urinary retention.
- ↑ risk of miscarriage or preterm delivery.
- May cause discomfort if very large.
- Large cysts may prevent engagement of the fetal head and predispose to malpresentation (rarely, may cause obstructed labour).

The complications are the same as in the non-pregnant state:

- torsion is most likely to occur at the end of the 1st trimester or in the puerperium (risk of torsion is between 3% and 25%)
- cyst haemorrhage may occur as a result of ↑ vascularity
- rupture (may follow impaction during labour).

Management of ovarian cysts in pregnancy

- ⚠ Acute complications should be treated by surgery at any gestation.
- Asymptomatic, non-enlarging cysts, cystadenomas, and dermoids should be managed conservatively.
- Cystectomy is performed in patients with:
  - symptoms or acute complications (torted, haemorrhagic, ruptured)
  - strong suspicion of malignancy
  - enlargement or large size (>8–10 cm).
- Elective surgery should be performed at 16–20 weeks:
  - risk of miscarriage is lower
  - access to the pedicle is easy.
- The choice of laparotomy or laparoscopy is dependent on:
  - risk of malignancy
  - urgency of the procedure
  - skills of the surgeon.
- The risk of miscarriage after emergency surgery for ovarian torsion can be as high as 22.2%.
- If a cyst causes obstruction of labour, delivery should be by CS and the cyst dealt with at the same time.

Malignancy and premalignancy of the genital tract in pregnancy: overview

- The incidence of cancer in pregnancy is about 1:6000 live births.
- This is much lower (about 50%) than in non-pregnant women, as fewer women would fall pregnant if they were aware of the diagnosis.
- The diagnosis may be delayed in pregnant women as symptoms such as vomiting, abdominal pain, backache, and feeling unwell are often attributed to the pregnancy itself.
- Treatment may be delayed in order to achieve fetal maturity; this is mostly guided by the woman's wishes.
- There does not appear to be any difference in the stage-for-stage survival and mortality figures and the prognosis.
- The recent CEMACH report introduced a new section on maternal deaths due to cancers.
- Overall, 28 cases were reported to the enquiry in the last triennium.
- Some cancers, particularly hormone-dependent ones, can grow rapidly in pregnancy but factors related to tumour growth in relation to the endocrine and physiological changes in pregnancy are still poorly understood.

Cervical carcinoma in pregnancy: diagnosis

This is the most common cancer of the genital tract to present in pregnancy, with an estimated incidence of 1:2000 pregnancies. There has been a decline in invasive carcinoma of the cervix in developed countries, which may be attributed to the cancer screening programme (see 📖 Chapter 22, 📖 p. 676).

Cervical screening and preinvasive disease

- The UK National Cervical Screening Programme ensures the majority of women have routine screening with appropriate referral.
- This allows women to delay pregnancy if they have had abnormal cytology.
- It may be more difficult to interpret a cytology result in a pregnant woman and consequently routine screening is deferred until >6 weeks postpartum.
- Where clinically indicated, referral for colposcopy should be made.
- At colposcopy it is more difficult to interpret changes in colour following application of acetic acid and iodine in pregnancy.
- Biopsy of the cervix can lead to brisk bleeding and, where possible, should be avoided in pregnancy.
- Risk of miscarriage or preterm labour following biopsy is low.
- If CIN is diagnosed by histology, repeat colposcopy is undertaken at 36 weeks and then 6–12 weeks postpartum.

▶ There is no evidence to suggest increased progression of preinvasive disease to invasive disease in pregnancy, hence the approach is generally conservative.

Presentation and diagnosis

⚠ Cervical carcinoma can present as recurrent bleeding in pregnancy in a woman not up to date with her smear tests.
- Pregnancy does not accelerate the progression of CIN to invasive disease.
- Prognosis may be dependent on the duration between diagnosis and treatment.
- Delaying treatment to achieve fetal maturity is not known to worsen prognosis.
- Of those women with cervical cancer in pregnancy, nearly 7% are diagnosed at the time of their pregnancy confirmation.
- Most women are asymptomatic at presentation (up to 65%).
- Diagnosis may follow the assessment of an abnormal smear or colposcopy.
- Colposcopy and cervical punch biopsy are safe in pregnancy.

▶ A large loop excision of the transformation zone (LLETZ) or knife cone biopsy carries a significant risk of haemorrhage and miscarriage
- Staging of the disease may be difficult when the uterus is enlarged:
  - avoid exposure of the fetus to ionizing radiation
  - MRI is safe in pregnancy.

Cervical carcinoma in pregnancy: management and prognosis

Management

Early invasive disease

* There is a risk of haemorrhage, infection, miscarriage, preterm labour, and prelabour rupture of membranes.
* 80% of pregnancies result in term deliveries and fetal survival is over 90%.

Stage 1a and b

* In the 1st and 2nd trimesters radical hysterectomy and lymphadenectomy may be performed with the fetus in utero.
* In late mid-trimester (>24 weeks) CS may be performed followed by radical hysterectomy and lymphadenectomy:
  * a classical section reduces the risk of encroaching on the tumour.
* There is little evidence to suggest any benefit, but if the patient presents in labour, an emergency CS may be performed to reduce dissemination of the disease.

Advanced disease

* Treatment should not be delayed.
* If the pregnancy is >24 weeks, management must be individualized according to the mother's wishes; baby should be delivered at an appropriate gestation, by classical CS, and radiotherapy instituted.

Prognosis (see Chapter 22, 📖 p. 689)

* There is no evidence to suggest that when early-stage disease is diagnosed in pregnancy, the prognosis is worse than for non-pregnant women.
* The 5-year survival in pregnant women with advanced disease is lower than for their non-pregnant counterparts:
  * this difference could be due to radiation dosimetry during or soon after pregnancy.

Ovarian cancer

- Only 2–3% of the ovarian tumours that require surgery in pregnancy are malignant. Nearly 1/3 of these are dysgerminomas, teratomas, or germ-cell tumours.

Presentation

- Most tumours are asymptomatic and discovered during viability USS.
- <25% are >10 cm.
- Some will present as abdominal pain due to a cyst accident:
  - torsion complicates 10–15% of tumours.

Management of ovarian cancer in pregnancy

- A cyst identified in the 1st trimester should be re-scanned at 14 weeks (most corpus luteal cysts involve by then):
  - if it has not ↑ to >5 cm, conservative management is appropriate
  - if >5 cm serial USS should be used to monitor any change in size or morphology (which may prompt surgery).
- Where there are signs of malignancy in the tumour:
  - surgery can be limited to unilateral oopherectomy but a complete staging must be performed
  - if staging at laparotomy is suggestive of spread beyond the ovary, or if histology determines the need for chemotherapy, a multidisciplinary approach is taken.

Chemotherapy in pregnancy

- There is limited evidence of safety or efficacy in pregnancy:
  - especially regarding bleomycin, etoposide, and cisplastin for germ cell tumours.
- Chemotherapeutics are teratogenic in the 1st trimester:
  - careful counselling regarding termination of the pregnancy should be undertaken.
- Each case has to be individualized, based on:
  - gestation
  - tumour histology
  - patient choice.
- Where there is evidence of extracapsular invasion, a total hysterectomy, bilateral salpingo-oopherectomy, and pelvic node sampling should be considered.

Vulval carcinoma

80% occur in those >65 years. Vulval intraepithelial neoplasia (VIN) is seen in younger women.

Presentation (see Chapter 22, 📖 p. 716)

- Symptoms are the same in pregnancy as the non-pregnant state.
- Most patients with pre-invasive disease are asymptomatic.
- Nearly 70% present with pruritus vulvae; 57% may present with a mass or an ulcer.
- Bleeding occurs in 25%.
- Diagnosis is made according to histological findings after colposcopic assessment, excision biopsy, and groin node sampling.

Management of vulval carcinoma in pregnancy

Pre-invasive disease (VIN)
- Treatment can be delayed until after delivery, when a wide local excision is usually sufficient.

Invasive disease
- Treatment is the same as for a non-pregnant woman
- If the pregnancy is 36 weeks or more, the baby should be delivered and treatment started:
  - there is no evidence on the best mode of delivery.
- If the wound on the vulva has healed there is no contraindication to a vaginal delivery.

Prognosis

- Generally 5-year survival is thought to be 80% if the groin nodes are negative, but ↓ to 40% when groin nodes are positive.
- There is little evidence that pregnancy worsens the prognosis.

Perinatal mortality: overview

The role of modern maternity care is to ensure a safe maternal and fetal outcome at childbirth. A system whereby lessons can be learnt from adverse outcomes using analysis of databases and audits should improve outcome.

The first body established to do this in the UK was the Confidential Enquiry into Maternal Deaths (CEMD) in 1952 and subsequently the Confidential Enquiry into Stillbirths and Deaths in Infancy (CESDI) in 1992. The aim of these organizations was to undertake on-going national surveys of perinatal and infant deaths, identify risks, and make recommendations to improve clinical practice.

The Confidential Enquiries into Maternal and Child Health (CEMACH) is the successor to these and looks into the maternal, perinatal, and child health issues with extensive lay and voluntary sector involvement.

From 1954 to mid 1990s, stillbirth and neonatal death rates in England and Wales fell steadily. In 1992 the gestation recognized for a stillbirth was decreased from 28 weeks to 24 weeks.

Definitions

- **Late fetal loss**: a child delivering between 22+0 and 23+6 weeks of gestation who did not, at any time after being delivered, breathe or show any other signs of life.
- **Stillbirth**: a child delivered after the 24th week of pregnancy and who did not, at any time after being completely expelled from its mother, breathe or show any other signs of life.
- **Early neonatal death**: death of a live-born baby occurring less than 7 completed days from the time of birth.
- **Late neonatal death**: death of a live-born baby occurring from the 7th day of life and before 28 completed days from the time of birth.
- **Stillbirth rate**: number of stillbirths per 1000 live births and still-births.
- **Perinatal mortality rate** (UK): number of stillbirths and early neo-natal deaths per 1000 live births and stillbirths.
- **Perinatal mortality rate** (WHO): number of late fetal losses, stillbirths, and early neonatal deaths per 1000 live births and stillbirths.
- **Neonatal mortality rate**: number of neonatal deaths per 1000 live births (may be adjusted to take into account babies with congenital abnormalities, then referred to as 'corrected neonatal mortality rate'.)

Classification of perinatal mortality

Causes of death are classified by the Extended Wigglesworth system and supplemented by the Obstetric Aberdeen classification.

Perinatal mortality surveillance data from 2004:

Stillbirth rates
- Unexplained antepartum deaths contributed to the largest proportion of deaths (>50%).
- Severe lethal/congenital malformations 15%.
- Antepartum haemorrhage 10%.
- Death from intrapartum causes 7%.
- Pre-eclampsia 4%.
- Maternal disorder 5%.
- Other specific causes 5%.
- Infection 2%.

✸ A newly developed classification system for stillbirth, Relevant Condition at Death (ReCoDe), has shown that the majority of the unexplained group are probably growth restricted (a problem masked by the current classification system).

Neonatal deaths
- Immaturity 49%.
- Congenital anomaly 22%.
- Intrapartum causes 11%.
- Infection 7%.
- Other specific causes 7%.
- Sudden infant death syndrome (SIDS) 3%.
- Unclassifiable 1%.

Stillbirth rates since 1954

1954	23/1000 total births
1997	5.3/1000 total births
2001	5.4/1000 live births
2002	5.7/1000 live births
2003	5.8/1000 total births
2004	5.7/1000 total births

Neonatal mortality rates since 1954

1954	18/1000 live births
1997	3.9/1000 live births
2003	3.7/1000 live births
2004	3.4 /1000 live births

Perinatal mortality: key findings

- The stillbirth rate remains high, at 5.7/1000 total births.
- 3/4 of stillbirths deliver after 28 weeks gestation.
- Multiple births have a 3.2 times higher stillbirth rate and 7.0 times higher neonatal death rate than singleton pregnancies.
- Stillbirth and neonatal death rates are higher in:
  - socially deprived areas
  - women of African-Caribbean, Asian, or other ethnic origin.
- Post-mortem rates have plateaued at 42% after a significant fall throughout the 1990s and early 2000s.

Risk factors for perinatal mortality include:

- Maternal age.
- Ethnicity.
- Social deprivation.
- Gestational age.
- Low birth weight.
- Multiple pregnancy.

Ethnicity as a risk factor

The stillbirth rates (SB) and neonatal mortality (NNM) rates were shown to be higher for babies of non-white mothers.
- Black mothers:
  - SB 2.8× and NNM 2.7× higher than Caucasian mothers.
- Asian mothers:
  - SB 2.0× and NNM 1.6× higher.
- Chinese and other minority ethnic mothers:
  - SB and NNM 1.9× higher.

Low birth weight as a risk factor

2/3 of all stillbirths and >70% of all neonatal deaths had a birth weight <2500 g, compared with only 7.6% of all live births.

Strategies for improving the understanding of risk factors

From 2005 onwards, CEMACH plans to develop a new reporting system of perinatal mortality data to provide a more comprehensive picture of the factors associated with perinatal deaths. Emphasis will be placed on:
- Identifying details in the 'unexplained' category.
- Place of delivery, place of death, and the effect of intrauterine and neonatal transfers.
- The inclusion of several more factors in the data collection that will give further insight into perinatal mortality and its causes.
- Better understanding of the causes by improving post-mortem rates.
- Strategies to improve care for women with social deprivation and ethnic minorities.

📖 CEMACH, Perinatal mortality 2005; www.cemach.org.uk

📖 Chief Medical Officer's Annual Report 2007, Chapter '500 missed opportunities' www.dh.gov.uk/en/Publicationsandstatistics/Publications/AnnualReports/

Maternal mortality: definition

The 9th and 10th revisions of the *International classification of diseases, injuries and causes* (ICD-9/10) define a maternal death as, 'death of a woman while pregnant or within 42 days of the end of the pregnancy, from any cause related to or aggravated by the pregnancy or its management, but not from accidental or incidental causes'.

Direct maternal deaths

- Result from obstetric complications of the pregnant state (pregnancy, labour, and puerperium), from interventions, omissions, incorrect treatment, or from a chain of events resulting from any of the above.

Indirect maternal deaths

- Arise from pre-existing disease or disease that developed during pregnancy and which was not due to direct obstetric causes but which was aggravated by the physiological effects of pregnancy and includes:
  - epilepsy
  - cardiac disease
  - diabetes
  - hormone-dependent malignancies.

ICD-10 also introduced new terms for maternal mortality:

Pregnancy-related death

- Death occurring in a woman while pregnant or within 42 days of termination of pregnancy, irrespective of the cause of the death (unlike maternal deaths, this includes accidental and incidental causes).

Late maternal death

- Death occurring between 42 days and 1 year after termination of pregnancy, miscarriage, or delivery that is due to direct or indirect maternal causes.

Coincidental (fortuitous) maternal death

- Includes accidental or incidental deaths, which would have happened even if the woman was not pregnant, and includes:
  - domestic violence
  - road traffic accidents.

Maternal mortality ratio (MMR)

This is defined as the number of direct and indirect maternal deaths per 100 000 live births.

The Confidential Enquiry into Maternal Deaths (CEMACH)

In 1949, the issue of reporting maternal deaths was raised at the 12th British Congress of Obstetrics and Gynaecology and this led to the establishment of an enhanced regional and national assessment by clinicians. A series of triennial reports were instituted to disseminate the findings and recommendations, with a view to reduce maternal deaths and to improve practice. In April 2003, the Confidential Enquiry into Maternal and Child Health (CEMACH) for England and Wales came into existence. It is an independent body funded by and reporting to, the National Patient Safety Agency (NPSA). The primary objective of CEMACH, as part of the Government's clinical governance objective, is to review mortality and improve maternal and child health. CEMACH assesses the causes and trends in maternal deaths and identifies avoidable and substandard factors that may have led to these deaths. Based on these findings it makes recommendations and suggestions concerning the improvement of clinical care.

Why is CEMACH important?

- Each year more than 20 million women experience ill health as a result of pregnancy, the lives of nearly 8 million are threatened, and over half a million women die as a result of pregnancy and childbirth.
- It is estimated that 88–98% of maternal deaths in the world are avoidable with timely and effective care.
- The reporting of such deaths and their causes is important in order to identify avoidable causes and institute recommendations to improve practice.
- The recent world estimate of overall MMR is around 400 per 100 000 live births:
  - in the UK during 2003–05 the MMR was 14:100 000.
- 432 maternal deaths were reported to the enquiry:
  - 132 direct maternal deaths
  - 163 indirect deaths
  - 55 coincidental deaths
  - 82 late deaths.
- Maternal death in the recent report is higher than in the previous triennium.
- In general the women who died:
  - appeared to be in poorer health
  - smoked more
  - Over half of those whose BMI was known, were overweight or obese.

📖 Saving mothers' lives. The 7th report on confidential enquiries into maternal deaths in the UK; CEMACH 2007. www.cemach.org.uk

Avoidable factors identified by the 7th CEMACH report

▶ The report commented on the number of health-care professionals who appear to be unable to identify and manage common medical conditions or potential emergencies outside their immediate area of expertise.

⚠ Resuscitation skills in the health-care professionals were also considered to be poor in an unacceptably high number of cases.

Care was hampered by a lack of communication between disciplines and agencies including:
• Poor or non-existent team working.
• Inappropriate delegation to junior staff.
• Inappropriate or too short consultations by phone.
• Lack of sharing of information including between the GP and the maternity team.
• Poor interpersonal skills.

⚠ This lack of sharing of information between various agencies was particularly noted with regard to self-harm and child protection issues.

'Top ten' CEMACH 2007 recommendations

• Preconception counselling should be provided for women with pre-existing serious medical or mental health problems, including obesity.
• Antenatal services should be accessible and welcoming.
• Women >12 weeks gestation on referral should be seen within 2 weeks.
• Immigrant women should have a full medical history and clinical assessment (including cardiovascular examination) at booking.
• All pregnant women with a systolic BP of ≥160 mm/Hg require antihypertensive treatment.
• Women must be advised that CS is not risk free and may cause problems in their current and future pregnancies.
• Service providers must ensure clinical staff learn from any critical events or serious untoward incidents in their NHS trust.
• Clinical staff must have improved training in identification and treatment of serious medical and mental health conditions as well as improved life support skills.
• Routine use of a national obstetric early warning chart.
• Guidelines are needed for the management of:
  • the obese pregnant woman
  • sepsis in pregnancy
  • pain and bleeding in early pregnancy.

Digested data in this topic is reproduced from *Saving mothers' lives*. The 7th report on Confidential enquiries into maternal deaths in the UK; CEMACH 2007, with the permission of the Confidential Enquiry into Maternal and Child Health www.cemach.org.uk

CEMACH: direct deaths I

Venous thromboembolism (VTE) (see 📖 Chapter 10, p. 386)

- There were 41 deaths from VTE during 2003–05:
  - 33 from pulmonary embolism (PE)
  - 8 from cerebral vein thrombosis.
- Risk factors were identified in 27 of the 41 women.

VTE: CEMACH Recommendations
- Urgent need for a guideline on the management of obese women.
- All women should be assessed for risk factors for VTE.
- Women with previous VTE should be offered thromboprophylaxis with LMWH.
- Care must be taken with phone consultations, as early symptoms of life-threatening embolism are generally mild.

Pre-eclampsia and eclampsia (see 📖 Chapter 2, p. 62)
- 18 deaths were recorded from hypertensive disease of pregnancy:
  - 10 from intracranial haemorrhage
  - 2 from cerebral infarction
  - 2 from multi-organ failure
  - 1 from massive liver infarction.

Pre-eclampsia: CEMACH recommendations
- Women with a systolic BP of ≥160mm/Hg need antihypertensives.
- Anaesthetists should anticipate ↑ BP at intubation with a general anaesthetic.
- Syntometrine® must not be used for hypertensive women (or those who have not had their BP checked).
- Fulminating pre-eclampsia occurs at term, and post-term, as well as pre-term.

Genital tract sepsis (📖 see Chapter 9, p. 352)

- Resulted in 18 direct deaths.
- 10 died after CS, all were overweight.
- Women with sepsis may present with a variety of symptoms such as abdominal pain, diarrhoea, vomiting, and pyrexia.

Sepsis: CEMACH recommendations
- All staff must be aware of the sign and symptoms of sepsis and critical illness.
- High dose broad-spectrum antibiotics should be started immediately without waiting for microbiology results.
- Sepsis may mimic placental abruption and must be considered.
- Sepsis should be considered in all recently delivered women who feel unwell and are pyrexial.

CEMACH 2003–5:Summary of direct causes of maternal death

- VTE (41).
- Hypertensive disease of pregnancy (18).
- Genital tract sepsis (18).
- Amniotic fluid embolism (17).
- Haemorrhage (14).
- Early pregnancy causes (14).
- Anaesthesia related (6).
- Genital tract trauma (3).
- Acute fatty liver (1).

Risk factors for genital tract sepsis identified by CEMACH

- Obesity.
- Diabetes or impaired glucose tolerance.
- Impaired immunity.
- Anaemia.
- Vaginal discharge.
- History of pelvic infection.
- History of group B streptococcal infection.
- Amniocentesis or other invasive procedures.
- Cervical cerclage.
- Prolonged spontaneous rupture of membranes (SROM).
- Vaginal trauma.
- CS.
- Wound haematoma.
- Retained products of conception after miscarriage or delivery.

Digested data in this topic is reproduced from *Saving mothers' lives*. The 7th report on Confidential enquiries into maternal deaths in the UK; CEMACH 2007, with the permission of the Confidential Enquiry into Maternal and Child Health www.cemach.org.uk

CEMACH: direct deaths II

Amniotic fluid embolism (AFE) (see Chapter 10, 📖 p. 394)
- 19 deaths were due to AFE (↑ number since the last report):
  - 2 were late deaths (survived the initial event but died weeks later).

AFE: CEMACH recommendations
- Many women will report premonitory symptoms including:
  - Breathlessness, chest pain, feeling cold, light-headedness, distress panic, paraesthesia, nausea and vomiting.
- In several cases the mother's condition was not recognized until it was too late.
- All cases of suspected or confirmed AFE should be reported to the National Amniotic Fluid Embolism Register at UKOSS.
- Attempts should be made to confirm AFE at post-mortem.

Haemorrhage (see Chapter 10, 📖 p. 377)
- 17 maternal deaths from haemorrhage were reported.
- 10 of the 17 women received less than optimal care.
- 3 were as a result of genital tract trauma.

Haemorrhage: CEMACH recommendations
- Regular training on identifying and managing maternal collapse.
- Use of an early warning scoring system to recognize occult bleeding.
- Seek early assistance from senior colleagues and those with greater gynaecological surgical experience.
- Management of placenta percreta requires a large multidisciplinary team.
- Guidelines for women refusing blood products must be made available to all staff as part of routine training.
- All women with previous CS must have their placental site determined and attempts made to diagnose accreta or percreta (MRI).

Early pregnancy deaths
- 14 deaths resulted from early pregnancy causes.
- 10 were due to ectopic pregnancy.
- 1 death was believed to result from an illegal abortion.

Early pregnancy: CEMACH recommendations
- GPs and A+E staff should be aware of the atypical presentation of ectopic pregnancy (such as diarrhoea, vomiting, and fainting).
- Medical management of ectopic should adhere to strict protocols.
- Women with OHSS should receive thromboprophylaxis.

Anaesthesia-related deaths
- 6 deaths were directly due to anaesthesia.
- 31 additional deaths were contributed by anaesthesia.
- 4 of the women were obese (2 were morbidly obese).

CEMACH: indirect causes of death

The most common cause of indirect maternal death was cardiac disease. This was even higher than deaths due to thromboembolism.

Cardiac disease in pregnancy (see 📖 Chapter 5, p. 184)

- 48 deaths were recorded that resulted from heart disease (↑ rate)
  - a further 34 women died later from cardiac disease but are included in the late deaths.
- The leading cause of death is now myocardial infarction (MI) and dissection of the thoracic aorta.
- 8% had congenital heart disease.
- Rheumatic mitral stenosis has re-emerged as a cause of maternal death.
- The ↑ appears to relate to the growing incidence of acquired heart disease related to poor diet, smoking, alcohol, and obesity.

Cardiac disease: CEMACH recommendations
- The possibility of rheumatic heart disease must be considered in immigrant women.
- Women at higher risk of developing cardiac disease in pregnancy should be advised of the risks before conception.
- Low threshold for investigating women with symptoms of MI or aortic dissection.
- If you not confident or competent about interpreting an ECG, you should show it to someone who is!

Deaths due to malignancy

- 81 deaths related to malignancy were reported (the ↑ is believed to reflect better follow-up).

Malignancy: CEMACH recommendations
- Women should be encouraged to examine their breasts regularly.
- Pregnancy is not a contraindication for appropriate radiological investigations.

Other indirect causes of death

- 87 other indirect deaths were recorded, including:
- Diseases of the central nervous system (34), including:
  - subarachnoid haemorrhage (11)
  - epilepsy (9).
- Infectious diseases (13) including:
  - HIV infection (1).
- Diseases of the respiratory system (9):
  - asthma (5).
- Endocrine disorders, including:
  - diabetes (4).

MI in pregnancy (see 📖 Chapter 5, p. 189)

- Ischaemic heart disease is now common.
- The risk is higher in older women and the age at childbirth is increasing.
- All the women who died had identifiable risk factors, including:
  - obesity
  - older age and higher parity
  - smoking
  - diabetes
  - pre-existing hypertension
  - family history of ischaemic heart disease.
- MI and acute coronary syndrome can have an atypical presentation in pregnancy (abdominal or epigastric pain and vomiting).
- There should be a low threshold for investigating symptoms especially in women with risk factors.
- There should also be a low threshold for emergency coronary intervention (such as angioplasty and stenting).
- Thrombolysis should not be withheld in the pregnant or puerperal woman.

Indirect deaths: some specific recommendations

- Increased awareness of the interaction of common medical conditions and pregnancy.
- All women with serious medical conditions should be referred to a specialist as early as possible.
- Facilities to allow communication between physicians and obstetricians such as a combined medical obstetric antenatal clinic.
- The consultant obstetrician should be informed about all sick pregnant inpatients, whether their problem is medical or obstetric.
- Units should have access to CT and MRI.
- Multiple attendances are signs of serious undiagnosed disease or social problems.
- Women with epilepsy have a risk of sudden death and should be warned of this before considering stopping their anticonvulsants.

Digested data in this topic is reproduced from *Saving mothers' lives*. The 7th report on Confidential enquiries into maternal deaths in the UK; CEMACH 2007, with the permission of the Confidential Enquiry into Maternal and Child Health www.cemach.org.uk

CEMACH: psychiatric illness and domestic abuse

Deaths from psychiatric illnesses (see 📖 Chapter 12, p. 436)

- There were 104 deaths recorded which were due to or associated with psychiatric causes:
  - 37 were due to suicide (↓ rate since last report)
  - 24 were due to substance misuse
  - 10 women died violently, including 5 murders.

Psychiatric causes: CEMACH recommendations

- Women referred to child protection services may actively avoid antenatal care, despite being at high risk.
- Extra vigilance is required if women have requested termination of pregnancy (TOP) but had to continue with the pregnancy.
- Women with drug and alcohol misuse should have multidisciplinary care which includes a psychiatrist, GP, and obstetric team
- Social and addiction services should be involved.
- Women with opiate addiction should be offered substitution therapy (methadone).
- Perinatal mental health team should provide care to all women at risk of mental illness.
- Should a woman require hospitalization in the postnatal period, a mother and baby unit is the appropriate place.
- Women with a past history of psychiatric illness should be counselled regarding the risk of recurrence after delivery and guidelines for the management of such relapses should be available in all trusts.

Domestic abuse

⚠ Domestic abuse is an important issue in obstetrics.
- 70 women who died from 'all causes' had features of domestic abuse:
  - most had self-reported domestic abuse
  - none had been routinely asked about it.
- 19 women were murdered by their partners:
  - 5 did not speak English; in all cases husbands acted as interpreters
  - all had at least 2 identifiable risk factors but none was referred for help or advice.

Domestic abuse: CEMACH Recommendations

- Enquiries about domestic violence should be routinely included in the social history.
- Women should be seen alone at least once during the antenatal period.
- Information about local agencies and emergency helplines should be displayed in suitable areas where women can have access to them.
- All health-care professionals should make themselves aware of the importance of domestic abuse.

Some indicators of domestic abuse in maternity care

- Late booking and /or poor or non-attendance at antenatal clinic.
- Repeat attendance at antenatal clinic, GP surgery, or A&E for minor injuries or trivial or non-existent complaints.
- Unexplained admissions.
- Non-compliance with treatment regimens or early self-discharge from hospital.
- Repeat presentation with depression, anxiety, self-harm, and psychosomatic symptoms.
- Injuries that are untended and of several different ages, especially to the neck, head, breasts, abdomen, and genitals.
- Minimalization of signs of abuse on the body.
- Sexually transmitted diseases and frequent vaginal or urinary tract infections and pelvic pain.
- Poor obstetric history:
  - repeated miscarriages or TOPs
  - stillbirth or pre-term labour
  - pre-term birth, IUGR, low birth weight
  - unwanted or unplanned pregnancy.
- The constant presence at examinations of the partner, who may be domineering, answer all the questions for her, and be unwilling to leave the room.
- The woman appears evasivse or reluctant to speak or disagree in front of her partner.

Digested data in this topic is reproduced from *Saving mothers' lives*. The 7th report on Confidential enquiries into maternal deaths in the UK; CEMACH 2007, with the permission of the Confidential Enquiry into Maternal and Child Health www.cemach.org.uk

Substance abuse and psychiatric disorders

Substance abuse in pregnancy

- The huge increase in drug and alcohol abuse in the UK since the 1980s has been disproportionately large in women of childbearing age.
- The prevalence of substance abuse is:
  - 4.7% for alcohol
  - 2.2% for drug dependence.
- It has a serious effect on the mother's health as well as consequences for fetal well-being.
- There is under-identification because of:
  - inadequate history taking
  - reluctance to admit to substance abuse
  - late booking
  - poor antenatal attendance.
- Poor communication between GPs, social services, midwives, and obstetricians is a hindrance to adequate care.
- In the last triennium, CEMACH reported 31 maternal deaths that were either directly or indirectly related to substance abuse:
  - social deprivation was a common factor
  - all but one pregnancy was unplanned.

Definitions relating to substance abuse

Problems associated with substance abuse are categorized in ICD-10 under the heading 'Mental and behavioural disorders due to psychoactive substance abuse'.

- **Harmful use**: a pattern of psychoactive substance use that is causing damage to physical or mental health.
- **Intoxication**: a transient syndrome due to recent substance ingestion that produces clinically significant psychological and physical impairment.
- **Dependence syndrome**: a cluster of physiological, behavioural, and cognitive phenomena in which the use of a substance or a class of substances takes on a much higher priority for a given individual than other behaviours that once had greater value.
- **Tolerance**: a homeostatic adaptation to chronic administration of a drug; to ameliorate longer-term toxicity and to allow the organism to continue functioning while chronically intoxicated.
- **Withdrawal**: a characteristic pattern of signs and symptoms (psychological and physical) that occur when a drug is stopped after a period of chronic administration, or an antagonist to the drug is given.

Morbidity and mortality in substance abusers

Coexisting psychiatric disorders

There is a close association between substance misuse and other mental illnesses such as personality disorder, depression, and anxiety.

Physical complications

- Substance misuse is often accompanied by a general neglect of health with nutritional deficiency, poor hygiene, and generalized immunosuppression.
- As well as direct pharmacological consequences from the substance there as risks from the route of administration.
  IV drug use may lead to:
- HIV infection.
- Hepatitis C (prevalence of between 50–80% in UK drug users) and hepatitis B (30–50%).
- Venous thrombosis.
- Subcutaneous abscesses.
- Bacterial endocarditis.
- Septicaemia (may be fungal).
- Poor venous access in an emergency situation.

Withdrawal effects

- Withdrawal symptoms can be distressing but are rarely life threatening.

Social damage

- May lead to problems with the employer and work-related accidents.
- Leads to financial strain with damaging effects on the family.
- Antisocial and criminal activities may arise from behavioural changes and the need for money.
- There may be child protection issues as a result of neglect or abuse.

Death

- There is a significant mortality (10–15% in opioid misusers over 10 years).
- Mostly accidental due to overdose.
- Suicide is also a frequent cause of death.
- Deaths from HIV and hepatitis infection are becoming more common.
- Approximately 60% of deaths in drug addicts are related to drug use itself.

Perinatal morbidity and mortality with substance abuse

Risks of the following are increased:
- Preterm birth and prematurity.
- IUGR.
- Low birth weight.
- Symptoms of withdrawal from drugs.
- Increased stillbirth and neonatal mortality.
- Sudden infant death syndrome.
- Physical and neurological damage from drugs or violence.
- Fetal alcohol syndrome.

Substance misuse in pregnancy: management

Maternal issues

CEMACH has emphasized the extent of this problem and made the following recommendations:

- To tailor proper antenatal and postnatal care, a detailed history that includes the use of illicit drugs, tobacco, and alcohol should be taken.
- Women using opiates should be prescribed substitution therapy (methadone).
- Women should not undergo opiate detoxification during pregnancy.
- Women on illicit drugs may be at risk of violence and abuse and have other complex social, psychiatric, and psychological problems.
- They should thus be handled very sensitively, with dignity, in full confidence and encouraged to attend for antenatal care.
- All patients should have a multidisciplinary care with the involvement of:
  - GP
  - social services
  - obstetric team (possibly including a specialist midwife)
  - local addiction services (possibly including a psychiatrist).
- Contraceptive advice should be offered where indicated.

Fetal issues

Most abusers will use more than one substance so there may be multiple risks to the fetus. By definition, this is a high-risk pregnancy. General considerations should include:

- Detailed anomaly USS:
  - consider the need for a later cardiac anomaly USS.
- Serial USS for growth and well-being:
  - ↑ risk of IUGR.
- Increased awareness of the ↑ risk of obstetric complications such as:
  - preterm labour
  - placental abruption.

Alcohol abuse

Alcohol abuse is defined as drinking that causes mental, physical, or social harm to an individual.

- Alcohol consumption by women has increased over the last 15 years.
- Excessive consumption of alcohol can lead to alimentary disorders such as liver damage, gastritis, peptic ulcer, oesophageal varices, and acute and chronic pancreatitis.
- Damage to the liver, including fatty infiltration, hepatitis, cirrhosis, and hepatoma is particularly important.
- Neurological damage such as peripheral neuropathy, epilepsy, and cerebellar degeneration, and cardiovascular complications such as hypertension and stroke are common.
- There may be child protection issues arising from potential neglect as well as direct harm.

Fetal alcohol syndrome

- There is evidence that this occurs in some children born to mothers who drink excessively (incidence of 0.5–5:1000 live births). The exact relationship between alcohol and birth defects is a complex one, but there is no known safe lower limit for alcohol consumption; current recommendations limit consumption to 1 unit per day. Women drinking ≥18 units/day have a 1 in 3 chance of fetal alcohol syndrome. It is characterized by pre- and postnatal retardation, developmental delay, and a characteristic craniofacial dysmorphism correlating with low IQ.

Features of fetal alcohol syndrome

- IUGR.
- Short stature.
- Developmental delay.
- Micro-ophthalmia.
- Short palpebral fissure.
- Short nasal bridge.
- Microcephaly with prominent forehead.
- Thin upper lip and small philtrum.
- Cleft palate.
- Maxillary hypoplasia.
- Gait abnormalities.
- Cardiac abnormalities.

Management of pregnancy in women abusing alcohol
- Attempt to reduce harm by:
  - counselling about risks and encouraging ↓ alcohol intake
  - encouraging antenatal attendance (ensure supportive, non-judgemental environment)
  - facilitating contact with support groups such as AA
  - facilitating contact with social services (for help with benefits and improve housing)
  - screening for domestic abuse
  - offering help with smoking cessation if required.
- Detailed anomaly USS.
- Serial USS to assess growth and fetal well-being.
- Multidisciplinary team management with involvement of:
  - paediatric team
  - anaesthetic team
  - social services
  - local specialist alcohol support workers.
- May need child protection case conference.

Drugs of abuse: opiates

Routes of administration

Opiates (including morphine, heroin, methadone, buprenorphine) may be taken by snorting (intranasally), smoking, SC ('skin popping'), orally, or IV.

Maternal effects of opiates

- Act on the opioid receptors distributed throughout the CNS.
- They have many physical effects including drowsiness, respiratory depression, nausea, hypotension, and papillary constriction.
- They act on pain receptors and may have significant mood-altering effects, producing a sensation of euphoria or intense pleasure.
- They are both physically and psychologically addictive.
- Withdrawal syndrome occurs within 4–12 hours after the last opiate dose, peaking at 48–72 hours and subsiding by the end of 7–10 days.
- Characteristic symptoms of withdrawal include myalgia, arthralgia, dysphoria, insomnia, agitation, diarrhoea, and shivering.
- Withdrawal is not life threatening.
- Annual mortality rate is about 1–2%, mostly due to overdose.

Effects of opiates on pregnancy

- Opiates are not known to cause any specific congenital abnormalities.
- Babies of mothers abusing opiates are at ↑ risk of:
  - IUGR
  - stillbirth
  - sudden infant death syndrome.
- Withdrawal usually occurs within 24 hours of birth; symptoms include:
  - irritability and exaggerated startle response
  - jitteriness and tremors
  - poor feeding
  - hypotonicity.

Methadone maintenance treatment

- Methadone has a longer half-life than heroin, resulting in a more stable plasma concentration and allowing once-daily administration.
- Women already on replacement may need their methadone dose ↑ due to the physiological plasma dilution effect of pregnancy.
- Starting methadone may help with risk reduction by:
  - ↓ the physical risks of injecting
  - stabilizing lifestyle
  - ↓ the financial burden of purchasing street drugs
  - improving contact with health-care professionals.
- Compliance with the treatment may:
  - ↓ neonatal mortality
  - ↑ birth weight.

⚠ These benefits can be lost if the mother also uses street drugs.
⚠ Withdrawal in pregnancy has a high risk to the fetus and should only be considered in highly motivated women with good social support.

Management of pregnancy in women abusing opiates

- Attempt to reduce harm by:
  - starting methadone
  - encouraging antenatal attendance (ensure supportive, non-judgemental environment)
  - facilitating contact with social services (for help with benefits and improve housing)
  - screening for domestic abuse
  - offering help with smoking cessation if required.

- Screening for STIs including HIV, hepatitis.
- Monitor injection sites for infection.
- Low threshold for antibiotics with symptoms of sepsis (may be atypical pathogens).
- High index of suspicion with any symptoms of VTE (may be unusual sites).
- Detailed anomaly USS.
- Serial USS to assess growth and fetal well-being.
- Multidisciplinary team management with involvement of:
  - paediatric team (baby will need admission to special care baby unit (SCBU))
  - anaesthetic team (IV access may be difficult)
  - social services
  - local specialist drug support workers.

- May need child protection case conference.

Drugs of abuse: cocaine

Routes of administration
- Intranasal is the major route.
- IV use either alone, or with heroin, has a high mortality rate.
- Smoking the freed alkaloid base as 'crack' is becoming common in the UK, especially in poor inner city areas.

Maternal effects of cocaine
- Inhibits the reuptake of neurotransmitters including dopamine.
- May result in euphoria, anorexia, verbosity, and sense of well-being.
- Also has stimulant effects from sympathetic overdrive.
- Deaths are mostly from accidents, cerebrovascular complications (intracranial bleed and emboli), and cardiac arrhythmias.

Effects of cocaine on pregnancy

- Teratogenicity:
  - microcephaly
  - cardiac defects
  - possible genitourinary, limb, and gut defects.
- Vasoconstriction may cause abnormal placentation, resulting in:
  - ↑ risk of pre-eclampsia
  - ↑ risk of abruption
  - IUGR.
- Down-regulation of myometrial β-adrenoreceptors may cause:
  - miscarrige
  - uterine irritability
  - preterm labour.
- Neonates:
  - a limited withdrawal syndrome may occur
  - occasionally show hypotension and cardiac arrythmias
  - are at ↑ risk of sudden infant death.

☙ Cocaine may have a detrimental effect on neurodevelopment, leading to developmental delay.

Management of pregnancy in women abusing cocaine

- Attempt to reduce harm by:
  - counselling about the risks and encouraging ↓ cocaine use
  - encouraging antenatal attendance (ensure supportive, non-judgemental environment)
  - facilitating contact with social services if needed
  - screening for domestic abuse
  - offering help with smoking cessation if required.
- Detailed anomaly USS
- Fetal cardiac USS at 23–24 weeks
- Serial USS to assess growth and fetal well-being
- Multidisciplinary team management with involvement of:
  - paediatric team
  - anaesthetic team
  - social services
  - local specialist drug support workers.
- May need child protection case conference.

Drugs of abuse: other stimulants

Amphetamine sulphate

Routes of administration
- Illicit amphetamine can be taken orally, intranasally, or IV.

Maternal effects of amphetamine
- Enhances the dopaminergic neurotransmitter system.
- The stimulant properties are dose related and characterized by sympathetic overdrive (tachycardia, sweating, dry mouth, tremor).
- Effects on pregnancy
- No proven syndrome of congenital abnormalities.
- Neonates occasionally show hyperactivity and poor feeding.

☙ May have similar risk of miscarriage, preterm labour, and IUGR as cocaine

Ecstasy (MDMA)

Mode of action
- Like amphetamines, it increases the release of dopamine and also releases 5-hydroxutryptamine (5-HT), which may account for its hallucinogenic properties.
- It is selectively neurotoxic to fine serotonergic neurons.

Routes of administration
- Most commonly taken as a capsule in a dose of about 50–150 mg.
- May also be injected or snorted.

Maternal effects
- Feelings of positive mood state, euphoria, sociability, and intimacy.
- Panic, paranoia, psychosis, and neuroses are also common and may extend to visual hallucinations, delusions, and suicidal feelings.

Effects on pregnancy
- Appears to have similar teratogenicity to cocaine, with a reported ↑ in:
  - cardiac defects
  - limb and gut abnormalities.
- Neonates occasionally show hyperactivity and poor feeding.

☙ May have similar risk of miscarriage, preterm labour, and IUGR as cocaine.

Management of pregnancy in women abusing stimulants

- Attempt to reduce harm by;
  - Counselling about the risks and encouraging ↓ drug use
  - Encouraging antenatal attendance (ensure supportive, non-judgemental environment)
  - Facilitating contact with social services if needed
  - Screening for domestic abuse
  - Offering help with smoking cessation if required
- Detailed anomaly USS
- If using ecstasy, consider fetal cardiac USS at 23–24 weeks
- Serial USS to assess growth and fetal well-being
- Multidisciplinary team management with involvement of;
  - Paediatric team
  - Anaesthetic team
  - Social services
  - Local specialist drug support workers
- May need child protection case conference

Drugs of abuse: sedatives and cannabis

Benzodiazepine and barbiturates

Since benzodiazepines first became available in the 1960s there have been many changes in the prescribing guidelines. Although the use of benzodiazepines as hypnotics has decreased, they are still prescribed as an anxiolytics.

Mode of action
- They act on GABA-A receptors and enhance their response to GABA.

Route of administration
- Given orally, bioavailability is almost complete, with peak plasma concentrations in 30–90 minutes.
- Highly lipid soluble and diffuses rapidly through the blood–brain barrier and placenta; appears in breast milk.
- IV or IM administration may lead to an unpredictable absorption rate.

Maternal effects
- Tolerance develops after 2–3 days and is marked by 2–3 weeks.
- Tachyphylaxis has been reported.
- Onset of withdrawal is about 2–3 days after stopping (depending on the drug) peaking at 7–10 days and abating by 14 days.
- Symptoms of sensory disturbance such as hyperacusis, photosensitivity, and abnormal body sensations are common.
- Anxiety symptoms and features of depression, psychosis, seizures, and delirium tremens are also seen.

Effects in pregnancy
- May cause increased congenital abnormalities, especially cleft lip and palate.
- Withdrawal symptoms in the baby include hypotonia, respiratory problems, and poor feeding.

Cannabis

Derived from the plant *Cannabis sativa*. It is consumed either as the dried plant in the form called marijuana or grass, or as the resin secreted by the flowers.

Mode of action
- Acts on the specific cannabinoid receptor (anandamide) in the CNS.

Route of administration
- Mostly smoked, often with tobacco, but may be ingested with food or in a herbal solution.

Maternal effects
- Like alcohol, it may cause either exhilaration or depression.
- It may also produce hallucinations and is an appetite stimulant.

Effects on pregnancy
- There is no definite evidence of teratogenicity.

Other drugs of abuse

Hallucinogens, lysergic acid diethylamide (LSD), mescaline

- Usually consumed orally as small squares of blotting paper soaked in LSD, the drug causes hallucinations and visual illusions without lowering consciousness
- Its action is mediated through the activation of the $5HT_2$ receptors.
- The physical actions of LSD are variable:
  - initially there is an increase in the heart rate and blood pressure with adverse myocardial and cerebrovascular effects.
  - However, overdosage does not have a significant physiological reaction.
- ☛ There may be a risk of miscarriage and congenital abnormalities among regular users.

Volatile substances ('glue sniffing')

- Volatile substance misuse is a widespread problem mainly in the younger population.
- The substances used are generally solvents and adhesives (hence the term 'glue sniffing').
- Toluene, acetone, petrol, cleaning fluids, and aerosols are usually inhaled.
- Most often this is associated with other addictions such as tobacco and alcohol.
- It can lead to sudden maternal death from acute intoxication due to respiratory depression and cardiac arrhythmias.
- ☛ Little is known about the effects in pregnancy.

Tobacco

⚠ This is the most common substance of abuse and leads to complications including:
- ↑ risk of miscarriage.
- ↑ risk of placental abruption.
- Low birth weight.
- ↑ risk of neonatal death and sudden infant death syndrome.

▶ Women should be advised to stop smoking, or at least cut down, in pregnancy.
- Help from specialist smoking cessation advisers should be available.
- Nicotine replacement therapy (patches or gum) may be used in pregnancy.

Antenatal psychiatric disorders: overview

Women of childbearing age carry a high burden of psychiatric disorders, particularly depression and anxiety. Although the rates of psychiatric disorder during pregnancy appear similar to rates at other times in the life cycle (5–10%) the consequences are complicated by the additional risks to mother and fetus. Women with existing mental disorder require particularly careful management during pregnancy.

The importance of screening

△ Mental illness is a leading cause of maternal death in the UK.
• The majority of these deaths are the result of suicide, which is itself most strongly associated with perinatal depression.
• Over half of suicides occur between 6 weeks prenatally and 12 weeks postnatally, emphasizing the importance of early detection of antenatal psychiatric disorder and suicidal ideation.
• Most psychiatric disorders in pregnancy go unrecognized and unrecorded in the absence of systematic screening.
• Past history of mental illness is the best predictor of psychiatric disorder in pregnancy.
• Routine screening should include:
  • Personal mental health history.
  • Other vulnerability factors, including substance misuse.
  • Family history of bipolar affective disorder (confers genetic vulnerability and a first episode is 7 times more likely to present in the immediate postnatal period).

Planning pregnancy with psychiatric disorders

Women suffering with recurrent and severe mental disorders who want to have children may benefit from pregnancy planning, as:
• Relapses are predicted by major life events.
• A medication holiday can be tried before conception, avoiding complications of relapse on pregnancy.
• Reproductive toxicology of essential medication can be minimized.
• Closer antenatal monitoring can be planned in advance.
• Contingency plans, including those for child protection, can be made with, and shared by, all the relevant agencies and care givers.

📖 Antenatal and postnatal mental health. Clinical management and service guidance. NICE Clinical Guideline 45. National Institute for Health and Clinical Excellence, 2007. www.nice.org.uk

Antenatal psychiatric disorders: specific disorders

The classification and symptoms of psychiatric disorders appear in the ICD-10.

Anxiety disorders

- Panic disorder, generalized anxiety disorder, and obsessive–compulsive disorder are all relatively common in pregnancy.
- Symptoms include pervasive or episodic fearfulness, avoidance, and autonomic arousal.
- Excessive reassurance seeking may be a presenting feature.
- Must identify any concurrent depression requiring treatment.
- Can be highly distressing and merit clinical attention, although evidence for an adverse effect on fetal outcome remains conflicting.
- High antenatal anxiety is a predictor for postnatal depression.
- Psychological management (including CBT) is preferable to anxiolytics but access within the timescale of pregnancy may be limited.

⚠ Benzodiazepine use should be avoided.

Bipolar affective disorder

- Affects ~1% of women of childbearing age.
- Characterized by severe episodes of depression or mania (elevated mood, excitability, irritability and over-activity) often associated with psychotic symptoms that can pose a significant risk to mother and fetus.
- Associated with a twofold higher risk of admission postnatally than at other times.
- Decision to stop medication in existing patients when pregnancy is discovered should be made only after a careful risk/benefit review.

⚠ Associated with a high suicide rate.

Schizophrenia

- Affects ~1% of women of childbearing age.
- Clinical features vary but include delusions, hallucinations, and abnormalities of affect, speech, and volition.
- Maintenance medication is usually required throughout pregnancy.
- A significant proportion of patients are unable to care for the child.
- The lifetime risk of schizophrenia for a child with one affected parent is in the order of 10%.

Eating disorders

- Bulimia nervosa affects 1% of women of childbearing age and anorexia nervosa 0.2%.
- Characterized by disturbances in eating behaviour and abnormalities in body image.
- Although anorexia nervosa is associated with reduced fertility and fecundity, patients with sub-threshold symptoms can become pregnant and require careful monitoring and management.
- Possible effects on fetal outcome include IUGR, low birth weight, prematurity, and a possible increase in congenital anomalies.

Depression

⚠ As common antenatally as it is postnatally.
- Characterized by:
  - low mood
  - lack of energy or increased fatigability
  - loss of enjoyment or interest in usual activities
  - low self-esteem
  - feelings of guilt, worthlessness, or hopelessness
  - poor concentration
  - change in appetite (leading to weight loss or gain)
  - suicidal ideation.
- Associated with an increased risk of suicide.
- Can be effectively treated with pharmacological and psychological therapy.

📖 ICD-10 Classification of mental and behavioural disorders, WHO, 1992.

Psychiatric medications

Anticonvulsant mood stabilizers

Carbamazepine
- Major malformation rate 2.2%
  - high rate of neural tube defects
  - others include craniofacial abnormalities and distal digit hypoplasia.
▶ Breast-feeding is not recommended.

Lamotrigine
- Major malformation rate 2.1%:
  - high rate of cleft palate.
▶ Caution with breast feeding.

Sodium valproate
- Major malformation rate 6%:
  - very high rate of neural tube defects
  - others include craniofacial abnormalities and distal digit hypoplasia
  - significant neurobehavioural toxicity (22% of exposed infants develop low verbal IQ).

Antidepressants
- No strong evidence of ↑ malformations with tricyclic drugs.
- Paroxetine may have an association with cardiac malformations.
- SSRIs in late pregnancy have been associated with ↑ incidence of persistent pulmonary hypertension in the infant.
- SNRIs are relatively untested and so are not recommended as first line drugs in pregnancy.

▶ Sertraline and paroxetine have particularly low concentrations in breast milk and are therefore recommended for breast-feeding mothers

Antipsychotics
- Older antipsychotics (such as haloperidol) are preferred because more data is available with no strong evidence of ↑ malformations.
- May be an effective alternative to mood stabilizers in women with bipolar affective disorder.

Benzodiazepines
- See 📖 p. 434.

Lithium
- 50% of women with bipolar affective disorder stabilized on lithium relapse within 40 weeks of stopping it.
- Early pregnancy—risk of Ebstein's anomaly lower than previously estimated at 0.05–0.1% against a background risk of 0.0005%.
- Late pregnancy—levels need to be measured more frequently as plasma volume and GFR increase.
- Labour—reduced vascular volume and potential dehydration necessitates frequent monitoring of level.
- Neonate—reported association with floppy baby syndrome, neonatal thyroid abnormalities, and nephrogenic diabetes insipidus

▶ Breast-feeding is not recommended.

Considerations for managing psychiatric medications in pregnancy

- ⚠ Any decision to stop psychiatric medication for women with serious mental health problems should be made in consultation with a specialist, bearing in mind that the period of maximum vulnerability has often passed by the time pregnancy is identified. For example, an estimated 50% of women with bipolar affective disorder maintained on lithium will relapse during a 40 week pregnancy if it is stopped.
- Most psychiatric drugs are not associated with a significant increase in fetal anomalies.
- The risks of a relapse of psychiatric disorder during pregnancy tend to be underestimated.
- The risks of continuing medication need to be considered in terms of:
  - early fetal exposure
  - late fetal expose
  - delivery and neonatal withdrawal
  - breast feeding
  - longer term neurobehavioural toxicity.

Postnatal depression

Over 10% of women are depressed in the postnatal period. Although the term 'postnatal depression' is both clinically useful and acceptable to women, there is no evidence that it is any different from depression at any other time in a woman's life. It should accordingly be taken seriously and not dismissed as a mild, self-resolving condition that does not require treatment. This is emphasized by recent evidence of a link between postnatal depression and infant developmental problems when there are associated difficulties in the mother–infant relationship.

Diagnosis

The key features of depression are (see Antenatal disorders, 📖 p. 439):
- Tearfulness.
- Irritability.
- Anxiety.
- Poor sleep.

It can easily be missed if specific enquiries are not made, especially with milder cases. New mothers with depression are often embarrassed by their feelings and reluctant to admit to sadness at a time when they feel they are expected to be happy.

Screening for depression

NICE suggests the following questions are used to screen for depression both antenatally and at 4–6 weeks and 3–4 months postnatally:
- During the past month, have you often been bothered by feeling down, depressed, or hopeless?
- During the past month, have you often been bothered by having little interest or pleasure in doing things?

If the woman answers 'yes' to both of these:
- Is this something you feel you need or want help with?

Other screening questionnaires like the Edinburgh Postnatal Depression Scale (EPDS) are also helpful in identifying postnatal depression, and are routinely used by health visitors in many services.

Treatment and recovery

Mild to moderate depression may respond to self-help strategies and non-directive counselling ('listening visits' by a health visitor). Moderate to severe depression usually requires treatment with antidepressant medication and/or psychotherapy (cognitive behavioural therapy). Breast feeding is not a contraindication for antidepressant treatment, but drugs with low excretion in breast milk, such as sertraline, are preferred.

Women who have experienced postnatal depression have a high (>70%) lifetime risk of further depression and a 25% risk of depression following subsequent deliveries. For this reason, women who present in pregnancy with a history of postnatal depression are likely to benefit from closer postnatal follow-up.

Postpartum 'baby blues'

Over 50% of women experience a brief period of emotional instability starting around 3 days after delivery and resolving spontaneously within 10 days, characterized by the following features:

- Tearfulness.
- Irritability.
- Anxiety.
- Poor sleep.

This usually responds to support and reassurance.

Puerperal psychosis

This is a commonly used term that describes a range of psychotic conditions presenting in the immediate postnatal period. Most cases are episodes of bipolar affective disorder, although severe unipolar depression, schizophrenia, and acute physical illness with associated organic brain syndrome can all present with psychotic symptoms.

Presentation

Puerperal psychosis presents rapidly (usually within 2 weeks of delivery) following approximately 1 in 500 births. The associated suicide rate is in the order of 5% and the infanticide rate is up to 4%. Prediction and prevention are therefore key service priorities.

> **Risk factors include:**
> - Personal history of bipolar affective disorder.
> - Previous episode of puerperal psychosis.
> - 1st-degree relative with history of puerperal psychosis.
> - 1st-degree relative with bipolar affective disorder.

High-risk patients

⚠ A woman with bipolar affective disorder, and a personal or family history of puerperal psychosis, has a 60% risk of puerperal psychosis.

High-risk patients should be referred to specialist perinatal mental health services antenatally, so an appropriate care plan can be developed and the use of prophylactic medication, following delivery, may be considered.

Treatment and recovery

- ⚠ Women presenting with puerperal psychosis need urgent psychiatric assessment and treatment.
- They should be admitted, because of the risks to both mother and baby (neglect as well as direct harm):
  - ideally this will be to a specialist mother and baby unit, where the maternal–infant relationship can be protected.

⚠ Any decision to admit a baby to a mother and baby unit must be child centred, and involve full consideration of the longer term possibility of the baby remaining with the mother if the mental health problems have been long-standing.

Puerperal psychosis is treated according to diagnosis. This may involve:
- Antidepressant or antipsychotic medication.
- Mood stabilizers.
- ECT.

Most patients presenting with puerperal psychosis make a full recovery but the 10-year recurrence rate (puerperal and non-puerperal) is up to 80% and the 10-year re-admission rate is of the order of 60%.

Gynaecological anatomy and development

Gynaecological history: overview

▶ Always introduce yourself and explain what you are going to do, as patients visiting a gynaecologist are often very nervous.

Personal information
- Name, date of birth, age.
- Relationship status.
- Occupation.
- Partner's details and occupation (relevant in infertility patients).

Current problem
- Description of the problem.
- Severity, duration, relationship to menstrual cycle.
- Aggravating and relieving factors.
- Any previous investigations or treatment.

Menstrual history
- Date of first day of last menstrual period (LMP).

⚠ **Always think:** is this patient pregnant?
Every woman you see (10–60 years old) should be considered potentially pregnant till proved otherwise—then you will not miss it!

- Age at menarche/menopause.
- Menstrual pattern (number of days bleeding/length of cycle).
- Amount and character of bleeding (flooding, clots).
- Any intermenstrual or postcoital bleeding.
- Any associated pain (dysmenorrhoea).
- Use of contraception and details.

Past obstetric history (see Chapter 1, 📖 p. 2)
All pregnancies must be recorded including miscarriages, ectopic pregnancies, TOPs, and molar pregnancies. Outcomes, gestation and mode of delivery, any complications, birth weight, and current health of child(ren) should all be documented.

Past gynaecological history
- History of any other gynaecological problems especially endometriosis, polycystic ovaries, subfertility, or previous gynaecological surgery.
- Date of last cervical smear and result.

Sexual history
- Dyspareunia: superficial or deep
- Sexually transmitted infections or pelvic inflammatory disease (PID).
- Any abnormal vaginal discharge.

Gynaecological history: other relevant details

Micturition
General enquiry—if urinary symptoms disclosed then explore:
- Frequency (day and night).
- Pain or burning sensation (dysuria).
- Urgency.
- Urinary incontinence (stress or urge).
- Haematuria.

Bowel habit
General enquiry—if bowel symptoms disclosed then explore:
- Regularity.
- Associated bloating, pain, or difficulty defecating.
- Use of laxatives.
- Any rectal bleeding.

Medical and surgical history
- Any medical conditions especially dibetes, hypertension, asthma, thromboembolism. Previous abdominal surgery is important.

Drugs and allergies
- Details of all medication (doses and duration of use).
- Allergies to medications and severity (anaphylaxis or rash?).
- Use of folic acid in pregnancy.

▶ Consider the risks for all drugs in relation to pregnancy (see Chapter 5, 📖 p. 258).
- Possible teratogenesis.
- Altered pharmacodynamics and pharmacokinetics.
- Toxicity in breast milk.

Family history
- Especially diabetes, hypertension, and thromboembolism when COCP or HRT use is being considered.
- Familial gynaecological cancers should always be considered as well as others with a genetic association including:
  - breast
  - bowel
  - prostate.

Social history
- Home conditions and relationships.
- Smoking.
- Occupation and conditions of work.
- Alcohol intake.
- Lifestyle issues such as use of recreational drugs.

Gynaecological examination

General examination
- Height and weight
- BMI (= weight (kg)/[height (m)]^2)
- General, e.g. signs of anaemia, thyroid disease.

Abdominal examination
- **Inspection:** skin quality, abdominal distension, surgical scars (umbilical—laparoscopy) or Pfannensteil, any visible masses.
- **Palpation:**
  - superficial palpation for guarding, tenderness, rigidity
  - deep palpation for any masses and if present determine if arising from the pelvis ('can I get below the mass?')
- **Percussion:** dull if the mass is solid, tympanitic if distended bowel, shifting dullness and fluid thrill in case of ascites.
- **Auscultation:** usually used postoperatively to detect bowel sounds.

Good practice for intimate examinations
- Full explanation of procedure and reasons for it should precede examination.
- Verbal consent should be obtained.
- A trained chaperone is mandatory (not partner or children).
- The patient must be able to undress and dress in privacy and cover herself at all other times.
- Any students or extra personnel present should be introduced and consent obtained for their presence.

Pelvic examination
- **All equipment must be ready** (speculum, KY jelly, swabs, cytobrush, pipelle, etc.) **before** the patient is exposed.
- **Position the woman:**
  - dorsal (most common in gynaecological outpatient setting)
  - lithotomy (used for vaginal surgery, the feet suspended from poles)
  - Sim's (used for examination of pelvic organ prolapse, modification of the left lateral).
- **Inspection:** describe any swelling, inflammation, skin changes, lesions or ulceration seen anywhere on the vulva. Do the same for the vagina and cervix once the speculum is passed.
- **Speculum examination:** see box, 🕮 opposite p. 449 for description of technique. Describe findings in vagina and on cervix.

▶ Don't forget to take any swabs required such as HVS or *Chlamydia*.
- **Bimanual vaginal examination(VE):** See box, 🕮 p. 449 for description of technique.

How to do a speculum examination
- Cusco's bivalve speculum is more frequently used but Sim's speculum may be used in the examination of pelvic organ prolapse.
- Use a warm and well-lubricated speculum.
- The labia minora must be adequately parted with the left hand.
- Insert the speculum upwards and backwards (direction of vagina).
- Advance into vagina fully (until it cannot be advanced any further).
- Directly visualize as you open the blades to expose the cervix.
- If cervix not seen: close blades, withdraw slightly, change direction and open again.
- Speculum removal: ensure the blades are open while sliding over cervix, avoiding trapping it—watch what you are doing!
- The blades should be closed at the introitus, not trapping any vagina.

How to do a bimanual vaginal examination (VE)
- The index and middle fingers of the right hand are introduced into the vagina (⚠ remember to use plenty of lubricant). The fingers of the left hand should be placed on the abdomen above the symphysis pubis and the uterus and adnexae are then palpated between the two hands (hence 'bimanual palpation').

Checklist for VE
- **Cervix:**
  - consistency
  - tenderness
  - external os (?open).
- **Uterus:**
  - axis (anteverted, axial, or retroverted)
  - size (equivalent to gestational weeks of a gravid uterus)
  - consistency (soft in a gravid uterus, firm, or hard with fibroids)
  - mobility (may be fixed in endometriosis when adhesions are present or with advanced malignancy).
- **Adnexae:**
  - normal ovaries are usually not palpable
  - any masses (cystic/solid) and describe approximate size.
- Tenderness is assessed by direct digital pressure into the fornices and cervical excitation elicited by moving the cervix laterally.

▶ Uterine masses usually move with cervix, ovarian masses do not.

▶ Obese patients are usually difficult to palpate, so an ultrasound examination of the pelvis may be of value.

Anatomy: female reproductive organs

See Chapter 1 📖, p. 10 for anatomy of the bony pelvis.

Vagina
- Fibromuscular tube, 7–10 cm long.
- The cervix enters through the anterior wall.
- In the resting state the anterior and posterior walls are opposed.

Uterus
- Approximately 8 × 5 × 3 cm in size (non-pregnant).
- Composed mainly of smooth muscle.
- Divided into the corpus and cervix uteri.
- Cylindrical and joins the uterine cavity at the internal os and the vagina at the external os.
- Anteverted in 80% of women (the remainder are retroverted or rarely axial).

Uterine (Fallopian) tubes
- 10 cm long; lie in the upper part of the broad ligament.
- Divided anatomically into:
  - isthmus (medial)—opens into the uterus at the ostia
  - infundibulum (lateral) with fimbrial end closely applied to the ovary
  - ampulla—in between (where fertilization takes place).

Ovaries
- Approximately 3 × 2 cm during reproductive years.
- Attached to the posterior surface of the broad ligament by the mesovarium.
- Situated in the ovarian fossa at the division of the common iliac artery (the ureter runs immediately underneath).

Supports of the uterus, vagina, and pelvic floor
- Middle:
  - transverse cervical ligaments (cardinal ligaments)
  - pubocervical ligament
  - uterosacral ligaments.
- Lower:
  - levator ani muscles and coccygeus
  - urogenital diaphragm
  - the superficial and deep perineal muscles with the perineal body.

▶ Defects and weaknesses of these supporting structures due to fascial tearing and denervation during parturition and surgery can cause organ prolapse and problems with urinary incontinence

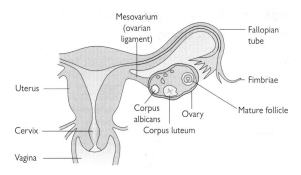

Fig. 13.1 Basic coronal view of the female pelvis. Adapted from Pocock G, Richards C. *Human physiology: the basics of medicine*, 2nd edn, OUP, 2004. By permission of Oxford University Press.

Anatomy: blood supply and relationship to other structures

Blood supply
Uterus
- The uterine artery:
  - branches from the internal iliac
  - runs behind the peritoneum to enter the lateral border of the uterus, through two layers of the broad ligament
  - anastomoses with the ovarian and vaginal arteries.
- The venous drainage is to the internal iliac vein.

Ovaries
- The ovarian arteries:
  - branches of the abdominal aorta from below the renal arteries.
- The right ovary drains directly into the inferior vena cava.
- The left ovary drains into the left renal vein.

Vagina
- Supplied by
  - vaginal artery
  - Inferior vesical artery
  - clitoral branch of the pudendal artery.

Urinary tract
Ureters
- Retroperitoneal throughout.
- Enter the pelvis in the base of the ovarian fossa.
- Run above the levator ani in the base of the broad ligament.
- Insert into the bladder posterolaterally.

⚠ The ureters are very close to the uterine artery near the lateral fornix and can be injured at hysterectomy.

Bladder
- Lies anterior to the uterus.
- 3 layers: serous (peritoneal), muscular (detrusor smooth muscle), and mucosa (transitional epithelium).
- Supplied by the superior and inferior vesical arteries (internal iliac artery).

Rectum
- Lies posterior to the uterus (separated from it by loops of small bowel lying in the pouch of Douglas).
- A thin rectovaginal septum separates the vagina and rectum.
- Supplied by superior, middle, and inferior rectal arteries (from the inferior mesenteric, internal iliac, and pudendal arteries respectively).

See Fig. 13.2.

Lymphatic drainage of the pelvic organs

- *Vulva and lower vagina* → inguinofemoral → external iliac nodes
- *Cervix* → cardinal ligaments → hypogastric, obturator, internal iliac → common iliac, and para-aortic nodes
- *Endometrium* → broad ligament → iliac and para-aortic nodes
- *Ovaries* → infundibulopelvic ligament → para-aortic nodes

⚠ Knowledge of lymphatic drainage is important when considering metastatic spread from genital tract cancer.

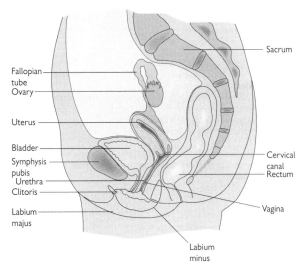

Fig. 13.2 Basic sagittal view of female pelvis demonstrating relationship to other pelvic organs. Adapted from Pocock G, Richards C. *Human physiology: the basics of medicine*, 2nd edn. OUP, 2004. By permission of Oxford University Press.

Anatomy: external genitalia

Perineum
- The area inferior to the pelvic diaphragm, can be divided into:
  - anterior urogenital triangle (pierced by the vagina and the urethra)
  - posterior anal triangle.
- The superficial and deep perineal fascias are continuous with the labia majora and are attached:
  - anteriorly to the pubic symphysis
  - laterally to the body of the pubis.
- The superficial perineal muscles are:
  - Superficial transverse perineus
  - Ischiocavernosus
  - Bulbocavernosus.

Vulva
The external genital organs are known collectively as the vulva and are composed of the mons pubis, labia majora and minora, and clitoris.
- **Labia majora:**
  - lateral boundary of the vulva from the mons pubis to the perineum.
- **Labia minora:**
  - anteriorly join to cover the clitoris
  - posteriorly form the fourchette.
- **Clitoris:**
  - composed of erectile tissue covered by a prepuce
  - supplied by a branch of the internal pudendal artery.
- **The vestibule:**
  - lies between the labia minora and the hymen
  - the urethra lies anterior in the vestibule
  - posteriorly and laterally lie the vestibular or 'Bartholin's' glands.

See Fig. 13.3.

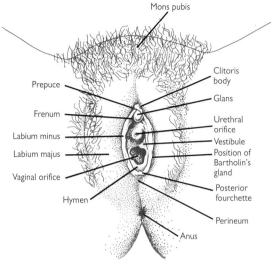

Fig. 13.3 External female genitalia. Reproduced from Collier J, Longmore M, Brinsden M. *Oxford handbook of clinical specialties*, 7th edn, OUP, 2006. By permission of Oxford University Press.

Malformations of the genital tract: overview

These congenital malformations range from asymptomatic minor defects to complete absence of the vagina and uterus. The prevalence is estimated to be as high as 3%.

Aetiology

They arise from failure of the paramesonephric (Mullerian) ducts to form, fuse in the midline, or fuse with the urogenital sinus:

- Complete failure to form:
  - Rokitansky syndrome (uterovaginal agenesis).
- Partial failure to form:
  - unicornuate uterus.
- Failure of the ducts to fuse together properly:
  - longitudinal vaginal septae
  - bicornuate uterus
  - uterus didelphus (complete double system).
- Failure to fuse with the urogenital sinus:
  - transverse vaginal septae.
- Remnants of the mesonephric (Wolffian) ducts may be present as lateral vaginal wall or broad ligament cysts:
  - these are usually trivial incidental findings and rarely of clinical significance.

⚠ Always look for renal and urinary tract anomalies (up to 40–50% coexistence).

Clinical features

Presentation often depends on whether it causes obstruction of menstrual flow.

- **Rokitansky syndrome**: painless 1° amenorrhoea, normal 2° sexual characteristics, absent vagina (dimple only).
- **Imperforate hymen**: cyclical pain, 1° amenorrhoea, bluish bulging membrane visible at introitus.
- **Transverse vaginal septum**: cyclical pain, 1° amenorrhoea, possible abdominal mass ± urinary retention due to haematocolpos, endometriosis due to retrograde menstruation.
- **Longitudinal vaginal septae and rudimentary uterine horns**: dyspareunia alone if no obstruction, but if one hemi-uterus is obstructed then increasing cyclical pain in the presence of normal menses ± abdominal mass and endometriosis.
- **Uterine anomalies** (bicornuate uterus, arcuate uterus, uterine septae): often asymptomatic, may present with 1° infertility, recurrent miscarriage, preterm labour, or abnormal lie in pregnancy (a causal relationship with these conditions is controversial).

Embryology of the female genital tract in a nutshell

- Genetic sex is determined at fertilization.
- Gender becomes apparent in the normal fetus by the 12th week of development.
- By the 6th week of life the following structures start to develop either side of the midline:
  - genital ridges (induced by primordial germ cells from the yolk sac)
  - mesonephric (Wolffian) ducts (lateral to the genital ridge)
  - paramesonephric (Mullerian) ducts (lateral to the mesonephric ducts).
- In the female fetus the mesonephric ducts regress.
- The paramesonephric go on to develop into:
  - the fallopian tubes (upper and middle parts)
  - uterus, cervix, and upper 4/5 of the vagina (this results from the lower part of the ducts fusing together in the midline).
- The lower 1/5 of the vagina develops from the sinovaginal bulbs of the urogenital sinus which fuses with the paramesonephric ducts.
- The muscles of the vagina and uterus develop from the surrounding mesoderm.

▶ Development of male genitalia is instigated by a single transcription factor encoded on the Y chromosome. In its absence the fetus will develop a female phenotype.

▶ The mesonephric ducts also sprout the ureteric buds (which go on to form the kidneys and ureters) and caudally develops into the trigone of the bladder. Hence the close association between genital tract and urinary tract abnormalities.

Malformations of the genital tract: management

Investigations

- A thorough history and examination are required.
- Abdominal and transvaginal ultrasound (± HyCoSy) are invaluable.
- Hysterosalpingograms (HSGs) are of limited use.
- MRI is the gold standard, especially if complex surgery is planned.
- Examination under anaesthetic ± vaginoscopy and hysteroscopy may be required.

⚠ Renal tract ultrasound ± intravenous urography should always be undertaken because of the high incidence of related renal tract abnormalities.

▶ If the uterus and upper vagina are absent, androgen insensitivity syndrome (46XY female) needs to be excluded by karyotyping, particularly if secondary sexual characteristics are only partially developed or absent.

Aims for the management of genital tract malformations

- Minor anomalies usually need nothing more than reassurance, particularly if an incidental finding, as most are of no clinical significance.
- Management should be a multidisciplinary approach involving psychological help for the patient and her parents as well as arranging correction of the anomaly.
- The aim of any treatment should be well defined.

- **Imperforate hymen:** easily corrected by a cruciate incision in the obstructive membrane.
- **Vaginal septae:** should be removed surgically. Obstructive uterine anomalies should also be surgically corrected or removed. This can commonly be performed laproscopically and/or hysteroscopically. These procedures can be technically difficult and should only be performed in centres with expertise in this area.
- **Rokitansky syndrome:** the creation of a functional vagina may be done by the use of vaginal dilators alone or a variety of surgical techniques. Timing should be related to when sexual activity is anticipated.
- Patients should be given access to information regarding their condition; support groups are often very helpful.

📖 Mayer Rokitansky Kuster Hauser syndrome support group: http://mrkhorg.homestead.com

---

Aims for the treatment of genital tract malformations

- Creation of a functional sexual conduit.
- Relief of menstrual obstruction and associated symptoms.
- Prevention of long term sequelae of endometriosis due to obstruction.
- Restoration or optimization of fertility wherever possible.

Disorders of sex development (DSD)

Sex determination occurs in the embryo with the female phenotype being the default setting. Male genitalia require testosterone to develop; the sex determining region (SRY) gene on the Y chromosome is principally responsible for development of the testis, which in turn secretes anti-Mullerian hormone (AMH) which causes regression of the paramesonephric ducts. If any part of this process fails, the resulting offspring may be genetically male but phenotypically female.

Causes of DSD, classified according to karyotype

46XX karyotype
- Virilizing forms of congenital adrenal hyperplasia.
- Maternal virilizing condition or ingested drug.
- Placental aromatase deficiency.
- True hermaphroditism.

46XY karyotype
- Androgen Insensitivity syndrome.
- Defects of testosterone biosynthesis (e.g. 17β-hydroxysteroid dehydrogenase deficiency).
- Pure gonadal dysgenesis (Swyer's syndrome).
- Partial gonadal dysgenesis 2° to single gene mutations.
- 5α-reductase deficiency.
- Leydig cell hypoplasia,

Abnormal karyotype
- Turner's syndrome—aneuploidy or mosaicism.
- X0/XY gonadal dysgenesis.

Later presentations of DSD
- DSD is not synonymous with ambiguous genitalia. Many conditions will present much later.
- Androgen insensitivity, Swyer's syndrome, and Turner's syndrome often present with 1° amenorrhoea.
- Although often associated with a degree of genital ambiguity 5α-reductase deficiency and 17β-hydroxysteroid dehydrogenase-3 deficiency may present with masculinization at puberty.

Ambiguous genitalia at birth

Genitalia are said to be ambiguous when their appearance is neither that expected for a girl nor for a boy. Incidence approximately 1:4000 births.

The extent ranges from mild clitoral enlargement to micropenis with hypospadias.

❶ Never guess the sex of a baby.

A full family history, drug history, and whether the mother has experienced any virilization during pregnancy should be ascertained.

Investigations

- Full assessment of the infant should occur looking for:
  - evidence of life-threatening salt-losing crisis (adrenal insuffiency), including hypovolaemia, hypoglycaemia, and hyperpigmentation.
  - △ U+Es are essential and must be sent urgently.
  - features of Turner's syndrome or other congenital anomalies
  - full inspection of genitalia carefully recording of position of orifices.
- Urgent serum 17-hydroprogesterone.
- 24 hour urine collection for steroid analysis.
- Karyotyping with urgent fluorescent in situ hybridization (FISH) for the Y chromosome.
- Ultrasound to locate gonads and presence of a uterus.
- Further investigations as deemed appropriate by the multidisciplinary team.

Corrective surgery

✒ Full disclosure is now advocated and parents should be fully informed of the risks of surgery over and above the usual risks of surgery and anaesthesia. These include:

- Surgery as an infant may not be definitive.
- Each episode of surgery increases the risk of damage to the sensitivity of the genitalia and dissatisfaction with sexual function in adult life.
- The child may one day want to be the opposite sex to that assigned, because of hormonal influences on the fetal brain.

The need for gonadectomy should be discussed openly regarding the risk of malignancy, especially for patients with gonadal dysgenesis (35% lifetime risk); with other conditions it may be advocated to prevent further virilization. In all cases parents should be given time to think.

The child should be given age and developmentally appropriate information regarding their condition at an early stage, with psychological support as required leading up to full disclosure so they can be involved in decisions regarding their care.

Coping with a child with ambiguous genitalia

- Keeping parents informed and psychologically supported at a very difficult time is of prime importance.
- Referral to a dedicated multidisciplinary team is essential.
- Pressure to decide on sex of rearing should not be allowed to interfere with giving time to allow parents to come to terms with their child's condition or reach the correct diagnosis.
- Parents must be full partners in allocation of sex of rearing.
- Access to relevant support groups is invaluable.

📖 Intersex Society of North America (ISNA) http://www.isna.org

📖 Androgen Insensitivity Syndrome Support Group (AISSG) http://www.aissg.org

Congenital adrenal hyperplasia (CAH)

- An autosomal recessive condition of enzyme defects in the adrenal steroidogenesis pathways leading to:
  - cortisol deficiency
  - ↑ACTH secretion with build up of cortisol precursors
  - ↑androgen production.
- 90% is due to deficiency of 21-hydroxylase.
- If severe, aldosterone production is also affected leading to salt wasting.
- Incidence ~ 1:14 000 births (carrier rate of 1:80).
- The gene responsible is *Cyp21*, located on chromosome 6 (but up to 20% cases have no mutation detectable).

Clinical features of CAH (46XX but appear male)

There is a wide spectrum of presentations including:
- Neonatal salt wasting crisis and hypoglycaemia.
- The commonest cause of ambiguous genitalia at birth, responsible for up to 50% cases (ranges from mild clitoral enlargement to a near normal male appearance).
- Childhood virilization, accelerated growth with early epiphyseal closure → restricted final height.
- Late-onset with hirsutism and oligomenorrhoea.

▶ Diagnosis is by detection of elevated plasma 17-hydroxyprogesterone levels and 24 hour urinary steroid analysis.

Fertility and CAH

- Menstrual irregularity occurs in:
  - ~30% of non-salt-losers
  - ~50% of salt-losers.
- Natural fertility:
  - ~60% women with non-salt-losing CAH
  - ~10% women with salt-losing CAH.
- Almost all have polycystic ovaries on ultrasound.
- Fertility treatment should be the same as for women without CAH.
- High levels of progesterone in poorly controlled CAH may be contraceptive by blocking implantation.

Management of CAH

- A multidisciplinary approach by paediatric urologists, endocrinologists, psychologists, and gynaecologists is required.
- Treatment requires replacement glucocorticoid to suppress ACTH and ↓ excess androgen production (whether dexamethasone, hydrocortisone, or prednisolone is used is a balance between risk of iatrogenic Cushing's syndrome and compliance, especially with teenagers).
- Salt-losing CAH requires fludrocortisone to replace aldosterone.
- Antiandrogens may be used to combat the effects of raised androgens with lower doses of glucocorticoids.
- In pregnancy requirement is ↑ for both mineralocorticoid and glucocorticoid (placental aromatase converts testosterone to oestradiol protecting the fetus from virilization and destroys excess therapeutic hydrocortisone).
- Prenatal diagnosis is available if a previous child has CAH:
  - dexamethsone is started with a positive pregnancy test (it crosses the placenta and suppresses the fetal adrenal ↓ the severity of ambiguous genitalia)
  - if CVS then shows the fetus is male or negative for the gene mutation, it can be stopped.

Surgery for ambiguous genitalia

- The aim of surgery is to improve the cosmetic appearance of the genital area and to provide potentially normal sexual function during adulthood.
- Feminizing genitoplasty is a very complex procedure that requires highly experienced surgeons in a specialized unit.

☛ There is no current consensus about the ideal timing for surgery. Traditionally surgery as an infant was advocated. Emerging evidence from research and adult patients has led some surgeons to limit surgery in infancy to a perineoplasty and defer vaginoplasty until adolescence.

- As there is a risk of damaging clitoral sensation with surgery consideration must be given to deferring clitoral surgery, especially in mild or moderate cliteromegaly.
- Vaginoplasty can be achieved by a variety of techniques including a 'pull-through' technique, skin flaps, skin grafts, or the use of bowel substitution. To avoid postoperative stenosis regular dilator use may be required. This is not recommended in children, so delaying surgery may be more appropriate.

Androgen insensitivity syndrome (AIS)

- Caused by a mutation in the androgen receptor gene causing resistance to androgens in the target tissues:
  - in the embryo the testis develops normally but the testosterone-dependent Wolffian structures do not
  - AMH is still secreted by the fetal testis, so regression of the Mullerian structures also occurs.
- It has an X-linked recessive pattern in 2/3 of cases (20% de novo mutation).
- If the mutation can be identified in a family then prenatal diagnosis can be offered with CVS.
- It can be complete (CAIS) or partial (PAIS).
- It is the commonest form of under-masculinization in an XY individual.
- Incidence of CAIS is thought to be about 1:20 000, that of PAIS is unclear.

Clinical features of AIS (46XY but appear female)

- CAIS individuals have:
  - female external genitalia
  - a short blind-ending vagina
  - absent uterus and fallopian tubes.
- Diagnosis may be made:
  - prenatally: fetal karyotype (XY) does not match female ultrasound findings
  - after birth: inguinal hernias or labial swellings are found to contain testes
  - at puberty: breast development is normal, pubic and axillary hair are scanty or absent, and menstruation fails to occur.
- PAIS includes a broad spectrum of under-masculinization from the severe with almost normal female phenotype and clitoral enlargement to morphologically normal male with hypospadias.
- The mildest form (MAIS) will not present till puberty with a high-pitched voice and gynaecomastia.

⚠ With CAIS physical appearance is feminine, as is core gender identity.

▶ Individuals with PAIS raised as female have a higher than average dissatisfaction with gender identity (some studies show >40% request gender reassignment).

▶ Diagnostic tests should include karyotype and pelvic ultrasound (to exclude Mullerian structures and locate testes).

Management of AIS

⚠ The lifetime risk for malignancy within the testes is thought to be about 2% and therefore there is no need for immediate gonadectomy.
- If CAIS is diagnosed before puberty the testes may be left in to allow natural puberty without the need for HRT in a child.
- After puberty:
  - gonadectomy should be offered because of the difficulty in monitoring intra-abdominal testes
  - HRT with oestrogens should be implemented
  - some may require testosterone replacement to feel their best.
- Bone mineral density should be checked as, even with good compliance to HRT, a degree of osteopenia is noted.
- Once sexual activity is anticipated then vaginal lengthening with the use of dilators should be offered.
- If dilators fail to help then consider vaginoplasty.

Coping with the diagnosis of AIS

- The patient should be referred to a multidisciplinary team experienced in the management of DSD.
- Input from a psychologist should be offered with an open door policy (disclosure may need to be repeated on subsequent visits).
- The clinician should offer to explain the condition to the patient's relatives or boyfriend.
- Information should be given regarding her diagnosis and referral to patient support groups offered.

📖 Androgen Insensitivity Syndrome Support Group (AISSG) http://www.aissg.org

Disorders of growth and puberty

Puberty is the development of secondary sexual characteristics in response to an ↑ in the pulsatile secretion of LH. In girls breast budding with accelerated growth is usually the first sign, followed by development of pubic and axillary hair, with menarche occurring ~2 years after breast budding. The average age for menarche is 12.7 years.

Precocious puberty

This is the onset and progression of signs of puberty before the age of 8 or menarche before the age of 10 years. Precocious puberty leads to early accelerated linear growth with premature epiphyseal closure resulting in restricted final height.

Causes of precocious puberty

- Central precocious puberty (CPP):
  - mostly idiopathic
  - congenital (e.g. cerebral palsy)
  - CNS space-occupying lesion.
- Peripheral precocious puberty (PPP):
  - 1° hypothyroidism
  - hormone-secreting ovarian cysts
  - McCune–Albright syndrome
  - late onset CAH (premature pubic hair).

Full history and examination
Should include documenting Tanner's stage and enquiring about:
- Cerebral palsy.
- Previous diagnosis of intracranial space-occupying lesion.
- Exposure to sex steroids.

Investigations
Should include:
- Bone age (from a hand radiograph).
- Cranial MRI.
- Pelvic USS.
- FSH/LH/Oestradiol/17-hydroxyprogesterone.
- Thyroid function tests.
- GnRH stimulation test.

Treatment
Should be for the underlying cause:
- If idiopathic CPP, injectable GnRH analogues are used as they:
  - have minimal side effects in children
  - enable achievement of normal final height
  - cause breast, uterine, and ovarian regression (so the child resembles its peers)
  - have no long term effect on bone mineral density in this age group
  - are safe to use for 4–5 years.

Tanner's stages

I Prepubertal, basal growth rate, no breast or pubic hair development.
II Accelerated growth, breast budding, sparse straight pubic hair.
III Peak growth velocity, elevation of breast contour, coarse, curly pubic hair spreading on to mons pubis, axillary hair.
IV Growth slowing, areolae form 2° mound, adult pubic hair type but no spread to inner thigh.
V No further increase in height, adult breast contour, adult pubic hair type and distribution.

▶ Menarche usually occurs in stage III or IV.

Delayed puberty and 1° amenorrhoea

Definition

The absence of menstruation and secondary sexual characteristics by age 14. 1° amenorrhoea also includes the absence of menstruation with normal secondary sexual characteristics by age 16 (see 📖 Chapter 14, p. 486).

> **Causes of delayed puberty include:**
> - Constitutional delay.
> - Chronic systemic disease/weight loss.
> - Hypothalamopituitary disorders (hypogonadotrophic hypogonadism, pituitary tumours).
> - Ovarian failure (Turner's syndrome, Swyer's syndrome, iatrogenic).

History

Should include details of:
- Chronic illnesses
- Anorexia
- Excessive exercise
- Family history of similar problems.

Examination

Should include assessment of:
- Height and weight.
- Pubertal (Tanner) stage.
- Visual fields (pituitary tumours).
- Hirsutism.
- Any stigmata of chronic disease.
- Signs of Turner's syndrome.

Investigations

- LH/FSH, testosterone, thyroid function tests and prolactin.
- Karyotype.
- Pelvic ultrasound or MRI if Mullerian anomaly suspected.
- Cranial MRI if prolactin >1500 mU/L.

⚠ hCG—never forget pregnancy as a cause of amenorrhoea, even 1°.

> **Management**
>
> - Referral to an appropriate specialist is critical.
> - Input may be required from endocrinologists, psychologists, and neurosurgeons.
> - Treatment will depend on the diagnosis.

▶ Puberty can be induced with low-dose oestrogen (oral or patches) and growth hormone. This is a specialist area for a paediatric endocrinologist.

Vaginal discharge: in childhood

Vaginal discharge is the commonest complaint in young girls and is often associated with itching or soreness. The history is usually from the carer but the child should be engaged in the conversation and asked questions about her complaint, which should include:

- Duration, frequency and quantity of the discharge.
- Colour and odour.
- Blood staining.
- Whether the child wipes 'front to back'.
- Use of bubble baths, soaps, washing powders.
- Previously tried creams or ointments.

Examination should be done carefully with the carer present. Frog-leg position or knee-chest position can be used and often seated in the mother's lap can be most reassuring for the child. A cotton-tipped swab may be used to collect a sample of discharge, for microbiological assessment, from the posterior vulva.

▶ If the discharge is bloodstained, particularly purulent, or profuse then examination under anaesthetic and vaginoscopy (and removal of any foreign body) are appropriate.

Differential diagnosis

- Vulvovaginitis.
- Foreign body (commonly small bits of toilet paper).
- Trauma (including sexual abuse).
- Rare tumours.
- Skin disease.

Vulvovaginitis

- Most common cause of vaginal discharge and soreness.
- Often occurs when she starts to be responsible for going to the toilet.
- Normally no specific organisms are isolated.
- Treatment is based on simple measures:
  - wiping front to back
  - avoidance of perfumed soaps, bubble bath, and biological washing powder for underwear
  - loose cotton underwear (avoid tights, leggings, and pants at night)
  - a simple emollient such as nappy cream may be helpful.

⚠ Antifungal, antibiotic, or steroid creams are unhelpful and may cause further irritation.

- If these measures are unhelpful, a short course of oestrogen cream may be beneficial.
- The symptoms always improve at puberty.

Sexual abuse

⚠ Always needs to be considered but it is an area fraught with difficulty. Seek senior advice if you have any concerns.

▶ Many chronically sexually abused girls show no signs on examination.

- Inspection of the hymen can be misleading for the inexperienced doctor as irregularities, notches, and hymenal tags can all be normal findings.
- If a sexually transmitted infection is detected in young girls it is normally an indicator of abuse but not always.
- If abuse is suspected the child should be referred to the lead doctor responsible for child protection.
- The child should be examined by the most experienced doctor available; if possible, refer to a local dedicated centre

If abuse is suspected

⚠ It is your duty to disclose confidential information if there is an issue of child protection.

⚠ If swabs are to be useful medico-legally, set protocols for a chain of evidence need to be followed, and seek senior advice urgently.

Vaginal discharge: in adolescence

Vaginal discharge in adolescents may be
- Physiological leucorrhoea requiring explanation only.
- A foreign body such as a retained tampon.
- Due to any of the infections that affect adult women (see Chapter 16, 📖 p. 522).

The adolescent consultation differs from that of an adult patient as obtaining a history may be more complicated. Usually the girl will be accompanied by a parent and unwilling to disclose information in front of them. It is important to give her an opportunity to talk to you away from her parent; this may be easily achieved by asking the parent to sit outside for the examination. Your manner should be frank and non-judgmental. She may need advice regarding contraception as well as treatment for her presenting complaint.

The girl may be very anxious about the examination and may be much more forthcoming with information once this is completed.

▶ Always explain what you are going to do, as this helps to allay anxiety.

The British Association for Sexual Health and HIV has specific guidelines for the treatment of infections and has a proforma for consultations with the under 16s.

📖 http://www.bashh.org

Sexually transmitted infections in adolescents
- The rates of sexually transmitted infections in teenagers are increasing rapidly.
- Teenagers are likely to have unprotected intercourse and are biologically more susceptible to infections than adults are.

⚠ The risk of pelvic inflammatory disease in a sexually active 15 year old may be up to 10 times that of a sexually active 25 year old.

⚠ Always remember that a teenager having consensual sex may also be the victim of abuse.

Dermatological conditions in children and adolescents

Many dermatological conditions affect children and may well present on the vulva. Children will generally present with itching and soreness, with skin changes being noticed by a carer. Adolescents may be slow to present due to embarrassment and uncertainty of what are normal changes associated with puberty.

Labial adhesions

- The labia minora stick together due to the hypo-oestrogenic state.
- Usually asymptomatic:
  - noticed at nappy changing or bathing by the carer
  - occasionally may be associated with soreness (if an element of vulvovaginitis is present).
- Resolves spontaneously at puberty with no long term problems.
- Treatment is oestrogen cream (pea-sized amount daily for up to 4 weeks):
  - useful if dysuria is present
  - reassuring for the carer to see the adhesions disappear
  - commonly reappear when treatment is stopped (should be explained before starting it)
- Surgery is not indicated.
- Ultrasound to check for mullerian structures can be offered for reassurance if the adhesions are severe.

Lichen sclerosus (see Chapter 22, 🕮 p. 666)

- Chronic inflammatory condition.
- Occurs in about 1:900 prepubertal girls.
- Usually presents with severe itching associated with dysuria and surface bleeding.
- Shiny, white crinkly plaques are classically distributed in a 'butterfly' pattern around the anogenital area.
- Diagnosis is usually by inspection alone in children.

⚠ Rubbing and scratching by the child leads to telangiectasia, purpura, fissures, and bleeding, wrongly leading to suspicions of sexual abuse.

- Can be associated with other autoimmune diseases (careful examination is required for other signs of illness).
- Treatment is symptomatic relief with the use of topical corticosteroids.
- Symptoms generally improve at puberty although the condition will still be present.
- Long-term follow up is required (association with squamous cell carcinoma in adulthood).

Other common dermatoses found in young people

Molluscum contagiosum
- Common in school age children.
- A pox virus usually causing shiny pale pink, oval papules on the trunk and limbs but anogenital spread is common.
- Destruction of the papules is painful and can lead to scarring so is not recommended.
- Resolves spontaneously in 6–18 months (but may take up to 3 years).

Irritant dermatitis
- Trigger factor is dependent on age group:
  - urine and faeces in infants.
  - bubble bath, soap, and sand in toddlers and young girls.
  - shampoo and shower gels in adolescents.
- Check no secondary infection with *Candida*.
- Advise avoidance of triggers and use of a simple barrier cream.

Threadworms
- Common in schoolchildren with poor hand hygiene.
- Worms migrate from the anus and cause anogenital itching.
- Skin is excoriated and sore and can have secondary infection.
- Treat with systemic antiparasitic (such as mebendazole) and a local barrier cream.
- Emphasize the need for improved hand washing to prevent re-infection.

Eczema and psoriasis
May present on the vulva as part of a generalized condition.

Vulval ulceration: differential diagnosis
- Aphthous ulcers
- Behçet's disease
- Lipshutz ulcer
- Herpes simplex (in a young child, consider the possibility of abuse).

Warts
- In sexually active teenagers HPV 6 and 11 are most common.
- In children common cutaneous warts (HPV 2) are found.
- Most will resolve untreated within 5 years (destructive treatments may be poorly tolerated in children but may be useful).

⚠ Sexual abuse should be considered in children with anogenital warts but vertical transmission can present up to 3 years of age and transmission can occur from existing warts on the child's fingers.

Gynaecological disorders: in adolescence

Following menarche there is a continuing change in pituitary-ovarian activity. regular ovulatory cycles usually establish soon, and if irregular cycles or menorrhagia persist then there is a high probability that there is an underlying disorder such as polycystic ovarian syndrome (PCOS) or dysfunctional uterine bleeding.

⚠ Do not assume that heavy, painful periods, irregular menses, or pelvic pain are a physiological part of adolescence.

Menstrual disorders (see 📖 Chapter 14, p. 486)

Amenorrhoea
- Eating disorders are common in this age group and, if missed, anorexia nervosa can have life-threatening complications.

⚠ Don't forget pregnancy—talk to the patient privately.

Oligomenorrhoea
- If persists after menarche up to 50% will continue to have irregular cycles
- Normal puberty is associated with an increase in insulin resistance:
  - if coupled with excessive adolescent weight gain consider PCOS
  - long-term risks of insulin resistance and endometrial hyperplasia are harder to get across to adolescents.
  - management should be symptom orientated with an anti-androgenic combined contraceptive pill (COCP) and advice regarding weight loss.

Menorrhagia
- Teenagers may not be aware of what is normal blood loss; try to get them to quantify loss in terms of pad soakage.
- The COCP is very useful in this age group.

Ovarian cysts (see Chapter 22)

All types that occur in adult women also occur in adolescents but with varying frequency.
- Simple unilateral, unilocular cysts are the most commonly found cysts in children and adolescents (most resolve spontaneously).
- Complex cysts/solid ovarian tumours are most likely to be germ cell in origin, most commonly benign cystic teratomas.

▶ Preservation of reproductive function should always be considered in children and adolescents undergoing treatment for ovarian masses whether benign or malignant.

⚠ 10% of ovarian tumours in children are malignant.
▶ Epithelial tumours account for less than 20% of ovarian cysts in children and adolescents.
▶ 3–5% of ovarian tumours in children are sex-cord tumours.

Pelvic pain (see Chapter 16)

Acute pelvic pain
- Adolescents may be more prone to torsion of the ovary or fallopian tube than older women and this should always be considered.

Chronic pelvic pain
- 1° dysmenorrhoea occurs in ~80% of adolescents.
  - Associated with an early menarche.
  - Has a significant effect on schooling, sleep, exercise, and family life.
  - Treat with NSAIDS and the COCP.
  - Pain unresponsive to NSAIDS/COCP should be investigated with transabdominal pelvic ultrasound and diagnostic laparoscopy.
- Endometriosis often presents atypically in adolescents and symptoms may be non-cyclical.
- Rare Mullerian anomalies (e.g. obstructed rudimentary horn) may present with pelvic pain of increasing severity and predispose to endometriosis:
  - if suspected, get an MRI.

⚠ Chronic pelvic pain is commonly reported in individuals who have suffered sexual abuse. Be aware of any signs of ongoing abuse.

Gynaecological cancers: in childhood

⚠ Extremely rare. All should be managed in a tertiary referral centre with links to the UK Children's Cancer Study Group (UKCCSG).

The most common is an ovarian germ cell tumour with the second being a vaginal embryonal rhabdomyosarcoma (sarcoma botryiodes).

Ovarian cancer in children

- Incidence 1.7/million in children under 15 years, 21/million in girls aged 15–19 years
- >80% germ cell tumours (most are dysgerminomas).
- Others include epithelial tumours (especially in the teens) and sex-cord stromal tumours (usually under 10 years).
- Present most commonly with pain, and an ovarian mass on pelvic ultrasound.
- Hormone-producing tumours may present with vaginal bleeding and or precocious puberty.
- Check hormonal profile and tumour markers (see Chapter 22, 📖 p. 694 for details of investigations and management).
- In childhood 1° treatment is surgery with chemotherapy if required (as childhood ovarian cancer is so rare the majority will be entered into trials).
- Prognosis is good for germ cell tumours, 5-year survival >85% for all stages.

Non-ovarian cancers in children

- The most common is vaginal embryonal rhabdomyosarcoma, but this is still extremely rare with an incidence of approximately 0.5/million girls.
- Most present before the age of 5 years with vaginal bleeding and classically a polypoid mass in the vagina.
- Examination under anaesthetic, biopsy, cystoscopy, and rectal examination are required for diagnosis usually performed by a paediatric urologist.
- Multi-agent chemotherapy is the mainstay of treatment.
- 5-year survival is approximately 82% overall.
- Clear cell adenocarcinomas of the cervix and vagina are now incredibly rare, as DES (a synthetic oestrogen) has not been used in pregnancy since the 1970s.

Fertility implications of childhood cancer

- Childhood cancer has a cumulative risk of ~1:650 by age 15.
- Most common are leukaemias.
- Advances in the treatment means there is an overall survival rate in excess of 70% leading to increasing numbers of young adults affected by the reproductive consequences.

Late effects of cancer therapy

Ovary

- Premature ovarian failure can be caused by radiotherapy or chemotherapy.
- A prepubertal ovary is more resistant to damage ($\uparrow$ reserve of primordial follicles).
- Can present as delayed puberty, secondary amenorrhoea, or premature menopause depending on:
  - age at time of treatment
  - dose of radiotherapy
  - chemotherapeutic agents used (some have no effect on ovarian function).

Uterus

Abdominal, pelvic, or total body irradiation (TBI) can damage uterine function causing reduced uterine volume, decreased elasticity of uterine musculature, and impaired vascularization. Successful pregnancies have been reported following radiotherapy but there is a risk of miscarriage, premature delivery, and intrauterine growth restriction. Chemotherapy does not seem to affect uterine function

Hypothalamus/pituitary

Cranial irradiation or TBI can lead to hypogonadotrophic hypogonadism. With high-dose cranial irradiation progressive compromise occurs, 60% having gonadotrophin deficiency 4 years after treatment. Even with low-dose cranial irradiation the presence of regular periods does not equate with fertility.

▶ Early referral is essential for these women if they present with subfertility.

Further malignancy

Up to 4% of childhood cancer survivors will develop a 2nd 1° malignancy within 25 years of the initial cancer. This is thought to be the carcinogenic effect of radiotherapy and certain alkylating agents.

Fertility preservation in cancer

⚠ Urgent referral to an specialist assisted reproduction centre for advice before commencing cancer therapy is essential.

Rapid advances are being made in this field. Current techniques offered are:

- Oophoropexy:
  - translocation of the ovaries to reduce the dose of radiation by shielding them behind the uterus or removing them out of the pelvis.
- Ovarian stimulation and cryopreservation of mature oocytes or embryos:
  - generally not suitable for paediatric patients.
- Harvesting and cryopreservation of ovarian tissue:
  - with the aim of future auto-grafting and restoration of fertility or in-vitro maturation of oocytes
  - selected centres have offered this since the 1990s but outcomes so far have been disappointing.

Chapter 14

Normal menstruation and its disorders

Physiology of the menstrual cycle

The menstrual cycle involves the coordinated hormonal control of the endometrium allowing pregnancy or regular shedding (periods). Peptide hormones from the hypothalamus and pituitary direct the ovary to produce steroid hormones (HPO axis), which in turn control the endometrium (see Figure 14.1). The process is complex and aspects of its initiation, control, and cessation are not fully understood. The average ages of menarche and menopause are 13 (falling) + 52 respectively. Day 1 of a cycle is the first day of fresh bleeding and this should always be clarified on history of last menstrual period (LMP).

Follicular phase

- Pulsatile release of GnRH from the hypothalamus → anterior pituitary to produce follicle stimulating hormone (FSH).
- FSH promotes follicular development in the ovary → recruitment of a dominant follicle.
- Granulosa cells in the follicle produce oestrogen → endometrial proliferation.
- ↑ oestrogen levels → negative feedback on the HP axis (via inhibin) to stop further FSH production.

Ovulation

Increasing oestrogen (positive feedback via activin) → altered hypothalamic GnRH pulsatility → pituitary production of luteinizing hormone (LH). The LH surge occurs 36 hours before ovulation.

Luteal phase

- The follicle collapses down to become the corpus luteum ('yellow body') which produces oestrogen and progesterone (from theca cells).
- Progesterone and oestrogen act on an oestrogen-primed endometrium to induce secretory changes → thickening and ↑ vascularity.
- The corpus luteum always has a fixed lifespan of 14 days before undergoing involution to become a corpus albicans ('white body'):
  - if implantation occurs, hCG 'rescue' of the CL allows continued production of progesterone to support the endometrium
  - in the absence of pregnancy, CL degeneration → a rapid fall in progesterone and oestrogen initiating menstruation.

Menstrual phase

- Rapid ↓ in steroids → shedding of the unused endometrium.
- Inflammatory mediators (PGs, ILs, and TNF) → vasospasm (24 hours) in the spiral arteries → hypoxia and devitalization of the endometrium.
- Vasodilatation and spiral artery collapse → loss of the layer and bleeding from vessels.
- The complex vascular changes, controlled by secondary messengers, also → natural haemostatic mechanisms including platelet plugs, the coagulation cascade and fibrinolysis.
- The endometrium is lost down to the basalis layer (up to 1/3 of menstrual loss is reabsorbed).
- All steroid hormones now at basal level, negative feedback is lifted and GnRH–FSH production can begin a new cycle.

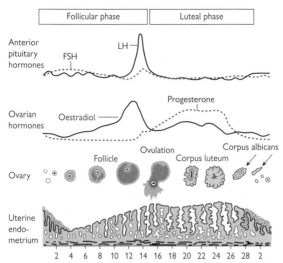

Fig. 14.1 The menstrual cycle. Reproduced from Sanders S et al. (eds) *Oxford handbook for the foundation programme*, OUP, 2005. By permission of Oxford University Press.

Normal cycle or pathological?

- Ovulatory cycles are usually 21–32 days with a basically regular pattern.
- A menstrual history with short or long cycles usually results from anovulation.
- Ovulatory cycles that vary do so due to the follicular phase (luteal phase is fixed).
- After menarche, cycles are often irregular for months or up to 5 years until maturation of the HPO axis reliably triggers ovulation.
- Perimenopausal periods are commonly irregular (usually ↑ cycle length) due to ovarian resistance to gonadotrophins and anovulatory cycles.
- Nearly all women will experience some menstrual irregularity in timing or flow at some stage—many are transient.

Bleeding and pain: what's normal?

- Bleeding can be 1–7 days with an average of 3–5 days.
- The reported amount of loss is highly variable.
- Periods described as 'heavy' should always be viewed as such.
- Pain is 'normal' (vasospasm and ischaemia) but is highly variable.

⚠ Pain interfering with normal functioning needs to be addressed.

⚠ Bleeding between periods (IMB) and after intercourse (PCB) is always abnormal.

Menstrual disorders: amenorrhoea

- **1° amenorrhoea** is lack of menstruation by age 16.
- **2° amenorrhoea** is an absence of menstruation for 6 months.

Diagnosis

History Emphasis on:
- Risk of pregnancy and type of contraceptive used.
- Galactorrhoea or androgenic symptoms (weight gain, acne, hirsutism).
- Previous genital tract surgery (intrauterine instrumentation or LLETZ).
- Issues with eating or excessive exercise.
- Drug use (esp. dopamine antagonists for psychiatric conditions).

Examination General, including:
- BMI <17 / >30, hirsutism, 2° sexual characteristics
- stigmata of endocrinopathies or Turner's syndrome
- evidence of virilization (deep voice, male pattern balding, cliteromegaly).
- **Abdominal:** may show masses due to tumours or genital tract obstruction.
- **Pelvic:** may show:
  - imperforate hymen
  - blind ending vaginal septum
  - absence of cervix and uterus.

Investigations for amenorrhoea

⚠ Pregnancy test.
- FSH/LH: ↑ in POF, ↓ hypothalamic causes (not useful in PCOS).
- Testosterone and SHBG are most useful for PCOS.
- Prolactin should always be tested.
- TFTs.
- Pelvic ultrasound:
  - can define anatomical structures; congenital abnormalities, Asherman's syndrome, haematometra, and PCOS morphology.
  - can indicate physiological activity; endometrial atrophy in POF.
- Karyotype if uterus absent or suspicion of Turner's syndrome.
- Specific tests for endocrinopathies where there is clinical suspicion.

Management Must be guided by the diagnosis and fertility wishes. Options include:
- Treat any underlying causes.
- Attain normal BMI.
- Cabergoline or surgery for hyperprolactinaemia.
- Cyclical withdrawal bleeds (COCP for PCOS).
- HRT for premature ovarian failure (POF).
- Relief of genital tract obstruction.
  - cervical dilation, hysteroscopic resection, incision of hymen.
- Specific treatment for endocrinopathies and tumours.

▶ Major congenital abnormalities, androgen insensitivity syndrome (AIS), etc. should be managed by multidisciplinary teams in specialist centres.

Common causes of amenorrhoea

Physiological causes

⚠ Pregnancy must always be excluded.

- Lactation.
- Menopause.

Iatrogenic causes

- Progestagenic contraceptives: Depo-provera®, Mirena IUS®, Implanon®, POP.
- Therapeutic progestagens, continuous COCP use, GnRH analogues, rarely danazol.

Pathological causes of amenorrhoea

- Hypothalamic:
  - Functional: stress, anorexia, excessive exercise, pseudocyesis
  - Non-functional: SOL, surgery, radiotherapy, Kallman's syndrome (1° GnRH deficiency).
- Anterior pituitary:
  - micro- or macroadenoma (prolactinoma) or other SOL
  - surgery
  - Sheehan's syndrome (postpartum pituitary failure).
- Ovarian:
  - Polycystic ovary syndrome (PCOS)
  - POF
  - resistant ovary syndrome
  - ovarian dysgenesis, especially due to Turner's syndrome (45X0).
- Genital tract outflow obstruction:
  - imperforate hymen
  - transverse vaginal septum
  - cervical stenosis
  - Asherman's syndrome (iatrogenic intrauterine adhesions).
- Agenesis of uterus and Mullerian duct structures:
  - sporadic or associated with AIS.
- Endocrinopathies:
  - hyperprolactinaemia
  - Cushing's syndrome
  - severe hypo/hyperthyroidism
  - CAH.
- Oestrogen- or androgen-secreting tumours:
  - usually ovarian or adrenal such as granulosa-thecal cell tumours and gynandroblastoma.

Menstrual disorders: oligomenorrhoea

When cycles are longer than 32 days they usually represent anovulation or intermittent ovulation. Transient oligomenorrhoea is common, ('stress' or emotionally related causes are often cited) and usually self limiting.

Causes

Similar to many of the causes of 2° amenorrhoea:
- PCOS is the commonest cause.
- Borderline low BMI.
- Obesity without PCOS.
- Ovarian resistance leading to anovulation, e.g. incipient POF, is rare but important,
- Milder degrees of hyperprolactinaemia need to be excluded as well as mild thyroid disease.

Management of oligomenorrhoea

What does the patient want? Regular periods or fertility?
- Provide reassurance.
- Treat any underlying causes as for amenorrhoea.
- It is not uncommon for no cause to be found, but serious pathology must be excluded.
- Attain normal BMI (weight loss or gain as appropriate).
- Provide regular cycles:
  - COCP or cyclical progestagens
  - for PCOS a minimum of 3 periods/year is recommended to ↓ the risk of endometrial hyperplasia due to unopposed oestrogen.
- Full fertility screening should be performed if ovulation induction is required.

Menstrual disorders: dysmenorrhoea

Pain is considered a normal symptom of menstruation. It is highly subjective and varies greatly between women. If a woman describes her periods as unacceptably painful, then they are!

- **1° dysmenorrhoea:** the pain has no obvious organic cause.
- **2° dysmenorrhoea:** the pain is due to an underlying condition.

Diagnosis

History

Should focus on

- Timing and severity of pain (including degree of functional loss):
  - commonly premenstrual pain ↑ in the first 1–2 days of bleeding, then easing.
- Pelvic pain and deep dyspareunia (may signify pelvic pathology).
- Previous history of pelvic inflammatory disease (PID) or sexually transmitted infections (STIs).
- Previous abdominal or genital tract surgery.

Examination

- Abdominal exam to exclude pelvic masses.
- Pelvic exam; cervical excitation, adnexal tenderness and masses.

Investigations

- STI screen (including *Chlamydia* swab).
- TVS; endometriomata, PID sequelae, fibroids, congenital abnormalities.
- Laparoscopy is usually reserved for women with TVS abnormalities, medical treatment failures or those with concomitant subfertility.

Management of dysmenorrhoea

- Appropriate reassurance and analgesia may be all that is required.
- Symptom control:
  - mefenamic acid 500 mg tds with each period effective
  - COCP to abolish ovulation
  - data on Mirena IUS ®demonstrates benefit.
  - paracetamol, hot-water bottles, etc. may be helpful for some.
- Treat any underlying causes:
  - endometriosis: COCP, progestagens, GnRH analogues
  - antibiotics for PID
  - relief of obstruction (usually surgical).
- Therapeutic laparoscopy—for above indications:
  - gold standard for diagnosis + management of endometriosis/ adhesions/complicated PID
- Hysterectomy is now rare for this indication alone.

▶ When no disease is identified or other management options have failed, then ovulation suppression by tricycling COCP or GnRH analogues for up to 9–12 months will limit the number of 'periods' and therefore pain.

1° dysmenorrhoea

Pain in the menstrual cycle is a feature of ovulatory cycles and is due to uterine vasospasm and ischaemia, nervous sensitization due to prostaglandins (PGs) and other inflammatory mediators, and uterine contractions. A maternal or sibling history of dysmenorrhoea is very common and the problem usually starts soon after menarche. Theories accounting for 1° dysmenorrhoea include:

- Abnormal PG ratios or sensitivity.
- Neuropathic dysregulation.
- Venous pelvic congestion.
- Psychological causes.

2° dysmenorrhoea

Underlying causes include:
- Endometriosis.
- Adenomyosis.
- Pelvic inflammatory disease (PID).
- Pelvic adhesions.
- Fibroids (though not always causal).
- Cervical stenosis (iatrogenic post LLETZ or instrumentation).
- Asherman's syndrome.
- Congenital abnormalities causing genital tract obstruction,
  e.g. non-communicating cornua.

▶ Pain clinic, psychological support, and self-help groups may be of benefit to some women who wish to maintain their fertility, especially when they have other pelvic pain symptoms.

Dysfunctional uterine bleeding (DUB): aetiology

Dysfunctional uterine bleeding (DUB) is a diagnosis of exclusion and is defined as any abnormal uterine bleeding in the absence of pregnancy, genital tract pathology, or systemic disease.

- Menorrhagia is the commonest symptom and DUB will ultimately be the cause in 50–60% of women with this symptom.
- Menorrhagia is responsible for 15–20% of gynaecological referrals.

△ Objective measures of blood loss >80 mL are clinically meaningless and should not be used outside research. If periods are reported as unacceptably heavy, then they are!

DUB at a glance

- Menorrhagia is the commonest gynaecological symptom you will see, and most of these women will have DUB.
- DUB is an umbrella term and is only diagnosed after exclusion of pathology.
- Women under 40 can safely be treated without investigation.
- TVS is the first line investigation if >40, failed medical therapy, or risk factors for endometrial disease.
- The majority of women will respond to medical therapy, especially tranexamic ± mefenamic acid
- The IUS is an excellent treatment that significantly reduces the number of women requiring surgery.
- Surgery should only be used in women who have completed their family and have had failed adequate medical therapy.
- MEA, balloon ablation or Novasure appear to be the easier to perform and should be offered before hysterectomy.
- Hysterectomy has higher morbidity and cost but is a guaranteed cure and long term satisfaction rates are high.

Aetiology

The exact causes of DUB are unknown. Proposed mechanisms at the endometrial level include:
- Abnormal PG ratios (+ other inflammatory mediators) favouring vaso-dilatation and platelet non-aggregation.
- Excessive fibrinolysis.
- Defects in expression/function of matrix metalloproteinases (MMPs), vascular growth factors, and endothelins.
- Aberrant steroid receptor function.
- Defects in the endomyometrial junctional zone.

The medical treatments tend to reflect the underlying pathologies (see, 📖 p. 494)

Dysfunctional uterine bleeding (DUB): diagnosis and investigations

Diagnosis

Symptoms

- Heavy and/or prolonged vaginal bleeding (with clots and flooding):
  - irregular, heavy periods usually occur at the extremes of reproductive life (postmenarche and perimenopausal).
- May be associated with dysmenorrhoea.
- Systemic symptoms of anaemia and disruption of life due to bleeding.
- A smear history and contraceptive use are vital information.

⚠ Totally erratic bleeding, intermenstrual bleeding (IMB), or postcoital bleeding (PCB) should prompt a search for cervical or endometrial pathology.

Clinical signs

- Anaemia
- Abdomino-pelvic examination is usually normal.

Differential diagnosis for DUB

- Submucous fibroids.
- Adenomyosis.
- Endometrial polyps, hyperplasia, or cancer.
- Very rarely, hypothyroidism or coagulation defects.

Investigations

⚠ Pregnancy should be excluded.
- FBC (Hb + MCV).
- Consider TFTs and clotting screen if clinically indicated.
- Cervical smears are not done opportunistically if smear history normal.
- STI screen including *Chlamydia* (important for IMB, PCB, or erratic bleeding).
- The risk of endometrial pathology <40 is very small so no further investigation required—treat and await clinical response.
- If >40, risk factors for endometrial disease, or no response:
  - TV USS—is good for identifying fibroids and polyps, and measuring endometrial thickness. The risk of endometrial pathology with a normal TV USS is small but it may be less accurate during menstruation.
  - hydro-sonography may be useful to identify or exclude polyps as the upper limit of 'normal' endometrial thickness is undefined in menstruating women.
  - pipelle endometrial biopsy to exclude endometrial hyperplasia or cancer
  - hysteroscopy and curettage (preferably outpatient) may be appropriate as above or if there is no response to initial medical treatment.

Dysfunctional uterine bleeding (DUB): medical management

Regular DUB

- **Antifibrinolytics:** tranexamic acid 1 g tds days 1–4 (40% ↓ in menstrual loss):
  - safe, non-hormonal, non-contraceptive
  - side effects: leg cramps, minor GI upset. Caution in cardiac disease.
- **NSAIDS:** mefenamic acid 500 mg tds days 1–5 (20–30% ↓ in loss and significant ↓ in dysmenorrhoea):
  - safe, non-hormonal/contraceptive.
  - side effects: GI upset incl. ulceration, renal impairment. Caution if asthmatic, CV disease, renal impairment, peptic ulcer.
- **COCP:** 20–30% ↓ loss and improvement in dysmenorrhoea:
  - provides contraception
  - for cautions + side effects see Chapter 19, 🕮 p. 596.
- **Oral progestagens** are of no benefit in regular menorrhagia.
- **Mirena IUS®:**
  - releases measured doses of levonorgestrel into the endometrial cavity for 5 years inducing an atrophic endometrium. Blood loss ↓ by up to 90% and ~30% will be amenorrheic at 12 months
  - provides contraception
  - side effects: insertional issues, irregular PV bleeding for first 4–6 months (usually abates); progestagenic side effects are rare due to minimal systemic absorption.

▶The IUS has caused a major ↓ in the number of hysterectomies performed for DUB.

Irregular DUB

- Tranexamic and mefenamic acid are useful to ↓ loss.
- COCP will also regulate an irregular cycle (safe up to the menopause if no other cardiovascular risk factors).
- Cyclical (days 5–26) Norethisterone 5 mg tds or medroxyprogesterone acetate 5–10 mg tds:
  - regulates cycle but little evidence to suggest ↓ in loss
  - side effects: bloating, headache.
- Mirena IUS®: as above.

Where first line therapy has failed, further medical treatment may be used in women who are very anaemic, bleeding continuously, having their life disrupted, or have cautions or contraindications to surgery
- GnRH analogues can achieve amenorrhoea quickly by inducing a medical menopausal state:
  - side effects: vasomotor symptoms and use limited to 6–12 months maximum due to bone loss.
- High-dose progestagens: medroxyprogesterone acetate 10 mg tds continuously will induce amenorrhoea but may be time-limited due to side effects as before.

Choice of management for DUB will depend on:

- Reproductive wishes and contraceptive needs.
- Whether periods are regular or irregular.

▶ Many women may just need reassurance that there is no serious cause.

▶ Anaemia should be corrected by treating the underlying cause of bleeding and using ferrous sulphate to replace lost iron stores.

Dysfunctional uterine bleeding (DUB): surgical management

Surgery should be reserved for the minority of women who fail to respond to medical management. Women have to be certain their families are complete before surgery.

Endometrial ablation

Destruction of the endoemtrium down to the basalis layer is effective for most women and should be offered to all women for consideration. Methods include: microwave (MEA), thermal balloon (Thermachoice) and Novasure (electrical impedance). Hysterocopic resection, or rollerball ablation, are now used much less often due to ↑ operative complications. Typical endometrial ablation results:
- 80%-90% of women are significantly improved
- 30% will become amenorrhoeic
- 20% will need a second procedure by 5 years.

Hysterectomy

Hysterectomy is the only guaranteed cure for DUB but RCTs have shown higher morbidity, longer recovery, and financial costs compared to endometrial ablation. Complications include haemorrhage; infection; and bladder, ureteric or bowel injury (<1%).

Long-term satisfaction rates for hysterectomy are generally high and regardless of method most women report improved sexual function—as one patient put it 'well, I now actually have sex now I'm not bleeding all the time'.

Current evidence regarding method of hysterectomy

- Vaginal hysterectomy is the route of choice over abdominal, where possible, as recovery, postoperative pain, and cost are reduced.
- Laparoscopic assisted vaginal hysterectomy (LAVH) takes longer than abdominal or vaginal, and has higher rates of urinary tract injury. No evidence supports routine use of this method.
- Subtotal hysterectomy is quicker and has a lower risk of bladder injury, but the possible improved sexual satisfaction rates are as yet unproven. There is a small risk of continuing light menstruation if residual endometrial cells are left, and women continue to require smear tests.

Premenstrual syndrome (PMS): overview

A working definition of premenstrual syndrome should include:
- Distressing psychological, physical, and/or behavioural symptoms.
- Occurrence during the luteal phase of the menstrual cycle (or cyclically after hysterectomy with ovarian conservation).
- Significant regression of symptoms with onset or during the period.

In general population 15% women are asymptomatic, 50% have mild PMS symptoms, 30% moderate, and 5–10% severe (up to 1 000 000 women in UK alone!)

Aetiology

Probable multiple aetiologies, but cyclical ovarian activity likely to be the central component (ovarian 'trigger' such as ovulation may initiate a cascade of events). A central increased responsiveness to a combination of steroids, chemical messengers (E2/serotonin, progesterone/GABA) and psychological sensitivity may play a part.

Diagnosis

Most women self diagnose. A detailed history can suggest a diagnosis of PMS but only prospective assessment can establish its true nature. A variety of symptom charts are available from the National Association of Premenstrual Syndrome, the national PMS charity at www.pms.org.uk.

Moderate–severe PMS involves disruption of interpersonal/work relationships, or interference with normal activities. DSM-IV diagnostic criteria (USA) for premenstrual dysphoric disorder (see text box below) are more specifically psychological but considered equivalent to severe PMS,

It is important to exclude organic disease and significant psychiatric illness. Perimenopausal women may have increasing premenstrual symptoms as well as menopausal symptoms.

📖 National Association of Premenstrual Syndrome www.pms.org.uk

---

DSM-IV criteria for premenstrual dysphoric disorder

≥5 symptoms present for most of the late luteal phase with remission within a few days of onset of menses and absence of symptoms in the week post menses. At least one symptom must be from first four:
- Markedly depressed mood, feelings of hopelessness or self-deprecation.
- Marked anxiety, tension (being 'on edge').
- Marked affective lability (e.g. feeling suddenly sad or tearful).
- Persistent and marked anger/irritability/increased conflicts.
- Decreased interest in usual activities (school, friends, hobbies).
- Subjective sense of difficulty in concentrating.
- Lethargy, easy fatiguability/lack of energy.
- Marked change in appetite, overeating, or specific food cravings.
- Hypersomnia or insomnia.
- Subjective sense of being overwhelmed or out of control.
- Other physical symptoms, such as breast tenderness or swelling, headaches, joint or muscle pain, a sense of 'bloating', weight gain.

Premenstrual syndrome (PMS): management

Hormonal

Progesterone and progestogens

A meta-analysis suggests no benefit of progesterone pessaries, suppositories, depot injections, or oral formulations

Ovulation suppression agents

- **COCP:** appears useful for some women. Yasmin® (drospirenone has better side effect profile) now has a licence for treatment of PMS.
- **Danazol:** 4 RCTs report benefit for PMS but there are significant masculinizing side effects. Treatment in luteal phase only is effective for breast tenderness.
- **Oestrogen:** transdermal oestrogen or implants at doses sufficient to suppress ovulation are not currently licensed but well established and accepted treatment of PMS. Oestradiol patch 100 micrograms twice weekly with a progestogen (cyclical basis). Implants generally makes them unsuitable for those who may wish to conceive.
- **GnRH analogues ± addback HRT** are of proven benefit for moderate to severe PMS but with a license for 6 months treatment only due to bone loss. Usually given with addback tibolone (fewer side effects and bone loss). 'GnRH test' useful for those considering hysterectomy and BSO for severe symptoms.

Non-hormonal

- **SSRIs/selective noradrenalin reuptake inhibitors:** a meta-analysis confirms benefit for continuous and luteal phase only treatment. No current licence in the UK so careful documentation is required as some women are reluctant to accept antidepressants. Side effects may be problematic.
- **Antidepressants:** tricyclics and anxiolytics have benefits for selected patients as indicated in at least 9 studies.

Surgery

Two trials have confirmed a benefit of removal of the ovarian trigger with the uterus to avoid the need for combined HRT as definitive treatment for severe PMS. However it is generally recommended that a 'GnRH test' is performed to ensure a benefit will be realized and/or another indication for hysterectomy is present.

📖 www.pms.org.uk

📖 www.bms.org.uk

Self-help techniques for managing PMS

Dietary alteration
Possible benefit with less fat, sugar, salt, caffeine and alcohol, frequent starchy meals, more fibre, fruit and vegetables, and 4 hourly small snacks.

Dietary supplements
- **Vitamin B6:** possible benefit for PMS symptoms and depressive symptoms.
- **Vitamin E:** studies small but promising.
- **Calcium:** 2 studies (1200–1600 mg) revealed some improvement in symptoms.
- **Magnesium:** appears most beneficial for premenstrual anxiety.
- **Evening primrose oil:** of value for mastalgia only.

Exercise
Moderate regular aerobic exercise promoting cardiovascular work is beneficial (3 controlled studies).

Stress reduction
Relaxation techniques, yoga, meditation, breathing techniques, and encouragement of healthier lifestyle may also help.

Complementary and alternative therapies used in PMS

- **Acupuncture:**
  - several RCTs show positive data for dysmenorrhoea.
- **Homeopathy:**
  - in a pilot study (n = 20), improvement in 90% compared to placebo.
- **Progesterone and wild yam:**
  - no benefit demonstrated in many studies.
- **Phytoestrogens:**
  - possible benefit for PMS symptoms (may be difficult to incorporate into a western diet).
- **Herbal remedies:**
  - 2 good trials confirm the benefit of *Vitex agnus castus* (20 mg once daily)
  - St John's wort may also be of value due to its action as a selective serotonin reuptake inhibitor SSRI; further studies awaited.
- **Mind–body:**
  - Aromatherapy, reflexology, photic stimulation, and magnotherapy may show some benefit but data are sparse.

Early pregnancy problems

Termination of pregnancy (TOP): overview

Around 186 000 terminations of pregnancy (TOP) are performed annually in England and Wales and 11 500 in Scotland. Over 98% of these are undertaken because of risk to the mental or physical health of the woman or her children. At least 1/3 of British women will have had a TOP by the time they reach 45 years of age.

UK law

Legislation varies throughout the world, with terminations remaining illegal in some countries.

The Abortion Act of 1967 legalized abortion in the UK and identified 5 categories, as follows:
- A: the continuance of the pregnancy would involve risk to the life of the pregnant woman greater than if the pregnancy were terminated.
- B: the termination is necessary to prevent grave permanent injury to the physical or mental health of the pregnant woman.
- C: the pregnancy has not exceeded its 24th week and the continuance of the pregnancy would involve risk, greater than if the pregnancy were terminated, of injury to the physical or mental health of the pregnant woman.
- D: the pregnancy has not exceeded its 24th week and the continuance of the pregnancy would involve risk, greater than if the pregnancy were terminated, of injury to the physical or mental health of any existing child(ren) of the family of the pregnant woman.
- E: there is a substantial risk that if the child were born it would suffer from such physical or mental abnormalities as to be seriously handicapped.

▶ Clauses A, B, and E have no time limit. Clauses C and D have a legal limit of 24 weeks.

Do doctors have an obligation to participate in TOPs?

According to the GMC, doctors must make sure their personal beliefs do not prejudice patient care. Doctors have the right to refuse to participate in TOPs on grounds of conscience but they should always refer the patient to another doctor who will help.

What about patients under 16?

Patients under 16 years should be encouraged to involve their parents but, provided they are considered to be competent, they can give their own consent.

Termination of pregnancy (TOP): methods

The method of TOP depends on the gestation of the pregnancy and the woman's choice. The procedures offered also vary from one centre to another.

Surgical

- *<7 weeks:* conventional suction termination should be avoided.
- *7–15 weeks:* conventional suction termination is appropriate, although, in some settings, the skill and experience of the practitioner may make medical TOP more appropriate at gestations >12 weeks.
- *>15 weeks:* dilatation and evacuation following cervical preparation; requires skilled practitioners (with necessary instruments and sufficiently large case load to maintain skills).
- Cervical preparation may be beneficial, particularly if the patient is <18 years or the gestation is >10 weeks. Possible regimes include:
  - misoprostol 400 micrograms PV 3 hours prior to surgery, or
  - gemeprost 1 mg PV 3 hours prior to surgery, or
  - mifepristone 600 mg po 36–48 hours prior to surgery.

Medical

- *<9 weeks:*
  - medical TOP, using mifepristone plus a prostaglandin is the most effective method of TOP in gestations <7 weeks. It is also an appropriate method for gestations 7–9 weeks.
- *9–13 weeks:*
  - medical TOP is an appropriate, safe, and effective alternative to surgery.
- *13–24 weeks:*
  - medical TOP with mifepristone followed by prostaglandin is appropriate, safe and effective in this group. Feticide should be considered in advanced gestations (>21 weeks).

Medications used in TOP

- *Mifepristone*: antiprogesterone which results in uterine contractions, bleeding from the placental bed, and sensitization of uterus to prostaglandins. It is used for medical TOP and may be used for cervical preparation prior to surgical TOP.
- *Misoprostol*: prostaglandin E1 analogue, used off-licence in medical TOP and for cervical preparation prior to surgical TOP. It stimulates uterine contractions.
- *Gemeprost*: prostaglandin E1 analogue. It is licensed for softening and dilatation of the cervix before surgical TOP in the first trimester and for therapeutic TOP in the second trimester.

📖 The care of women requesting induced abortion. RCOG Evidence-based clinical guideline Number 7. www.rcog.org.uk

Termination of pregnancy (TOP): management

Considerations before TOP

- **Counselling/support:** women should receive verbal advice and written information. Patients who may require additional support or counselling (evidence of coercion, poor social support, psychiatric history) should be identified and additional care offered.
- **Blood tests:**
  - Hb
  - blood group and antibodies
  - if clinically indicated, HIV, HBV, HCV, haemoglobinopathies.
- **Cervical smear:** if indicated.
- **Ultrasound scan:** is not a prerequisite in all cases but is necessary in cases where the gestation is in doubt or an ectopic pregnancy is suspected.
- **Prevention of infection:** a strategy for minimizing the risk of postabortion infection is important. This may include screening for lower genital tract infections such as *Chlamydia* (with treatment and contact tracing if positive).

Prophylactic antibiotic regimes used for TOP include:

- Metronidazole 1 g PR at time of TOP:
  - plus doxycycline 100 mg PO BD for 7 days, commencing on day of TOP
- Metronidazole 1 g PR at time of TOP:
  - plus azithromycin 1 g PO on day of TOP.

Following TOP

- Anti-D should be given to all Rh-negative women undergoing medical or surgical TOP (250 IU ≤20 weeks; 500 IU >20 weeks).
- Provide written patient information, which should include:
  - symptoms which may be experienced following TOP
  - symptoms requiring further medical attention
  - contact numbers.
- Follow-up within 2 weeks of TOP.
- Refer for further counselling if required.
- Discuss and prescribe/provide contraception.

Complications of TOP
- Bleeding (1:1000).
- Genital tract infection (10%).
- Uterine perforation (surgical TOP: 1–4:1000).
- Uterine rupture (mid-trimester medical TOP: <1:1000).
- Cervical trauma (surgical TOP: 1:100).
- Failed TOP (surgical: 2.3:1000; medical: 1–14:1000).
- Retained products of conception (1:100).
- Small increased risk of miscarriage or preterm delivery in subsequent pregnancies.
- Psychological sequelae.

📖 About abortion care: what you need to know. RCOG Information for patients. www.rcog.org.uk

📖 The care of women requesting induced abortion. RCOG Guideline 2004

📖 Family Planning Association. www.fpa.org.uk Tel 0845 3101334

📖 BPAS abortion care. www.bpas.org Tel 0845 7304030

📖 Marie Stopes International UK. www.mariestopes.org.uk Tel 0845 3008090

Bleeding in early pregnancy and miscarriage

Bleeding in early pregnancy may be associated with:
- Miscarriage.
- Ectopic pregnancy.
- Gestational trophoblastic disease.

Miscarriage
- Miscarriage is common, occurring in 15–20% of pregnancies.
- Defined as the expulsion or removal of a pregnancy, embryo, or fetus at a stage of pregnancy when it is incapable of independent survival:
  - includes all pregnancy losses before 24 weeks
  - the vast majority are before 12 weeks.

Early pregnancy assessment units (EPAU)

- Transvaginal ultrasonography and serum hCG estimations are invaluable in the diagnosis of early pregnancy problems.
- These should be readily available in dedicated EPAUs.
- These units allow for timely assessment, with easy access from the community, improved continuity of care and fewer admissions.

Anti-D prophylaxis (see Rhesus isoimmunization, Chapter 3, 📖 p. 133)

Anti-D should be given to all non sensitised rhesus-negative patients in the following circumstances:
- <12 weeks (250 IU IM):
  - uterine evacuation (medical and surgical)
  - ectopic pregnancies.
- >12 weeks:
  - all women with bleeding (250 IU IM before 20 weeks and 500 IU IM after 20 weeks).

Table 15.1 Classification, diagnosis, and management of miscarriage

	Clinical	USS findings	Management
Threatened miscarriage	Bleeding ± Abdominal pain Closed cervix	Intrauterine gestation sac Fetal pole Fetal heart activity	Anti-D if >12 weeks or heavy bleeding or pain
Complete miscarriage	Bleeding and pain cease Closed cervix	Empty uterus Endometrial thickness <15 mm	Anti-D if >12 weeks Serum hCG to exclude ectopic if any doubt Review if bleeding persists >2 weeks and consider endometritis or retained products of conception
Incomplete miscarriage	Bleeding ± Pain Open cervix	Heterogenous tissues ± Gestation sac Any endometrial thickness	Expectant/medical/ surgical Anti-D if >12 weeks or heavy bleeding or pain or medical/ surgical management
Missed miscarriage /Early fetal demise	± Bleeding ±Pain ± Loss of pregnancy symptoms Closed cervix	Fetal pole>6mm with no fetal heart activity Gestation sac diameter >20mm with no fetal pole or yolk sac	Expectant/medical/ surgical Anti-D if >12weeks or medical/surgical management
Inevitable miscarriage	Bleeding ± Pain Open cervix	Intrauterine gestation sac ± Fetal pole ±Fetal heart activity	Expectant/ medical/ surgical Anti-D if >12weeks or heavy bleeding or pain or medical/ surgical management
Pregnancy of uncertain viability	± Bleeding ±Pain Closed cervix	Intrauterine gestation sac <20 mm with no fetal pole or yolk sac Fetal echo with CRL<6 mm with no fetal heart activity	Rescan in 1 week Anti-D if heavy bleeding or pain
Pregnancy of unknown location	± Bleeding ±Pain Closed cervix	Positive pregnancy test Empty uterus No sign of extrauterine pregnancy	Serial serum hCG assay (48 hours apart) to exclude ectopic pregnancy Anti-D if heavy bleeding ● Consider serum progesterone level

Miscarriage: management

Expectant management
- Appropriate in those women who are not bleeding heavily.
- It is highly effective for women with an incomplete miscarriage.
- In women with a intact sac, resolution may take several weeks and may be less effective.
- Patients should be offered surgical evacuation at a later date if expectant management is unsuccessful.

⚠ Women should be warned that passage of pregnancy tissue may be associated with pain and heavy bleeding and 24-hour telephone advice and facilities for emergency admission should be available.

Medical
- Prostaglandin analogues (gemeprost or misoprostol) are used, administered orally or vaginally, with or without antiprogesterone priming (mifepristone).
- Bleeding may continue for up to 3 weeks after medical uterine evacuation.
- 24-hour telephone advice and facilities for emergency admission should be available.

Surgical management
- An ERPC (evacuation of retained products of conception) should be performed in patients who:
  - have excessive or persistent bleeding
  - request surgical management.
- Suction curettage should be used.

Complications of ERPC

- Infection.
- Haemorrhage.
- Uterine perforation.
- Retained products of conception.
- Intrauterine adhesions.
- Cervical tears.
- Intra-abdominal trauma.

⚠ Uterine and cervical trauma may be minimized by administering prostaglandin (misoprostol or gemeprost) before the procedure.

Psychological sequelae

- Miscarriage is usually very distressing.
- Women should be offered appropriate support and counselling.
- Written information may be useful.

📖 The management of early pregnancy loss. RCOG Guideline No.25 www.rcog.org.uk

Post-miscarriage counselling: patient's FAQs

What did I do to cause it?
Nothing. It was not stress at work, carrying heavy shopping, having sex, or any of the other reasons women worry about Sadly, miscarriages happen in about 20% of pregnancies.

If I had had a scan earlier could you have stopped it happening?
No, we might have found out it was happening sooner but we could not have stopped it. There is no effective treatment available to stop a 1st-trimester miscarriage.

How bad will the pain be if I opt for expectant management?
It will be like very severe period pain which comes to a peak when the tissue is being passed and then settles down shortly afterwards. Ibuprofen, paracetamol, or codeine should help and may be taken. If the pain is very bad you should contact the hospital for advice.

What is heavy bleeding?
Soaking more than 3 heavy sanitary pads in under 1 hour or passing a clot larger than the palm of your hand. If you bleed heavily you should seek medical attention urgently.

How long will I bleed for?
It should gradually get less and less but may be up to 3 weeks after the miscarriage before the bleeding stops completely.

Do I need bed rest afterwards?
No, not necessarily, but obviously it can be physically (and emotionally) draining so a few days off work may help. You can return to normal activities as soon as you feel ready.

How long will the pregnancy test remain positive?
hCG is excreted by the kidneys and it can take up to 3 weeks after a miscarriage for it all to be removed from the blood stream and a pregnancy test to record as negative.

How long before we can try again?
There is no good evidence that the outcome of a subsequent pregnancy is effected by how soon you conceive after a miscarriage. As long as you have had either a period or a negative pregnancy test since you miscarried, you can try again as soon as you feel physically and emotionally ready.

Does this make me more likely to have another miscarriage?
There are a very small number of women who will have recurrent miscarriages but for the vast majority the next time they get pregnant they will face the same odds; 20% risk of miscarriage and 80% chance of a baby.

📖 Association of Early Pregnancy Units. www.earlypregnancy.org.uk

📖 Miscarriage Association. www.miscarriageassociation.org.uk

Ectopic pregnancy: diagnosis

- **Definition:** implantation of a conceptus outside the uterine cavity
- **Incidence:** 11:1000 pregnancies and is increasing.
  - 98% are tubal; the remainder are abdominal, ovarian, cervical or rarely in Caesarean section scars
  - due to early presentation, with the advent of EPAUs, most women with EP are clinically very well.
- **Symptoms** (see text box on p. 511):
  - often asymptomatic, e.g. unsure dates
  - amenorrhoea (usually 6–8 weeks)
  - pain (lower abdominal, often mild and vague, classically unilateral)
  - vaginal bleeding (usually small amount, often brown)
  - shoulder tip pain (diaphragmatic irritation from intra-abdominal blood)
  - collapse (if ruptured).
- **Signs:**
  - often have no specific signs
  - uterus usually normal size
  - cervical excitation and tenderness occasionally
  - adnexal tenderness
  - adnexal mass very rarely
  - peritonism (due to intra-abdominal blood if ectopic ruptured).

△ There is no evidence to suggest that examining patients may lead to rupturing the ectopic. It is more important to examine them so you do not miss significant abdominal or pelvic tenderness.

△△ includes: threatened or complete miscarriage, bleeding corpus luteal cyst, ovarian cyst accident, and pelvic inflammation.

Investigations

- TV USS, to establish the location of the pregnancy, the presence of adnexal masses or free fluid:
  - a good EPAU will positively identify EP on TVS in 90% of cases rather than the absence of an intrauterine gestation.

△ At a serum hCG level of ≥1500 IU, a viable intrauterine pregnancy should be seen with TV USS (discriminatory zone). However, there is considerable variation in normal IUPs and this is a guide only—care is needed to avoid harming an early IUP. The rate of change is more important than any one value (see below).

- **Serum progesterone** is helpful to distinguish whether a pregnancy is failing: <20 nmol/L is highly suggestive of this, whether EP or IUP.
- **Serum hCG**, repeated 48 hours later:
  - the rate of rise is important
  - a rise of ≥66% suggests an intrauterine pregnancy
  - a suboptimal rise is suspicious of an ectopic pregnancy.
- **Laparoscopy:** gold standard but should only be necessary for clinical reasons or in a minority where a diagnosis cannot be made (remember TV USS should pick up 90%!)

Risk factors for ectopic pregnancy

May be present in 25–50% of patients:
- History of infertility or assisted conception.
- History of PID.
- Endometriosis.
- Pelvic or tubal surgery.
- Previous ectopic (recurrence risk 10–20%).
- IUCD in situ.
- Assisted conception, especially IVF.
- Smoking.

⚠ Symptoms of ectopic pregnancy

- Tend to have a poor positive predictive value to help discriminate between intra- and extrauterine pregnancy.
- All women with a positive pregnancy test should therefore be considered to have an ectopic pregnancy until proved otherwise.

⚠ An ectopic pregnancy is a life-threatening condition

- In the latest CEMACH (2003–2005) report, 10 women died from ruptured ectopic pregnancy—most because of lack of recognition.
- A high index of suspicion is essential.

Ectopic pregnancy: management

Expectant and medical management are safe options even with a diagnosed EP if there are strict selection criteria:

- Clinically stable.
- Asymptomatic or minimal symptoms.
- hCG, initially <3000 IU (can be tried >3000 IU but less successful).
- EP <3 cm and no fetal cardiac activity on TV USS.
- No haemoperitoneum on TV USS.
- Fully understand symptoms and implications of EP.
- Language should not be a barrier to understanding or communicating the problem to a third party (such as phoning an ambulance).
- Live in close proximity to the hospital and have support at home.
- You deem the patient will not default on follow-up.

Expectant

- With a falling hCG level and fulfilling the above criteria
- Requires serum hCG initially every 48 h till repeated fall in level; then weekly until <15 IU.

Medical

- Methotrexate is given intramuscularly as a single dose of 50 mg/m².
- hCG levels should be measured at 4 and 7 days and another dose of methotrexate given (up to 25% of cases) if the ↓ in hCG is <15% on days 4–7.

▶ Women should be given clear, written information about adverse effects and the possible need for further treatment.

▶ They should avoid sexual intercourse during treatment and use reliable contraception for 3 months after, as methotrexate is teratogenic.

⚠ All women managed expectantly or medically should be counselled about the importance of compliance with follow-up and should be within easy access of the hospital.

⚠ There is no level of hCG at which rupture cannot occur even when it is falling—symptoms and the clinical parameters are always more important than blood tests and scans!

Surgical

- Laparoscopy is preferable to laparotomy as it has shorter operating times and hospital stays, ↓ analgesia requirements and ↓ blood loss.

⚠ In haemodynamically unstable patients, laparotomy is more appropriate, as it is quicker.

- Salpingectomy is preferable to salpingotomy when the contralateral tube and ovary appear normal:
  - there is no difference in subsequent intrauterine pregnancy rates, but salpingectomy is associated with lower rates of persistent trophoblast and recurrent ectopic pregnancy.

⚠ In the presence of visible contralateral tubal disease, laparoscopic salpingotomy is appropriate.

❶ Remember Anti-D in Rh-negative patients.

⚠ Treatment of the haemodynamically unstable patient

Resuscitation
- 2 large-bore IV lines and IV fluids (colloids or crystalloids).
- Cross match 6 units of blood.
- Call senior help and anaesthetic assistance urgently.

Surgery
- Laparotomy with salpingectomy once the patient has been resuscitated.

Role of the early pregnancy assessment unit (EPAU)

- The EPAU allows for outpatient management of stable patients with early pregnancy problems, including ectopic pregnancies.
- There should be direct access for GPs and A&E staff.
- Facilities for transvaginal ultrasound scanning and hCG estimations.
- Dedicated EPAU staff provide continuity of care.

Side effects of methotrexate include

- Conjunctivitis.
- Stomatitis.
- Gastrointestinal upset:
  ⚠ many women will experience abdominal pain, which can be difficult to differentiate from the pain of a rupturing ectopic.

Less common sites for ectopic pregnancy

- Cervical, ovarian, CS scar, and interstitial pregnancies need expert input as there are no universally agreed ways to treat them.
- Generally preference is for medical treatment with surgical reserved for clinical need.
- Refer to a regional EPAU.

📖 Tubal pregnancy management. RCOG Guideline No. 21. www.rcog.org.uk

Pregnancy of unknown location (PUL)

Definition: Where there is no sign of an intrauterine pregnancy, ectopic pregnancy or retained products of conception in the presence of a positive pregnancy test or serum hCG >5 IU/L.

- This is the first diagnosis in 10% of EPAU attenders.
- The possible outcomes can be:
  - early IUP
  - Failing PUL
  - ectopic pregnancy (10% of PULs)
  - persisting PUL
  - very rarely an alternative source of hCG (such as a secreting ovarian or CNS tumours).

⚠ Even if the history is highly suggestive of a complete miscarriage having occurred, classify as a PUL unless you have seen POC, or TVS evidence of an IUP. 5–10% of 'complete miscarriages' diagnosed on history alone with an empty uterus on scan will in fact be ectopic pregnancies!

- **Presentation:**
  - asymptomatic
  - PV bleeding
  - abdominal pain.
- **Management:**
  - the symptoms and clinical parameters of the patient are the most important factors as for ectopic pregnancy
  - women with significant pain, tenderness, or a haemoperitoneum usually need laparoscopy
  - if the patient is well and stable then serum progesterone and hCG at the first visit and again after 48 hours.

Interpreting these results

- If progesterone <20 nmol/L:
  - likely failing pregnancy
  - repeat hCG in 7 days.
- If hCG ≥66% rise from 0–48 hours:
  - likely IUP
  - rescan in 10–14 days.
- If rise in serial hCG <66% or plateauing:
  - possible ectopic
  - close monitoring with serial hCG and TVS until diagnosis made or hCG <15 IU/L.
- If hCG plateauing or fluctuating:
  - persistent PUL after 3 consecutive samples with no diagnosis
  - methotrexate.
- If initial hCG >1500 IU/L
  - probable ectopic pregnancy
  - consider all management options depending upon clinical need.

⚠ All the same principles and criteria of expectant and medical management of ectopic pregnancies apply equally to PULs.

Recurrent miscarriage: overview

Definition as 3 or more consecutive, spontaneous miscarriages occurring in the first trimester with the same biological father. They may or may not follow a successful birth.

- Incidence is 1–2% and half of these are unexplained.

Risk factors

Advanced maternal age and increasing number of miscarriages are 2 independent risk factors.

Causes

- **Antiphospholipid syndrome (APS):** this is the most important treatable cause and is present in 15% of women with recurrent miscarriages. APS is defined as the presence of anticardiolipin antibodies or lupus anticoagulant antibodies with any criteria listed below:
  - 3 or more consecutive fetal losses before the 10th week of gestation
  - 1 fetus at 10 weeks gestation or older
  - 1 or more preterm births of a morphologically normal fetus at ≤ 34 weeks gestation associated with severe pre-eclampsia or placental insufficiency.
- **Genetic:** in 3–5% of couples, one of the partners carries balanced reciprocal or Robertsonian translocations. The carrier is phenotypically normal but 50–75% of their gametes will be unbalanced.
- **Fetal chromosomal abnormalities:** these can be incompatible with life. As the number of pregnancies ↑ the prevalence of chromosomal abnormality ↓ and the chance of recurring maternal cause ↑.
- **Anatomical abnormalities:** the frequency of congenital uterine abnormalities (uterine septae and bicornuate uterus) in the general population is unknown. In women with recurrent loss prevalence is estimated to be between 2% and 38%.
- **Fibroids** are present in up to 30% of women but their effect on reproductive outcome is controversial. Submucosal and intramural are thought to be more causative.
- **Thrombophilic disorders:** pregnancy is a hypercoaguable state. Gene mutations in factor V Leiden and factor II prothrombin G20210A have been associated with recurrent miscarriage.
- **Infection:** the evidence for this remains speculative. There is an inconsistent link to bacterial vaginosis.
- **Endocrine disorders:** their prevalence in patients with recurrent miscarriage is similar to that in general population. Well-controlled diabetes and thyroid disease is not a risk factor for recurrent miscarriage.
- **Cervical weakness** based on history of late miscarriage preceded by spontaneous rupture of membranes or painless cervical dilatation is a rare cause of recurrent loss and difficult to associate clearly with recurrent miscarriage.

Recurrent miscarriage: management

Investigations
- Parental blood for karyotyping.
- Cytogenetic analysis of products of conception (at time of miscarriage).
- Pelvic USS.
- Thrombophilia screening.
- Lupus anticoagulant (LA): (dRVVT/ aPTT).
- Anticardiolipin antibodies (aCL).
- Screening for bacterial vaginosis during early pregnancy in women with second trimester miscarriage is advisable.
- Cervical weakness is diagnosed on history alone and may be over-diagnosed as there is no objective testing in the non-pregnant state.

▶ There is insufficient evidence for asymptomatic women to be routinely tested for thyroid disease, thyroid antibodies, diabetes and hyperprolactinaemia.

▶ TORCH screening is unhelpful.

Management
At least 35% of couples with recurrent miscarriage will have lost pregnancies by chance and fall into the unexplained group. They have 75% chance of a successful pregnancy next time with no therapeutic intervention if offered supportive care alone in the setting of a dedicated EPAU.
- Empirical treatment in the unexplained miscarriage group is unnecessary and should be avoided.
- Patient with recurrent miscarriage should be seen in a dedicated clinic and be offered supportive care in early pregnancy.
- Surgical intervention for intrauterine (uterine septum) or uterine fibroids may be beneficial in highly selective cases.
- In women with APS, future live birth rate is significantly improved from 40% with low dose aspirin (75 mg) alone to 70% with combination therapy of aspirin and heparin together:
  - these should be commenced as soon as the viability of fetus is confirmed in first trimester up to late 3rd trimester.
- Cervical cerclage may be offered to an extremely select group after meticulous consideration of the diagnosis.
- Genetic referral for parental karyotype abnormalities or fetal chromosomal abnormality.
- Proven bacterial vaginosis in mid-trimester loss in previous pregnancy may indicate regular vaginal swabs along with rotating prophylactic antibiotics like clindamycin and amoxicillin up to 3rd trimester.

Other strategies which have been tried for recurrent miscarriage

- Lifestyle factors which have **not** been proven to effect the outcome of a pregnancy include:
  - bed rest
  - smoking cessation
  - reducing alcohol intake
  - losing weight.
- Steroids do not improve the live birth rate of women with recurrent miscarriage associated with APS and may ↑ significant maternal and fetal morbidity
- Other treatments which have been suggested for recurrent miscarriage but which are not backed by clinical evidence include;
  - oestrogen or progesterone supplementation
  - paternal white cell immunization
  - intravenous immunoglobulin
  - trophoblastic membrane infusion
  - human chorionic gonadotrophins
  - vitamin supplementation.

Hyperemesis gravidarum

Nausea and vomiting in pregnancy is common, occurring in at least 50% of pregnant patients. Hyperemesis gravidarum is excessive vomiting in pregnancy. It is rare, with an incidence of 1/1000.

Patients with multiple or molar pregnancies are at increased risk, due to high levels of hCG.

Diagnosis

- **Symptoms and signs:** 1st trimester of pregnancy, vomiting, weight loss, muscle wasting, dehydration, ptyalism (inability to swallow saliva), hypovolaemia, electrolyte imbalance, behavior disorders, haematemesis (Mallory–Weiss tears).

Investigations for suspected hyperemesis gravidarum

- Urinalysis to detect ketones in urine.
- MSU to exclude UTI.
- FBC ($\uparrow$HCT).
- U&E ($\downarrow$K$^+$, $\downarrow$Na$^+$, metabolic hypchloraemic alkalosis).
- LFT ($\uparrow$transaminases, $\downarrow$albumin).
- USS to exclude multiple and molar pregnancies and confirm viable intrauterine pregnancy.

Complications

- **Maternal risks:** liver and renal failure.

$\triangle$ Hyponatraemia and rapid reversal of hyponatraemia leading to central pontine myelinosis.

$\triangle$ Thiamine deficiency may lead to Wernicke's encephalopathy.

- **Fetal risks:** intrauterine growth restriction (IUGR).

$\triangle$ Fetal death may ensue in cases with Wernicke's encephalopathy.

Treatment

- Admit if not tolerating oral fluid.
- IV fluids (NaCl or Hartmann's; avoid dextrose-containing fluids as they can precipitate Wernicke's encephalopathy).
- Daily U&Es—replace K$^+$ if necessary.
- Keep NBM for 24 hours, then introduce light diet as tolerated.
- Antiemetics (regular or PRN) if no response to IV fluid and electrolyte replacement alone—consider metoclopramide 10 mg/8 h PO/IM/IV or cyclizine 50 mg/8 h PO/IM/IV or prochlorperazine 12.5 mg IM/IV tds or 5 mg PO tds.
- Thiamine (thiamine hydrochloride 25–50 mg PO tds or thiamine 100 mg IV infusion weekly).
- If vomiting is protracted and unresponsive to fluids and antiemetics, consider a trial of corticosteroids (prednisolone 40–50 mg PO daily in divided doses or hydrocortisone 100 mg/12 h IV).

Genital tract infections, and pelvic pain

Vaginal discharge

A commonly reported symptom, which may be physiological or pathological. It may sometimes appear to be disproportionately distressing.

Causes of increased vaginal discharge

Physiological
- Oestrogen related—puberty, pregnancy, COCP.
- Cycle related—maximal mid-cycle and premenstrual.
- Sexual excitement and intercourse.

Pathological
- Infection (usually sexually transmitted).
- Malignancy (any part of the genital tract).
- Foreign body (retained tampon or postpartum swab).
- Atrophic vaginitis (often blood-stained).
- Cervical ectropion or endocervical polyp.
- Fistulae (urinary or faecal).

History
- Duration (recent change in discharge?).
- Colour (clear, white, green, bloody).
- Consistency (watery, mucoid, frothy, curd-like).
- Amount (is a panty liner or pad required?).
- Associated symptoms (itching, burning, dysuria).
- Relationship of discharge to menstrual cycle.
- Precipitating factors (pregnancy, contraceptive pill, sexual excitement).
- Hygiene practices (douches, bath products, talcum powder).
- Sexual history (risk factors for sexually transmitted infections).
- Allergies.
- Medical history (diabetes, genital tract carcinoma).
- History of smear tests.

Examination
- Abdominal (masses, pain, tenderness).
- Speculum:
  - appearance of vulva and vagina (red, fissured, rash, excoriations)
  - appearance of discharge
  - cervix (inflammation, ectropion, evidence of carcinoma).
- Bimanual examination (masses, adnexal tenderness, cervical excitation).

Investigations
These will depend on the setting of the consultation, e.g. fresh wet mount with immediate microscopy may be readily available in a genitourinary (GUM) clinic but not in gynaecology outpatients.
- Endocervical swab for gonorrhoea (Amies transport medium).
- High vaginal swab (Amies transport medium).
- Endocervical swab for *Chlamydia* (urine testing may be available).
- Cervical smear.
- Vaginal pH measurement.
- Saline wet mount and Gram staining.
- 10% KOH wet mount ('whiff' test).
- Colposcopy.

Table 16.1 Typical characteristics of common causes for vaginal discharge

	Colour	Consistency	Odour	Vulval Itching	Treatment
Physiological	Clear/white	Mucoid	None	None	Reassure
Candida infection	White	Curd-like	None	Itching	Anti-fungal
Trichomonal infection	Green/grey	Frothy	Offensive	Itching	Metronidazole
Gonococcal infection	Greenish	Watery	None	None	Antibiotics
Bacterial vaginosis (BV)	White/grey	Watery	Offensive	None	Metronidazole
Malignancy	Bloody	Watery	Offensive	None	According to disease
Foreign body	Grey or bloody	Purulent	Offensive	None	Remove object
Atrophic vaginitis	Clear/blood-stained	Watery	None	None	Topical oestrogen
Cervical ectropion	Clear	Watery	None	None	Cryotherapy

Sexually transmitted infections (STIs)

STIs tend to 'hunt in packs'. Therefore, if one infection is identified, it is important to screen for all the rest. This is often best managed in a GUM clinic where there are facilities for on-site microscopy and Gram staining. Also, diagnosis of a STI is often an emotive issue as patients may be very concerned about confidentiality and the perceived associated stigma. The GUM clinic has a multidisciplinary team including health advisers who usually have a nursing background and are specially trained to work with issues relating to sexual health, including STIs. They are able to provide counselling and support, as well has assistance with contact tracing.

▶ Confidentiality within GUM clinics is even more stringent than in other parts of the NHS. The notes are kept separately from hospital notes and the patient's GP is not routinely informed of their attendance. This is a requirement defined by statute in the Venereal Diseases Act of 1917.

Risk factors for STIs

Known risk factors are:
- Multiple partners.
- Young adults (15–24 years old).
- Pregnancy before 20 years of age.
- Previous termination of pregnancy.
- History of previous STI.
- Abnormal cervical cytology.
- Involvement in the commercial sex industry.

Sexual history

If a STI is suspected it is important to take a full history including a sexual history. This must be performed in a sensitive and non-judgemental manner, and should include the following details:
- Last sexual intercourse:
  - gender of partner
  - type of sexual intercourse (oral, vaginal, anal)
  - contraception used (condoms, hormonal, none)
  - details of partner (long-term, casual traceable, non-traceable)
  - symptoms in partner
  - date of last sexual intercourse (may impact on timings of tests).
- Previous sexual partner/s:
  - same questions as above
  - details of all partners for at least the last 3 months.
- History of previous STIs.
- Date of last smear.
- Travel history including sexual encounters abroad.
- Risk factors for blood-borne viruses (IV drug use, etc.).
- Assessment of competency if under 16 years old (Fraser competence).

📖 http://www.bashh.org/guidelines

Chlamydia

Epidemiology
- *Chlamydia trachomatis*—obligate intracellular parasite.
- Commonest sexually transmitted infection (STI) in the UK.
- Nearly 110 000 cases were reported in 2005.
- Identified as an important cause of tubal infertility.

Symptoms
May present with increased vaginal discharge secondary to cervicitis but is usually asymptomatic and therefore is often only found by screening, on contact tracing, or when the complications present.

Diagnosis
- Endocervical swabs (requires specific medium for PCR).
- Urethral swabs.
- Urine for PCR (becoming more widely available).

Complications of *Chlamydia* infection
- Pelvic inflammatory disease (10–30% of infections result in PID).
- Perihepatitis (Fitz-Hugh–Curtis syndrome).
- Reiter's syndrome (more common in men):
  - arthritis
  - urethritis
  - conjunctivitis.
- Tubal infertility.
- ↑ risk of ectopic pregnancy.

Treatment
- Azithromycin 1 g single dose (>90% effective).
- Doxycycline 100 mg bd for 7 days.
- Contact tracing and treatment of partners.
- Abstinence until partner is treated and antibiotics completed.

Screening for *Chlamydia*

The National Chlamydia Screening Programme is being rolled out across the UK from 2006. It is part of the Department of Health's Sexual Health Strategy, and will employ the more acceptable urine test. The target population is women under 24 years of age.

📖 http://www.dh.gov.uk/PolicyAndGuidance/HealthAndSocialCareTopics/SexualHealth

Implications in pregnancy
Chlamydial infection appears to have some association with:
- Preterm rupture of membranes and premature delivery.
- Low birth weight.
- Postpartum endometritis.
The risks to the baby are of:
- Neonatal conjunctivitis (30% within the first 2 weeks).
- Neonatal pneumonia (15% within the first 4 months).

Herpes simplex

Epidemiology
- DNA virus—*Herpes simplex* type 2 (genital) and type 1 (oral).
- HSV type 1 is responsible for up to 30% of genital lesions.
- 2nd most common STI in the UK.
- Nearly 20 000 primary attacks were reported in 2005.

Symptoms
Primary HSV infection is usually the most severe and often results in:
- Flu-like illness.
- Inguinal lymphadenopathy.
- Vulvitis and pain (may be severe enough to cause urinary retention).
- Small, characteristic vesicles on the vulva.

Recurrent attacks are thought to result from reactivation of latent virus in the sacral ganglia and are normally shorter and less severe. They can be triggered by many factors including:
- Stress.
- Sexual intercourse.
- Menstruation.

Diagnosis
Usually made on the history and appearance of the typical rash. However, viral culture of vesicle fluid is the gold standard. Acute and convalescent antibody levels may sometimes prove helpful.

Complications of HSV infection
- Meningitis.
- Sacral radiculopathy—causing urinary retention and constipation.
- Transverse myelitis.
- Disseminated infection.

Treatment
There is no cure for genital herpes. Treatment with aciclovir is thought to be effective in reducing the duration and severity of the primary attack if given within 5 days of onset of symptoms. Simple analgesia and ice packs may help ease the pain. The use of condoms is recommended unless there is a history of herpes in both partners.

Implications in pregnancy
See Chapter 4, p. 162.

Gonorrhoea

Epidemiology

- *Neisseria gonorrhoeae*—intracellular Gram-negative diplococcus.
- 3rd most common STI in the UK.
- >19 000 cases were reported in 2005.
- >20% of strains now resistant to ciprofloxacin.

Symptoms

May present with a greenish vaginal discharge 2–7 days after intercourse, but is usually asymptomatic and therefore often only found by screening on contact tracing, or when the complications present.

Diagnosis

- Endocervical swabs (Amies charcoal transport medium).
- Urethral swabs.
- Rectal swabs (transmucosal spread)—if symptomatic.
- Pharyngeal swabs—if symptomatic.

Complications of gonococcus infection

- Pelvic inflammatory disease (~15% of infections result in PID).
- Bartholin's or Skene's abscess.
- Disseminated gonorrhoea may cause:
  - fever
  - pustular rash
  - migratory polyarthralgia
  - septic arthritis.
- Tubal infertility.
- ↑ risk of ectopic pregnancy.

Treatment

- The same antibiotics as are recommended for treating gonorrhoea in pregnancy:
  - ceftriaxone 250 mg IM (single dose)
  - cefixime 400 mg oral (single dose)
  - spectinomycin 2 g IM (single dose).
- Contact tracing and treatment of partners.
- Refrain from sexual intercourse until partner is treated.

Implications in pregnancy

- Gonorrhoea is associated with:
  - preterm rupture of membranes and premature delivery
  - chorioamnionitis
  - postpartum endometritis.
- The risks to the baby are of:
  - ophthalmia neonatarum (40–50%).

http://www.bashh.org/

Syphilis

Epidemiology
- *Treponemum pallidum*—spirochaete.
- Relatively rare STI in the UK, but steadily increasing.
- Nearly 3000 cases were reported in 2005.
- Infection occurs in 3 stages: primary, secondary, and tertiary syphilis.

Symptoms
Primary syphilis
- 10–90 days post infection.
- Painless, genital ulcer (chancre)—may pass unnoticed on the cervix.
- Inguinal lymphadenopathy.

Secondary syphilis
- Occurs within the first 2 years of infection.
- Generalized polymorphic rash affecting palms and soles.
- Generalized lymphadenopathy.
- Genital condyloma lata.
- Anterior uveitis.

Tertiary syphilis
- Presents in up to 40% of people infected for >2 years:
- Neurosyphilis—tabes dorsalis and dementia
- Cardiovascular syphilis—commonly affecting the aortic root.
- Gummata—inflammatory plaques or nodules.

Diagnosis
- Venereal Diseases Research Laboratory (VDRL) carbon antigen test or rapid plasma reagin test (RPR) are recommended for screening.
- Smear from the primary lesion may demonstrate spirochaetes on dark field microscopy.
- Fluorescent treponemal antibody absorption test (FTA-abs)—reported to be the most sensitive.

Complications
- Tertiary syphilis (see above).

Treatment
Treatment choice depends on compliance and penicillin allergy.
- Regimens used in order of preference are:
  - procaine penicillin G 750 mg IM for 10 days (used in pregnancy), or
  - benzathine penicillin 2.4 MU single dose IM (used in pregnancy), or
  - doxycycline 100 mg BD PO for 14 days (contraindicated in pregnancy), or
  - erythromycin 500 mg QDS PO for 14 days (used in pregnancy).
- Contact tracing (potentially over several years).
- Refrain from sexual intercourse until partner is treated.

Implications in pregnancy (see Chapter 4, 📖 p. 165)
- Preterm delivery.
- Stillbirth.
- Congenital syphilis.

Trichomonas

Epidemiology
- *Trichomonas vaginalis*—flagellated protozoan.
- Relatively common STI in the UK.
- Cervix may have a 'strawberry' appearance from punctate haemorrhages (2%).

Symptoms
Asymptomatic in 10–50% but may present with:
- Frothy, greenish, offensive smelling vaginal discharge.
- Vulval itching and soreness.
- Dysuria.

Diagnosis
- Wet smear will identify up to 80% of cases.
- Culture remains the gold standard (Diamond's TYM culture medium).

Complications
- There is some evidence that *Trichomonas* infection may enhance HIV transmission.

Treatment
- Metronidazole 2 g orally in a single dose, or
- Metronidazole 400–500 mg twice daily for 5–7 days.

This should be avoided in the first trimester of pregnancy.
- Contact tracing and treatment of partners.
- Refrain from sexual intercourse until partner is treated.

Implications in pregnancy
- *Trichomonas* is associated with:
  - pre-term delivery
  - low birth weight.
- *Trichomonas* may be acquired perinatally, occurring in 5% of babies born to infected mothers.

Human papillomavirus (HPV)

Epidemiology
- DNA virus, many subtypes.
- Subtypes 6 and 11 cause genital warts (condylomata acuminata).
- Subtypes 16 and 18 are associated with CIN and cervical neoplasia.
- 25% of people presenting with warts have other concurrent STIs.
- Over 81 000 cases were reported in 2005.

Symptoms
The vast majority of HPV infections are asymptomatic. Genital warts may cause localized skin irritation or catch on clothing, or an individual may just find their presence embarrassing.

Diagnosis
HPV infection is often diagnosed by the characteristic appearance on cervical cytology (smear tests) or colposcopy (whitening on topical application of acetic acid). Genital warts are usually identified by the clinical appearance of the lesion. Biopsy of cervical warts may be required to exclude neoplasia.

Complications
Increasing evidence is becoming available of the causative association between persistent infection with HPV 16 and 18 and high-grade CIN and cervical neoplasia. Smoking and immunosuppression both affect viral clearance thereby increasing the risk.

Treatment for genital warts
Treatment is aimed at destroying the visible wart and may be physical or pharmacological. There is a high rate of recurrence due to the latent virus in the surrounding epithelial cells.
- Podophyllin paint applied weekly (contraindicated in pregnancy).
- Podophyllotoxin solution applied twice daily, 3 days a week for 4 weeks (contraindicated in pregnancy).
- Trichloroacetic acid (repeated weekly).
- Cryotherapy (with liquid nitrogen).
- Surgery (excision or diathermy).

Implications in pregnancy
Genital warts tend to grow rapidly in pregnancy but usually regress again after delivery. Excision is not usually recommended at any gestation as they are extremely vascular and tend to cause significant bleeding.

Routine vaccination
In October 2007 the Department of Health announced plans to introduce routine HPV vaccination for all 12–13 year old girls in the UK. This should be in place by late 2008.

Bacterial vaginosis (BV)

Epidemiology
- Bacterial vaginosis is caused by an overgrowth of mixed anaerobes, including *Gardnerella* and *Mycoplasma hominis,* which replace the usually dominant vaginal lactobacilli.
- It is not sexually transmitted. About 12% of women will experience BV at some point in their lives but what triggers it remains unclear. However, BV is reported to be more common with:
- Termination of pregnancy.
- Intrauterine contraceptive devices (IUCD).
- Pelvic inflammatory disease (PID).

Symptoms
It may be asymptomatic but usually presents with a profuse, whitish grey, offensive smelling vaginal discharge. The characteristic 'fishy' smell is due to the presence of amines released by bacterial proteolysis and is often very distressing to the woman.

Diagnosis
- Increased vaginal pH >5.5.
- 'Whiff test'—characteristic fishy smell on adding 10% potassium hydroxide to the discharge.
- Microscopic detection of 'clue cells' (squamous epithelial cells with bacteria adherent to their walls).

Complications
It has been associated with an increased risk of pelvic infection after gynaecological surgery.

Treatment
Bacterial vaginosis may resolve spontaneously and even if successfully treated has a high recurrence rate. However, most women prefer it to be treated.
- Metronidazole 400 mg orally twice daily for 5 days, or
- Metronidazole 2 g (single dose).
- Clindamycin 2% cream vaginally at night for 7 days.

Implications in pregnancy
It is associated with an ↑ risk of:
- Mid-trimester miscarriage.
- Preterm rupture of membranes.
- Preterm delivery.

Candidiasis (thrush)

Epidemiology

Candidiasis is caused by infection with a yeast-like fungus, the most common being *Candida albicans*. It is not sexually transmitted. About 70% of women will experience it at some point in their lives and 20–40% of women are chronic carriers. Predisposing factors are those which alter the vaginal microflora and include:
- Antibiotics.
- Pregnancy.
- High dose COCP.
- Diabetes mellitus.
- Anaemia.

Symptoms

It may be carried asymptomatically but usually presents with:
- Vulval itching and soreness.
- Thick, curd-like, white vaginal discharge.
- Dysuria.
- Superficial dyspareunia.

Diagnosis
- Characteristic appearance of:
  - vulval and vaginal erythema
  - vulval fissuring
  - typical white plaques adherent to the vaginal wall.
- Culture from HVS or LVS.
- Microscopic detection of spores and pseudohyphae on wet slides.

Complications

It is unlikely to cause any significant complications unless the woman is severely immunocompromised.

Treatment
- As so many women are chronic carriers, candidiasis should only be treated if it is symptomatic.
- Clotrimazole 500 mg pessary ± topical clotrimazole cream, or
- Fluconazole 150 mg (single dose)—contraindicated in pregnancy.

Other simple measures may help to decrease recurrent attacks, such as:
- Wearing cotton underwear.
- Avoiding chemical irritants, e.g. soap and bath salts.
- Wiping the vulva from front to back.

Implications in pregnancy
- It is very common in pregnancy with no apparent adverse effects.
- Topical imidazoles are not systemically absorbed and are therefore safe at all gestations.

Pelvic inflammatory disease (PID): overview

Definition
PID is infection of the upper genital tract.

Incidence
The exact prevalence is hard to ascertain as many cases may go unde-tected, but is thought to be in the region of 1–3% of sexually active young women.

Causes
It is most commonly caused by ascending infection from the endocervix but may also occur from descending infection from organs such as the appendix. There are multiple causative organisms, but the most common sexually transmitted infections are *Chlamydia*, trachomatis and *Gonococcus*. Anaerobes and endogenous agents, either aerobic or facultative, may also be responsible.

History and examination
- A full gynaecological history including sexual history is necessary.
- An abdominal examination is required to elicit the site and severity of the pain.
- Speculum and vaginal examination should be performed to assess for adnexal masses, vaginal discharge or cervical excitation.

Risk factors for PID
- Age <25.
- Previous sexually transmitted infections.
- New sexual partner/multiple sexual partners.
- Uterine instrumentation such as surgical termination of pregnancy and intrauterine contraceptive devices.
- Postpartum endometritis.

Protective factors
- These include the use of barrier contraception, the Levonorgestral-releasing system (Mirena IUS) and the COCP.

Pelvic inflammatory disease (PID): diagnosis and treatment

Signs and symptoms

PID may be relatively asymptomatic, the diagnosis only being made retrospectively during investigation of subfertility. The following symptoms are suggestive of PID:
- Lower abdominal pain.
- Cervical excitation.
- Adnexal tenderness.
- Temperature >38°C.
- Vaginal discharge.
- Dyspareunia.

Investigations
- Endocervical and high vaginal swabs.
- WCC and CRP may be elevated.
- USS may be indicated if a tubo-ovarian abscess is suspected.
- Laparoscopy is the gold standard for the diagnosis of PID, however, it is invasive and usually only performed if a tubo-ovarian abscess is suspected.

Treatment

⚠ Negative swabs do not exclude PID, therefore early treatment is preferable.

Multiple antibiotic regimes are required to cover all potential causative organisms (see 📖 p. 533).
- Most patients can be treated in an outpatient setting.
- Patients should be reviewed after 72 hours to ensure adequate response to treatment.
- Inpatient treatment may be required if:
  - a surgical cause has not been excluded
  - symptoms are severe
  - there has been failure to respond to outpatient management
  - a tubo-ovarian abscess is suspected.
- Contact tracing and treatment of partners is essential.
- Intercourse should be avoided during the course of treatment.
- If there is USS evidence of a tubo-ovarian abscess, drainage may be required either by ultrasonic guided aspiration or at laparoscopy.

Complications of PID
- Tubo-ovarian abscess.
- Fitz-Hugh–Curtis syndrome.
- Recurrent PID.
- Ectopic pregnancy.
- Infertility.

Outpatient management of PID

- Oral ofloxacin 400 mg bd + oral metronidazole 400 mg bd for 14 days, **or**
- IM ceftriaxone 250mg or IM cefoxitin 2g immediately + oral probenecid 1 g followed by oral doxycycline 100 mg bd + metronidazole 400 mg bd for 14 days.

▶ Doxycycline and metronidazole are commonly used in clinical practice but there are no clinical trials to support their effectiveness.

Inpatient management of PID

- IV cefoxitin 2 g tds + IV doxycycline 100 mg bd, followed by oral doxycycline 100 mg bd + oral metronidazole 400 mg bd for a total of 14 days, **or**
- IV clindamycin 900 mg tds + IV gentamicin 2 mg/kg loading dose followed by 1.5 mg/kg tds, followed by either oral clindamycin 450 mg qds for a total of 14 days or oral doxycycline 100 mg bd + oral metronidazole 400 mg bd for a total of 14 days, **or**
- IV ofloxacin 400 mg bd + IV metronidazole 500 mg tds for a total of 14 days.

📖 Management of acute pelvic inflammatory disease. RCOG Guideline 32. www.rcog.org.uk

Acute pelvic pain

⚠ Acute pelvic pain in a woman of reproductive age with a positive pregnancy test is an ectopic pregnancy until proven otherwise.

Diagnosis
- History:
  - pain—site, nature, radiation, aggravating/relieving factors.
  - LMP.
  - contraception.
  - recent unprotected sexual intercourse (UPSI)
  - risk factors for an ectopic pregnancy (see Chapter 15, 📖 p. 511)
  - vaginal discharge or bleeding
  - bowel symptoms
  - urinary symptoms
  - precipitating factors (physical and psychological).
- Examination:
  - is she haemodynamically stable?—risk of bleeding from ectopic
  - abdomen—does she have an acute abdomen?, masses?
  - pelvic—are discharge, cervical excitation, adnexal tenderness, masses present?

Investigations
- Urinary/ serum hCG.
- MSU.
- Triple swabs (high vaginal, cervical, and endocervical *Chlamydia*).
- FBC, G and S (X-match if ectopic suspected), CRP.
- Pelvic USS—transvaginal or abdominal as appropriate.
- Abdominal X-ray (± contrast), CT, MRI as appropriate.
- Diagnostic laparoscopy.

Treatment:
- Resuscitate if necessary.
- Analgesia.
- Specific treatment will depend on cause of pain.
- Avoid unnecessary laparoscopy, especially in a woman with a history of chronic pain.

Gynaecological causes of acute pelvic pain

- Early pregnancy complications:
  - ectopic pregnancy (see Chapter 15, 📖 p. 510)
  - miscarriage (see Chapter 15, 📖 p. 508)
  - ovarian hyperstimulation syndrome (see Chapter 17, 📖 p. 578).
- PID (see 📖 p. 531).
- Ovarian cyst accident:
  - torsion
  - haemorrhage
  - rupture.
- Adnexal pathology:
  - torsion of fallopian tube/ parafimbrial cyst
  - salpingo-ovarian abscess.
- Mittelschmerz (German: *Mittel* = middle, *Schmerz* = pain).
- Pregnancy complications (see Chapter 2, 📖 p. 88):
  - fibroid degeneration
  - ovarian cyst accident
  - ligament stretch.
- Primary dysmenorrhoea (see Chapter 14, 📖 p. 490).
- Haematometra/haematocolpos.
- Non-gynaecological causes.
- Acute exacerbation of chronic pelvic pain.

Non-gynaecological causes of acute pelvic pain

Gastrointestinal
- Appendicitis.
- Irritable bowel syndrome.
- Inflammatory bowel disease.
- Mesenteric adenitis.
- Diverticulitis.
- Strangulation of a hernia.

Urological
- Urinary tract infection (UTI).
- Renal/bladder calculi.

Chronic pelvic pain (CPP): gynaecological causes

Definition

Intermittent or constant pelvic pain in the lower abdomen or pelvis of at least 6 months' duration, not occurring exclusively with menstruation or intercourse and not associated with pregnancy.

⚠ CPP is a symptom, not a diagnosis.

Prevalence

- Annual prevalence in women aged 15–73 is 38/1000 (asthma: 37/1000, back pain: 41/1000).
- Many women do not receive a diagnosis even after many years and multiple investigations.

Causes

Endometriosis
See Chapter 17.

Adenomyosis:

- Characterized by the presence of ectopic endometrial tissue in the myometrium.
- Often occurs after pregnancy, particularly after CS or TOP (breaches the integrity of the endometrial/myometrial junction).
- Initially causes cyclical pelvic pain and menorrhagia, but can worsen until pain is present daily.

Adhesions:

✦ It is still debated whether adhesions cause pelvic pain or are an incidental finding associated with other causes of pain.
- Two distinct adhesive disorders exist which are associated with pain:
  - *trapped ovary syndrome*: after hysterectomy the ovary becomes trapped within dense adhesions at the pelvic side wall
  - *ovarian remnant syndrome*: a small piece of ovarian tissue, not removed during oophorectomy becomes embedded within adhesions.
- Both of these can cause cyclical pain.

Pelvic venous congestion:

- Dilated pelvic veins, believed to cause a cyclical dragging pain.
- Worst premenstrually and after prolonged periods of standing and walking.
- Dyspareunia is also often present.

📖 The initial management of chronic pelvic pain. RCOG Guideline 41. www.rcog.org.uk

Chronic pelvic pain (CPP): non-gynaecological causes

Gastrointestinal causes

Irritable bowel syndrome (IBS)

- Common, occurring in ~20% women of reproductive age.
- Can cause dyspareunia.
- Can present with cyclical exacerbations, but may coexist with other pelvic pathology such as endometriosis.

Constipation

- Common cause of pelvic pain that is easily treated.

▶ Opiate analgesics should not be prescribed for CPP without a laxative.

Hernia

- Abdominal or pelvic hernias may cause pain.
- Rare hernias (such as obturator) should also be considered (lump with a cough impulse felt on VE).

Urological causes

Interstitial cystitis (IC)

- Inflammatory disorder causing pain, urinary symptoms and dyspareunia.
- Can be diagnosed on cystoscopy.
- Cyclical exacerbations can occur and pain is often relieved by voiding.
- May coexist with other pathologies.
- Recurrent UTIs with negative cultures ↑ suspicion.

Urethral syndrome

- Mild suprapubic pain associated with frequency and dysuria.
- Aetiology is not known but possibly due to a chronic low grade infection of the paraurethral glands ('female prostatitis').

Calculi

- May occasionally trigger a chronic pain cycle.

Musculoskeletal causes

Fibromyalgia

- Widespread pain especially in the shoulders, neck, and pelvic girdle.
- It is characterized by tender points and a reduced pain threshold.
- Often shows cyclical exacerbations.

Trigger points

- Discrete, focal, hyperirritable area in a taut band of skeletal muscle.
- Exact aetiology is unknown, but the pain can persist even after the underlying pathology has resolved.

Neurological causes

Nerve entrapments
- Trapped in fascia or a narrow foramen or in scar tissue after surgery.
- Classically results in pain and/or dysfunction in the nerve distribution.
- After 1 Pfannenstiel incision, 3.7% will have pain in the scar due to this.

Neuropathic pain
- Results from actual damage to the nerve (surgery, infection, or inflammation).
- Classically described as shooting, stabbing or burning.

Psychological associations with CPP

- A number of studies have shown that women with CPP have an increased number of negative cognitive and emotional traits, although it is not known whether these are a cause or a consequence of the pain.
- A history of abuse (physical, sexual, and psychological) is also associated with CPP, but may not be revealed at the first consultation.

Chronic pelvic pain (CPP): diagnosis

History
As for acute pelvic pain, but also including:
- A detailed history of the pain, including events surrounding its onset, site, nature, radiation, time course, exacerbating and relieving factors, and any cyclicity.
- A sexual history and future fertility wishes should be explored (it may be possible to discuss abuse at this point).
- Patients' beliefs (or 'fantasies') and concerns about the cause of the pain.

Examination
- Abdomen:
  - As for acute pelvic pain, but also looking for altered sensation and trigger points.
- Internal:
  - speculum if indicated, but may not be appropriate if history of vaginismus or pain secondary to difficult smear or abuse
  - 1- then 2-finger vaginal examination, looking for tension/trigger points in pelvic floor, adnexal tenderness/mass, cervical tenderness.
- Rectal:
  - only if indicated (strong suspicion of rectal endometriosis).

▶ The examination itself may be therapeutic. It is the time at which the woman is most vulnerable and new information is often revealed. The clinician should look for behavioural and emotional clues and pursue any leads that may be given.

Investigations
⚠ Be careful not to over-investigate initially.

Investigations should be guided by the history and examination findings.

Pain diary
A detailed pain diary can help both clinician and woman make connections which had not previously been noted.

Therapeutic trial of GnRH analogues
- With clearly cyclical pain, a trial of a GnRH analogue (GnRHa) can be a useful diagnostic tool:
  - women requesting a total abdominal hysterectomy with bilateral salpingo-oopherectomy (TAH & BSO) can be reassured that it may be a successful treatment if their pain is relieved with a GnRHa
  - if their pain persists on GnRHa treatment, they should be counselled that TAH & BSO is unlikely to remove their pain and other causes for it should be explored.

Chronic pelvic pain (CPP): treatment

Treatment needs to address both perpetuating and causative factors and is often best done within a multidisciplinary team. Success is more likely if treatment fits within the woman's own belief system.

Analgesia

- An analgesic ladder should be used to obtain appropriate pain relief.
- Pre-emptive analgesia for predictable cyclical exacerbations may prevent emergency admissions.
- Opiates may be required for severe, acute exacerbations, but if needed regularly, referral to a dedicated pain clinic should be made.
- Neuropathic treatments such as amitriptyline, gabapentin and pregabalin can be useful, as can topical capsaicin on abdominal (but **not** vulval) skin.

Hormonal treatments

- Both gynaecological and non-gynaecological causes can respond well.
- The COCP, progestagens, danazol and GnRH analogues are all effective but with different side effect profiles.
- Local disease may be controlled with a levonorgestrel-releasing system (Mirena IUS®).

⚠ If pain is improved with a GnRHa then this can be combined safely with low-dose HRT for at least 2 years.

Physiotherapy

▶ As many as 75% of women attending CPP clinics have musculoskeletal disorders, and dramatic results can often be obtained with physiotherapy.

Psychological therapy

- Psychosocial and psychosexual issues are often perpetuating factors.
- Exploring these in a non-threatening environment can both improve the pain experience and help develop a pain management plan.
- With negative psychological features, more specific treatments such as cognitive behavioural therapy may be useful.

Surgery

⚠ Patients with a chronic pain condition are more likely to develop postoperative pain and negative laparoscopies can reinforce abnormal health beliefs and psychological traits.

⚠ Surgery should be a second line investigation/treatment.
- There are instances when surgery (including hysterectomy) is necessary to treat disease or for investigations such as fertility concerns.
- Adequate postoperative analgesia must be provided.

Complementary therapies

- A variety of complementary therapies can produce good results and should be encouraged if the woman suggests them.
- Support groups can also give reassurance.

Subfertility and reproductive medicine

Polycystic ovarian syndrome (PCOS): overview

Background
- PCOS is the most common endocrine disorder in women.
- It is responsible for 80% of all cases of anovulatory subfertility.
- Estimated prevalence is 6–10% of women of childbearing age.
- The USS evidence of polycystic ovaries (PCO) is common (20–30% women).

Rotterdam criteria for diagnosing PCOS

Requires the presence of 2 out of the following 3 variables:
- Irregular or absent ovulations (cycle > 42 days).
- Clinical or biochemical signs of hyperandrogenism:
  - acne
  - hirsutism
  - alopecia.
- Polycystic ovaries on pelvic USS:
  - ≥12 antral follicles on one ovary
  - Ovarian volume >10 mL.

Aetiology
The pathogenesis of PCOS is not fully known. Given its heterogeneity, it is likely to be multifactorial. There is hypersecretion of LH (increased frequency and amplitude of LH pulses) in ~60% of PCOS patients (LH stimulates androgen secretion from ovarian thecal cells). An elevated LH:FSH ratio is often seen but this is not needed for the diagnosis. The following factors have been implicated:
- Genetic (familial clustering).
- Insulin resistance with compensatory hyperinsulinaemia (defect on insulin receptor).
- Hyperandrogenism (elevated ovarian androgen secretion).
- Obesity:
  - BMI> 30 kg/m^2 in 35–60% of women with PCOS
  - central obesity
  - worsens insulin resistance.

Investigations
- Basal (day 2–5): LH, FSH, TFTs, prolactin, and testosterone.
- If hyperandrogenisim:
  - dehydroepiandrosterone sulfate (DHEAS)
  - androstenedione
  - sex hormone binding globulin (SHBG).
- Exclude other causes of secondary amenorrhoea.
- Pelvic USS.

Examination
- BMI.
- Signs of endocrinopathy/hirsutism/acne/alopecia.

Long-term health consequences of PCOS

- Obesity, insulin resistance, and metabolic abnormalities including dyslipidaemia are all risk factors for ischaemic heart disease, though long-term studies in PCOS are not proven.
- Type II diabetes is a known risk of obesity and insulin resistance, and pregnant women with PCOS are at increased risk of gestational diabetes (📖 p. 236).
- Long periods of secondary amenorrhoea, with resultant unopposed oestrogen, is a risk factor for endometrial hyperplasia and, if untreated, endometrial carcinoma.

Polycystic ovarian syndrome (PCOS): management

The options should focus on the main concern of the woman.

Lifestyle modification This is the cornerstone to managing PCOS in an overweight women. Even a modest weight loss (5%) can improve symptoms. Weight loss through diet (dietitian; information leaflets) and exercise should be encouraged, and patients should feel supported.

Improving menstrual regularity
- Weight loss.
- Combined oral contraceptive pill (COCP).
- Metformin.

Controlling symptoms of hyperandrogenism
- Cosmetic (depilatory cream/electrolysis/shaving/plucking).
- Anti-androgens such as eflornithine (Vaniqua®) facial cream, finasteride, or spironolactone:
  - can be used to help with acne and hirsutism
  - can take 6–9 months to improve hair growth
  - avoid pregnancy (feminizes a male fetus).
- COCP:
  - reduces serum androgen levels by increasing SHBG levels
  - co-cyprindiol (dianette®) combines ethinylestradiol and cyproterone acetate
    providing a regular monthly withdrawal bleed and beneficial anti-androgenic effects.

Subfertility (see Ovulation induction, 📖 p. 570)
- Weight loss alone may achieve spontaneous ovulation.
- Ovulation induction with antioestrogens or gonadotrophins.
- Laparoscopic ovarian diathermy.
- IVF if ovulation cannot be achieved or does not succeed in pregnancy.

⚠ Women with PCOS who undergo IVF are at increased risk of ovarian hyperstimulation syndrome (see OHSS, 📖 p. 578)

Insulin sensitizers
- Metformin has been most widely used (not licensed for this in the UK):
  - may help regulate menstrual cycles and achieve ovulation
  - is no better than lifestyle modification
  - does not significantly improve hirsutism, acne, weight loss despite lowering androgen levels and improving insulin sensitivity.

➤ Data on the benefit of metformin in PCOS are conflicting and this may be as a result of variations in study populations, degree of obesity and differing definitions of the syndrome.

Psychological issues
PCOS can be difficult to manage and patients may require additional motivation. Symptoms can be distressing and result in low self-esteem. It is therefore important to manage patients sensitively, and to adopt a holistic approach incorporating all members of the multidisciplinary team.

Hirsutism and virilization: overview

Background

Vellus hair (prepubertal, unpigmented, downy hair) is irreversibly trans-formed into **terminal hair** (pigmented, coarse) through either increased free androgen or increased sensitivity of 5-α reductase (conversion of testosterone to the more potent dihydrotestosterone) in the skin. In women testosterone originates either directly from the ovaries (25%) and adrenal glands (25%) or from peripheral conversion of androstenedione or dihydroepiandrostenedione (-sulphate), which are produced in the ovaries and adrenal glands (50%). Testosterone is bound to SHBG (80%) and albumin (19%). In women, only 1% is free (active). Luteinizing hormone (LH) stimulates ovarian theca cells and adrenocorticotrophic hormone (ACTH) the adrenal glands to synthesize androgen.

Hirsutism

- Hirsutism is the presence of excessive facial and body hair in women.
- It is caused by an increase of systemic or local androgen resulting in a male hair growth pattern.
- The incidence of hirsutism is estimated to be around 10% in developed countries.
- Most commonly found in patients with PCOS together with acne, alopecia, and acanthosis nigricans.
- Even mild forms of hirsutism are often felt unacceptable by the patient and may cause mental trauma.
- Should also not be confused with hypertrichosis, which is a very rare, androgen-independent disorder.
  - hypertrichosis can involve vellus, lanugo, and terminal hair occupying the entire body surface including the face ('werewolf appearance')
  - congenital forms have been described (usually more severe)
  - can caused by drugs (phenytoin, ciclosporin, glucocorticoids), hypothyroidism, and anorexia nervosa.

Virilization

- Can be distinguished from hirsutism by the presence of:
  - clitoromegaly
  - balding
  - deepening of the voice
  - male body habitus.
- Is relatively rare and usually secondary to androgen-producing tumours or congenital adrenal hyperplasia (CAH).

Causes of hirsutism

- Ovary:
  - polycystic ovarian syndrome 95%
  - androgen-secreting tumours <1%
  - luteoma <1%.
- Adrenal gland:
  - congenital adrenal hyperplasia <1%
  - Cushing's syndrome <1%
  - androgen-secreting tumours <1%
  - acromegaly 1%
- External causes:
  - iatrogenic hirsutism <1%
  - drugs with androgenic effects (anabolic steroids, danazol, testosterone) <1%

Reasons for increased androgen levels

- Reduced SHBG levels:
  - hyperinsulinemia
  - liver disease
  - androgens
  - hyperprolactinemia
  - hypothyroidism.
- Increased production:
  - tumours
  - enzyme defects (including CAH)
  - Cushing's syndrome
  - hyperinsulinemia
  - increased LH levels stimulate theca cells.
- External androgen sources:
  - androgens
  - progestogens with androgenic potential
- Increased 5-α reductase sensitivity:
  - insulin growth factor-1 in patients with insulin resistance or hyperinsulinaemia.

Hirsutism and virilization: clinical appearance and investigations

Women mostly present with coarse and pigmented (terminal) hair in the face (upper lip, chin), chest, abdomen, back, and thighs. Ethnic differences in the severity of hair growth are common. Fair-skinned white women show less hair growth, while Mediterranean women have the greatest amount of terminal hair. Genetic differences in the activity of 5-α reductase seem to correlate with the severity of disease. Hirsutism is often accompanied by seborrhoea, acne, and male pattern alopecia.

History
- Age:
  - children with non-classical CAH
  - pregnant women with luteoma.
- Rate of onset of symptoms:
  - rapid onset of severe symptoms may indicate an androgen-producing tumour.
- Menstrual cycle:
  - oligo- or amenorrhoea.
- Genetic factors:
  - PCOS
  - enzyme deficiencies
  - type II diabetes.
- Drugs:
  - COCPs with androgen effects
  - drug abuse (body builders).
- General health and other symptoms:
  - Cushing's
  - acromegaly
  - liver disease.

Physical examination
- Exclude hypertrichosis.
- Signs of virilization should prompt a search for an androgen-producing tumour.
- BP:
  - ↑ with Cushing's and acromegaly
  - ↓ in hypothyroidism and CAH.
- Look for acanthosis nigricans:
  - marker of insulin resistance and hyperinsulinemia
  - skin grey-brown, velvety appearance mainly in the neck, axillae, vulva, and groin.

Ferriman–Gallwey Score to grade hirsutism

- Nine locations are evaluated and each receives a score between 0 (no growth) and 4 (complete hair cover):
  - Upper lip.
  - Chin.
  - Chest.
  - Upper abdomen.
  - Lower abdomen.
  - Upper back.
  - Lower back.
  - Upper arms.
  - Thighs.
- A score >8 is considered androgen excess.

◆ This score is subjective, difficult to compare between different ethnic groups and has a reduced validity in pre-treated women. It is therefore usually reserved for clinical studies.

Investigations for hirsutism

- Testosterone:
  - measure of ovarian and adrenal activity.
- DHEAS:
  - measure of adrenal activity.
- OGTT:
  - in women with indication of hyperinsulinemia/insulin resistance.
- 17-OHP:
  - to rule out CAH, if indicated.

▶ TVUSS to visualize polycystic ovaries is not necessary to diagnose PCOS in a woman with hirsutism and oligo-/amenorrhoea.

▶ Investigations to rule out rare causes of hirsutism such as Cushing's syndrome and acromegaly should be undertaken if clinically indicated.

Hirsutism: first-line treatment

Treatment is aimed at the underlying cause (especially important for the non-ovarian causes such as Cushing's or CAH).

- Lifestyle changes aiming at weigh reduction in women with PCOS.
- COCP:
  - treatment of choice in women not trying to conceive
  - progestational component: (LH suppression; 5α-reductase inhibition)
  - oestrogenic component: (SHBG ↑)
  - ethinylestradiol + cyproterone acetate (co-cyprindion Dianette®) licensed in UK for facial hirsutism (not for contraception!)
- Medroxyprogesterone acetate:
  - if COCP is contraindicated
  - LH suppression (less than OCP)
  - SHBG ↓ (counter productive)
  - testosterone clearance ↑ (induction of liver enzymes)
  - overall, similar results to COCP.

▶ Discontinue treatment after 1–2 years to observe if ovulatory cycles occur. Suppression of testosterone will last for 6–12 month after discontinuation in anovulatory patients.

Cosmetic approaches

- Hair removal will only be permanent if the dermal papilla is destroyed.
- Non-permanent approaches such as shaving or waxing do not worsen hirsutism.

Permanent measures

Laser

- 694–1064 nm.
- Uses melanin in hair bulb as chromophore.
- Heat causes papillar destruction.
- Works best on fair-skinned women with dark hair.
- Dark-skinned patients at higher risk of dermal damage (scarring and discomfort as more energy is needed).

Electrolysis

- Fine probe inserted into skin.
- Short-wave radio frequency causes heat, thereby destroying dermal papilla.
- Only permanent measure approved by FDA.

Non-permanent measures

- Local chemical depilatories (not for face).
- Bleaching.
- Waxing.
- Tweezing.
- Mechanical epilators.

Hirsutism: second-line treatment

- **Spironolactone** (50–200 mg daily, ↓ to 25–50 mg qds after few weeks):
  - aldosterone antagonist (diuretic)
  - inhibits ovarian/adrenal androgens
  - competes for androgen receptor in skin
  - inhibits 5α-reductase in skin
  - slow onset (at least 6 months)
  - hyperkalaemia possible (watch renal function)
  - add contraceptive as may cause feminization of male fetus.
- **Cyproterone acetate** (2 mg plus 35 micrograms ethinyl estradiol in co-cyprindiol (Dianette®)):
  - progestational agent with antiandrogenic potency
  - inhibits LH secretion and binds competitively to androgen receptor
  - best after 3 months of treatment
  - side effects: fatigue, oedema, weight gain, loss of libido, mastalgia.
- **Finasteride** (5 mg daily):
  - inhibits 5α-reductase (type II>type I; type I in skin, therefore limited potency for hirsutism and alopecia)
  - few side effects
  - best after 6 months
  - teratogenic: contraception needed.
- **Flutamide** (250 mg daily):
  - non-steroidal antiandrogen
  - best after 6 months, also for treatment of alopecia
  - hepatotoxicity (monitor liver enzymes regularly)
  - add contraceptive as may cause feminization of male fetus.
- **Eflornithine hydrochloride** (cream topically bd):
  - inhibits ornithine decarboxylase, responsible for hair growth
  - reduces speed of hair growth and hair becomes less coarse
  - works within 8 weeks, but quick recurrence after cessation
  - may worsen acne (obstructing pilosebaceous glands)
  - recommended for postmenopausal hair growth on upper lip.
- **GnRH agonists** (depot prescriptions):
  - suppress gonadotrophins, thereby suppressing ovarian androgens
  - should be combined with add-back HRT
  - expensive and equally effective as other approaches.

Last resort treatment

- Ketoconazole (400 mg daily):
  - antifungal agent
  - reduces androgen levels by inducing hepatic cytochrome P450 metabolic pathways
  - hepatotoxicity (monitor liver enzymes regularly)
  - loss of scalp hair
  - abdominal pain.

⚠ Most of the drugs mentioned are not licensed for this indication. Cyproterone acetate/ethinylestradiol, and eflornithine are the exceptions.

Hirsutism and the menopause

About 17% of patients are menopausal, mainly with facial hirsutism.

Treatment
- Eflornithine cream.
- Spironolactone.
- Cyproterone acetate with HRT (not ethinylestradiol).
- Estradiol + drospirenone HRT.

Endometriosis: overview

Endometriosis is the presence of endometrial-like tissue outside the uterine cavity. It is oestrogen dependent, therefore mostly effects women during their reproductive years. If the ectopic endometrial tissue is within the myometrium itself it is called **adenomyosis**.

Aetiology

The exact aetiology remains unknown, various theories exist but none accounts for all aspects of endometriosis.

- Retrograde menstruation with adherence, invasion, and growth of the tissue (Sampson):
  - most popular theory; however, >90% show menstrual blood in pelvis at time of menstruation.
- Metaplasia of mesothelial cells (Meyer).
- Systemic and lymphatic spread (Halban).
- Impaired immunity (Dmowski).

Incidence of endometriosis

General female population	10–12% (estimated)
Infertility investigation	20–30%
Sterilization	6%
Chronic pelvic pain investigation	15%
Dysmenorrhea	40–60%

Typical presentation of endometriosis (often combination)

- Infertility.
- Pain (often chronic pelvic pain):
  - cyclic or constant (ectopic endometrial tissue undergoes same cycle, causing repeated inflammation, which may result in the formation of adhesions)
  - severe dysmenorrhoea (can be due to adenomyosis)
  - dyspareunia (deep; indicates possible involvement of uterosacral ligaments)
  - dysuria (involvement of bladder peritoneum or invasion into bladder)
  - dyschezia and cyclic pararectal bleeding (for rectovaginal nodules with invasion of rectal mucosa)
  - chronic fatigue.

⚠ Pain symptoms are often non-specific, resulting in the delay of the diagnosis by up to 12 years.

▶ In 2–50% of cases there are no symptoms!

Location of endometriosis

Common sites:
- Pelvis (most common):
  - pouch of Douglas
  - uterosacral ligaments
  - ovarian fossae
  - bladder
  - peritoneum.

Rare sites:
- Lungs.
- Brain.
- Muscle.
- Eye.

▶ Endometriosis has been described in girls prior to menarche, and in men.

Appearance of endometriosis

- Peritoneal endometriotic lesions:
  - appear as minuscule (powder burn) to 1–2 cm lesions (red, bluish, brown, black, white; vesicular, cystic, petechial)
- Ovarian endometriotic cysts:
  - endometriomas can be >10 cm in size
  - usually filled with brownish fluid ('chocolate cysts'; old blood and tissue)
  - often associated with local fibrosis.
- Deep infiltrating endometriosis:
  - rectovaginal nodules can frequently result in fibrosis of the surrounding tissue and often have a solid appearance.

📖 Women's Health Specialist Library. www.library.nhs.uk/womenshealth/

📖 The investigation and management of endometriosis. RCOG Guideline 24 www.rcog.org.uk

Endometriosis: diagnosis

History
- Menstrual cycle.
- Nature of the pain:
  - site
  - relationship to cycle (mid cyle/dysmenorrhoea)
  - deep dypareunia.
- Haematuria or rectal bleeding during menstruation.

Examination
- Bimanual pelvic examination for:
  - adnexal masses (endometriomas) or tenderness
  - nodules/tenderness in the posterior vaginal fornix or uterosacral ligaments
  - fixed retroverted uterus
  - rectovaginal nodules.
- Speculum examination of vagina and cervix (rarely, lesions may be visible).

Investigations
- Transvaginal USS:
  - endometriomas
  - possibly for endometriosis of urinary bladder or rectum.
- Laparoscopy with biopsy for histological verification
  - especially important for deep infiltrating lesions
  - positive is confirmative, negative does not rule it out
  - endometriomas >3 cm should to be resected to rule out malignancy (rare).
- Laparoscopy should not be performed within 3 months of hormonal treatment (leads to underdiagnosis).
- Indications for laparoscopy:
  - NSAID-resistant lower abdominal pain/dysmenorrhea
  - pain resulting in days off work/school or hospitalization
  - pain and infertility investigation.
- It is good practice to document the extent of disease (photos or DVD).
- MRI, IVU, or barium enema (to assess extent of rectovaginal, bladder, ureteric, or bowel involvement).
- Serum CA125 is sometimes elevated with severe endometriosis but there is no evidence that it is a useful screening test for this condition.

Grading of endometriosis

The current system (Revised American Society of Reproductive Medicine classification, rASRM 1996) classifies the extent of endometriosis on a point system, taking into account:
• Location:
    • peritoneal
    • ovarian
    • pouch of Douglas.
• Size
    • <1 cm
    • 1–3 cm
    • >3 cm
• Depth of infiltration:
    • superficial
    • deep.
• Adhesions
    • filmy or dense
    • extent of enclosure (<1/3; 1/3–2/3, >2/3)
    • colour and form.

The points are added up and the stage of endometriosis is graded accordingly:
• Stage I   Minimal endometriosis   (1–5 points)
• Stage II Mild endometriosis   (6–15 points)
• Stage III Moderate endometriosis   (16–40 points)
• Stage IV Severe endometriosis   (>40 points)

❦ This value of system is highly controversial because of its subjectivity. The severity of disease has not been shown to have any correlation with the severity of pain. It may be of value in infertility prognosis and management.

Endometriosis: treatment

The approach should be determined by:
- Reason for treatment (pain or fertility).
- Side effect profile.
- Cost-effectiveness of each drug.

▶ All drugs are equally effective in relieving pain and are associated with up to 50% recurrence after approximately 12–24 months after stopping.

▶ It is acceptable to treat women empirically with progestagens or COCP without a laparascopic diagnosis. It is unclear whether it is preferable to take the COCP conventionally or over 3 months continuously (tri-cycling). NSAIDs are effective and may be used with hormonal drugs.

▶ Severe cases of endometriosis should be referred to a centre with expertise in advanced laparoscopic surgery.

Treatments for pain

Medical treatment
See Table 17.1.

Surgical treatment
- No RCTs have compared medical vs surgical treatment.
- There are no data supporting preoperative hormonal treatment.
- Postoperative 6 months treatment with GnRH analogues is effective in delaying recurrence at 12 and 24 months (not the case with COCP).
- Coagulation, excision, or ablation are the recommended surgical techniques and should be done by laparoscopy.
- As a last resort hysterectomy may be considered in patients with severe, treatment refractory dysmenorrhoea:
  - if performed, bilateral oophorectomy should be considered with add-back HRT.

Treatments for subfertility

Medical treatment
- No benefit in hormonal treatment (?–ve effect as delays ovulation).
- NSAIDs have been shown to inhibit ovulation when taken at mid cycle (probably through suppression of necessary PG production).

Surgical treatment
- Spontaneous pregnancy rate after surgical removal of endometriotic lesions is probably ↑ in minimal/mild endometriosis.
- Unclear efficacy for moderate/severe disease as no RCTs exist.
- Endometriomas (≥3 cm) should be removed:
  - best by cystectomy rather than drainage to ↓ recurrence rates.

▶ Fertility-sparing surgery should be the goal, to increase chance of spontaneous conception. However, in moderate to severe disease, IVF may be the treatment of choice.

Table 17.1 Medical treatment for pain from endometriosis

Drug	Applications/duration	Effect	Side effects
COCP	21 days with 7 day break or tricyclic Long term	Ovarian suppression	Headaches Nausea DV Stroke
Medroxy-progesterone acetate or other progestagens	Orally or IM/ SC injection (depot) Long term	Ovarian suppression	Weight gain Bloating Acne Irregular bleeding Depression
Gonadotropin releasing ormone (GnRH) analogues	SC/IM injection or nasal spray 3–6 months (if longer only with 'add-back' HRT)	Ovarian · suppression	Loss of bone density (reversible) Hot flushes Vaginal dryness Headaches Depression
Levonorgestrel-releasing IUD	Intrauterine Long term (change every 5 years if age <40)	Endometrial suppression; sometimes ovarian suppression	Irregular bleeding Spontaneous expulsion
Danazol	Oral 6 months (longest experience)	Ovarian suppression	Acne Hirsutism Irreversible voice changes
Aromatase inhibitors	Oral Probably 6 months (not licensed)	Local oestrogen suppression in endometrial lesions	Ovarian cysts Loss of bone density (reversible)

Gonadotrophin releasing hormone (GnRH) in health and disease

Biochemistry
- GnRH is a decapeptide synthesized in the hypothalamus.
- Released in a pulsatile manner in both males and females.
- Acts on G-protein coupled receptors in the anterior pituitary.
- Has a short half-life ($t_{1/2}$) of 2–4 minutes.

Physiological functions
The frequency and amplitude of the GnRH pulses are more important than absolute hormonal levels. During the fetal and neonatal periods GnRH is involved in normal development. The amplitude of pulsatile release is then decreased during childhood until puberty. It is not known what factor(s) trigger the increased frequency and amplitude of secretion seen during puberty, but this results in the release of gonadotrophins (high-frequency pulses of luteinizing hormone (LH) and low-frequency pulses of follicle stimulating hormone (FSH)) from the anterior pituitary gland and subsequently sex steroids from the ovary. A complex system of positive and negative feedback loops between GnRH, LH, FSH, progesterone and oestrogen regulate the normal menstrual cycle (see Chapter 14, p. 484).

Congenital GnRH deficiency
- Congenital hypothalamic hypogonadism is usually only diagnosed in females when a delay in puberty is noted, as female infants are phenotypically normal.
- When associated with an absence of the sense of smell (anosmia) it is known as **Kallman's syndrome**.
- It can be difficult to distinguish hypothalamic hypogonadism from delayed puberty; however, in the former pubic hair is present as adrenarche occurs normally and children are usually of normal height for their age.

Acquired GnRH deficiency
Acquired GnRH deficiency can be due to:
- Damage to the hypothalamus by:
  - trauma
  - tumour.
- Disruption of the hypothalamic–pituitary axis can occur secondary to:
  - intense physical training
  - anorexia nervosa.

GnRH as a treatment
- Pulsatile intravenous infusions of GnRH can be used to induce puberty and ovulation with a congenital deficiency.
- If deficiency is acquired, it is more usual to use oestrogen and progesterone on a long-term basis, or LH/FSH to induce ovulation.

Gonadotrophin releasing hormone (GnRH) agonists and antagonists

The short half-life of natural GnRH restricts its pharmacological use to i.v. pulsatile use. However, longer acting GnRH analogues (agonists) or receptor antagonists can be used to induce a temporary, reversible menopausal state as a treatment for a number of conditions.

GnRH analogues

- A number of different GnRH analogues exist, including:
  - goserelin acetate (Zoladex)
  - leuprorelin acetate (Prostap)
  - nafarelin (Synarel).
- Administration:
  - subcutaneous injection (daily, monthly or 3-monthly)
  - intranasally
  - intravaginally.
- They produce a prolonged activation of the GnRH receptor, resulting in an initial ↑ in FSH and LH secretion:
  - this may cause a worsening of symptoms ('initial flare')
- Continued activation of the receptor leads to ↓ LH/FSH secretion:
  - serum estradiol levels are suppressed by approximately 21 days
  - remain at similar levels to postmenopausal women with continued dosing.
- Indications and adverse effects are shown in text boxes, p. 565.
- Adequate barrier contraception should be used during treatment as there is a theoretical risk of teratogenicity and miscarriage.

Bone mineral density (BMD)

- Up to 6% BMD may be lost after the first 6 months treatment.
- If treatment is to be continued for longer than 3–6 months, the use of 'addback' HRT is recommended:
  - combined GnRH agonist and HRT addback has been shown to be safe for a period of up to 2 years
  - small ongoing studies suggest that longer term use will also be safe.
- Resumption of menstruation and return of fertility occur soon after stopping treatment.

GnRH antagonists

GnRH antagonists, such as cetrorelix, bind to receptors without activation and therefore do not cause an initial worsening of symptoms. They are currently licensed for assisted conception protocols and are used experimentally in endometriosis treatments. However, their effect on BMD and other side effects are similar to agonists.

Indications for GnRH analogue treatment

- Pre-surgery:
  - endometrial thinning prior to ablation/resection
  - fibroid shrinkage prior to myomectomy/hysterectomy.
- Endometriosis.
- Adenomyosis.
- Assisted reproduction:
  - pituitary down-regulation prior to superovulation.
- Diagnostic tool in chronic pelvic pain (see Chapter 16, 📖 p. 540).
- Breast cancer.
- Prostate cancer.

Adverse effects of GnRH agonists/antagonists

- Hot flushes.
- Mood swings.
- Vaginal dryness.
- Abnormal vaginal bleeding.
- Decreased libido.
- Breast swelling/tenderness.
- ↑ LDL ↓ HDL.
- Insomnia.
- Headaches.
- Loss of bone mineral density.
- Alterations in eyesight.
- Initial flare (agonists only).
- Bruising at injection site.

Female subfertility: overview

- Subfertility is very common, with 1 in 6 couples seeking specialist help.
- ~84% will achieve a pregnancy in 1 year of regular unprotected sexual intercourse (UPSI):
  - this ↑ to 92% after 2 years.
- Referral for specialist advice should be considered after at least 1 year of trying, though in certain situations prompt investigations and referral may be recommended:
  - female age >35 years
  - known fertility problems
  - anovulatory cycles
  - severe endometriosis
  - previous PID
  - malignancy.
- Couples should be treated on an individual basis, as there is not necessarily a right answer as to when investigations and treatment should start.
- The management of subfertility aims to correct any specific problem which may or may not be diagnosed.

Causes of subfertility

• Ovulation disorder	21%
• Tubal factor	15–20%
• Male factor	25%
• Unexplained	28%
• Endometriosis	6–8%
• Sexual dysfunction	4–5%

Causes of anovulation

Primary ovarian failure
- Premature ovarian failure.
- Genetic
  - Turners' syndrome (45X0; hypergonadotrophic hypogonadism).
- Autoimmune.
- Iatrogenic
  - surgery
  - chemotherapy.

Secondary ovarian disorders
- PCOS.
- Excessive weight loss or exercise.
- Hypopituitarism:
  - tumour
  - trauma
  - surgery.
- Kallman's syndrome (anosmia; hypogonadotrophic hypogonadism).
- Hyperprolactinaemia.

Female subfertility: diagnosis

History
It is vitally important to take a relevant and careful history in a sensitive manner, however embarrassing this may be for you. Couples are often seen together and sometimes it can be difficult to ask about sensitive issues; if necessary, each partner can be seen alone, though this not ideal. Also ask if a cervical smear is needed and about breast examinations.
- Age.
- Duration of subfertility and coital frequency.
- Menstrual cycle regularity and LMP (?pregnant).
- Pelvic pain (dysmenorrhoea; dysparuenia).
- Cervical smear history.
- Previous pregnancies.
- History of ectopic pregnancy.
- Previous tubal or pelvic surgery.
- Previous or current STIs.
- Previous pelvic inflammatory disease (PID).
- Coital frequency.
- Any relevant medical or surgical history.
- Drug history (any prescription drugs that may be contraindicated in pregnancy and ask about recreational drug use).
- Smoking.
- Number of units alcohol/week.
- Folic acid.

Clinical examination
- General examination:
  - BMI
  - signs of endocrine disorder: hyperandrogenism (acne, hair growth, alopecia), acanthosis nigricans (see PCOS); thyroid disease (hypo- and hyperthyroidism); visual field defects (? prolactinoma).
- Pelvic examination:
  - exclude obvious pelvic pathology (adnexal masses, uterine fibroids, endometriosis [painful, fixed uterus], vaginismus)
  - cervical smear
  - *Chlamydia* screening.

Investigations
- Primary care:
  - *Chlamydia* screening
  - baseline (day 2–5) hormone profile including FSH (high in POF; low in hypopituitarism), LH, TSH, prolactin, testosterone
  - rubella status
  - mid-luteal progesterone level (to confirm ovulation >30 nmol/L)
  - semen analysis (see Male subfertility, p. 000).
- Secondary care:
  - This assessment should ideally take place within a specialist clinic with appropriately trained multidisciplinary staff. The history should be confirmed with the couple and any missing details checked.

Assessment of tubal patency

- Hysterosalpingogram (HSG):
  - easily done
  - good sensitivity and specificity
  - can be uncomfortable
  - may have false-positive results (suggesting tubal blockage due to spasm).
- Laparoscopy and dye test:
  - day-case procedure which can be combined with a hysteroscopy to assess the uterine cavity if necessary
  - 'gold standard'
  - pelvic pathology (endometriosis, peritubular adhesions) can be diagnosed and treated
  - requires general anaesthetic
  - carries surgical risks.
- Hysterocontrast-salpingography (HyCoSy):
  - ultrasound with galactose-containing contrast medium
  - similar sensitivity to HSG
  - no radiation exposure.

Female subfertility: management

Management depends on duration and possible cause of subfertility. Couples should be informed of their options and given relevant evidence-based advice so they can make an informed choice.

Lifestyle modification
- Healthy diet.
- Stop smoking/recreational drugs.
- Reduce alcohol consumption.
- Regular exercise.
- Folic acid.
- Avoid timed intercourse (every 2–3 days).
- Avoid ovulation induction kits/basal temperature measurements (no evidence of success, and stressful).

Ovulation induction
- PCOS is the most common cause of secondary amenorrhoea and is responsible for 75–80% of anovulatory subfertility. Correction of the specific problem such as hyperprolactinaemia or excessive weight may be enough.
- Weight loss/gain as appropriate.
- Anti-oestrogens (e.g. clomifene 50 mg days 2–6):
  - ↑ endogenous FSH levels via negative feedback to pituitary
  - 8–10% multiple pregnancy
  - Side effects (hot flushes, mood labiality)
  - clomifene limited to 12 cycles maximum (? possible link to ovarian cancer)
  - needs ultrasound monitoring (abandon cycle if over-response).
- Gonadotrophins or pulsatile GnRH:
  - used for low oestrogen/normal FSH or clomifene-resistant PCOS
  - injections
  - expensive
  - multiple pregnancy risk
  - ultrasound monitoring (abandon cycle if over-response)
  - more easily titrated.
- Laparoscopic ovarian diathermy:
  - aims to restore ovulation in patients with PCOS
  - Effect lasts 12–18 months if successful
- Insulin sensitizers (metformin 500 mg tds):
  - used in women with PCOS
  - may achieve spontaneous ovulation
  - can be combined with clomifene to increase efficacy
  - recent conflicting data
  - not licensed
  - weight loss is more effective.
- Surgery:
  - preferably laparoscopic.
  - treat endometriosis (laser/diathermy/excision).
  - tubal surgery (microsurgery/adhesiolysis).
- Assisted reproduction (IUI, IVF, oocyte donation).

Psychological issues

Subfertility and its management can be very distressing. Some treatments have side effects and are not guaranteed to be successful. The stress of this and disappointment of failed treatment needs to be addressed. Couples should be offered counselling before and after treatment, along with information regarding patient support groups.

📕 www.rcog.org.uk

📕 www.nice.org.uk

Male subfertility

Accounts for 20–25% cases of subfertile couples. Investigation should start in primary care after 1 year, or earlier if history of genital surgery, cancer treatment, or previous subfertility. Trend of declining sperm concentration is not affecting global fecundity but there is increasing 'testicular dysgenesis syndrome' with an increase in cryptorchidism, testicular cancer, and hypospadias. Normal male fertility is dependent on normal spermatogenesis, erectile function, and ejaculation.

Normal semen analysis (WHO criteria)

- Volume > 2mL.
- Concentration > 20×10^6/mL.
- Motility >50% forward.

Azoospermia: No sperm in ejaculate.

Oligozoospermia: Reduced number of sperm in ejaculate.

Investigations

- FSH: elevated in testicular failure.
- Karyotype: exclude 47XXY.
- Cystic fibrosis screen: CBAVD.

Management

- Treat any underlying medical conditions.
- Address lifestyle issues (↓ alcohol, stop smoking).
- Review medications:
  - antispermatogenic (alcohol, anabolic steroids, sulfasalazine)
  - antiandrogenic (cimetidine, spironolactone)
  - erectile/ejaculatory dysfunction (α or β blockers, antidepressants, diuretics, metoclopramide)
- Medical treatments:
  - gonadotrophins in hypogonadotrophic hypogonadism
  - sympathomimetics (e.g. imipramine) in retrograde ejaculation
- Surgical:
  - relieve obstruction
  - vasectomy reversal.

⚠ Surgical treatment of varicocele does not improve pregnancy rate and is therefore not indicated.

- Sperm retrieval:
  - from postorgasmic urine in retrograde ejaculation
  - surgical sperm retrieval from testis with 50% chance of obtaining sperm (greater if FSH is normal).
- Assisted reproduction:
  - IUI (intrautertine insemination)
  - ICSI (intracytoplasmic sperm injection).
- Donor sperm.
- Adoption.

Pathogenesis of male subfertility

- **Semen abnormality (85%):**
  - idiopathic oligoasthenoteratozoospermia (OATS)
  - testis cancer
  - drugs (includiing alcohol, nicotine)
  - genetic
  - varicocele.
- **Azoospermia (5%):**
  - pretesticular: anabolic steroid abuse; idiopathic hypogonado-trophic hypogonadism (HH); Kalmann's, pituitary adenoma
  - non-obstructive: cryptorchidism, orchitis, 47XXY, chemo-radiotherapy
  - obstructive: congenital bilateral absence of the vas deferens (CBAVD), vasectomy, *Chlamydia*, gonorrhoea).
- **Immunological (5%):**
  - antisperm antibodies
  - idiopathic
  - infection
  - unilateral testicular obstruction.
- **Coital dysfunction (5%):**
  - mechanical cause with normal sperm function
  - ejaculation normal (hypospadias, phimosis, disability)
  - retrograde ejaculation (diabetes, bladder neck surgery, phenothiazines)
  - failure in ejaculation (MS, spinal cord/pelvic injury).

Assisted reproduction: IVF and ICSI

Assisted reproductive technologies (ART) refer to all fertility treatments in which sperm and oocytes are handled with the aim of achieving pregnancy. It includes in vitro fertilization (IVF), intra-cytoplasmic sperm injection (ICSI), pre-implantation genetic diagnosis (PGD), egg donation, and surrogacy.

In vitro fertilization (IVF)

Indications may include:
- Tubal disease.
- Male factor subfertility.
- Endometriosis.
- Anovulation.
- ↓ fecundity observed with ↑ maternal age.

Success is dependent on many factors including:
- Duration of subfertility:
  - ↓ success with ↑ duration.
- Age:
  - pregnancy rates are highest between 25 and 35 with a steep decline thereafter
  - elevated basal FSH levels may indicate a poor response to ovarian stimulation.
- Previous pregnancy:
  - higher chance of successful IVF outcome.
- Previous failed IVF cycles:
  - ↓ success.
- Presence of hydrosalpinx or intramural fibroid:
  - ↓ success.
- Smoking and ↑ BMI:
  - ↓ success.

Intracytoplasmic sperm injection (ICSI)

- A single sperm is injected into the ooplasm of the oocyte in ICSI.
- Used for men with severely abnormal semen parameters.
- May also be tried when failed fertilization has occurred in IVF cycles.
- Higher fertilization rates are obtained if the selected sperm exhibit some motility, but otherwise there are no strict selection criteria.
- Has greatly ↑ the success of IVF with severe male factor subfertility.
- Sperm may be retrieved from ejaculate or surgically from the epididymis or testes.
- Men with severe oligozoospermia should have karyotype and cystic fibrosis screening prior to ICSI.

There are concerns regarding transmission of genetic mutations when using ICSI. Sperms containing oxidatively induced DNA damage are capable of fertilizing oocytes. There is an increased incidence of Y chromosome deletions on subfertile men and this may be further propagated by transmission to the offspring born by ICSI resulting in infertility.

IVF: how it's done

▶ In preparation, HFEA consents and 'Welfare of the Child' issues must be considered.

- Down-regulation of the ovaries using GnRH analogues from day 21 (luteal phase) of the previous cycle:
  - alternatively in antagonist cycles ('short protocol') GnRH antagonists are co-administered with gonadotrophins during ovarian stimulation.
- Ovarian stimulation with recombinant FSH or human menopausal gonadotrophins:
  - response is monitored by transvaginal USS.
- Follicular maturation by administration of hCG, when significant mature-size follicles are seen on USS.
- Transvaginal oocyte retrieval by needle-guided aspiration (36 hours later).
- Sperm sample collected (or thawed if frozen), prepared and cultured with oocytes overnight.
- Fertilization checks of embryos,
- Embryo transfer by a fine catheter through cervix on day 2–3 (cleavage stage):
  - a maximum of 2 embryos are transferred in women under 40 and current debate on move to single embryo transfer given increased neonatal morbidity/mortality and ensuing costs of multiple pregnancy
  - blastocyst transfer may be considered.
- Surplus embryos may be cryopreserved for future frozen embryo replacement cycles.
- Luteal support given in form of progestogens.
- Pregnancy test 2 weeks later.

Assisted reproduction: other techniques

Preimplantation genetic diagnosis (PGD)
- Aims to reduce the recurrence of genetic risk in couples known to carry a heritable genetic condition.
- Many couples are fertile, but IVF allows embryo biopsy, single cell diagnosis and the transfer of unaffected embryos to the woman.
- Biopsies are usually done at cleavage stage and PCR or fluorescent in-situ hybridization (FISH) used for genetic diagnosis.

Intrauterine insemination (IUI)
- Couples who may benefit include those with:
  - mild male factor subfertility
  - minimal/mild endometriosis
  - unexplained subfertility
  - coital difficulties.
- Sperm is prepared and placed into the uterus to aid conception.
- The lower threshold for sperm concentration suitability for IUI has been suggested as a total motile count of >10 M/mL.
- NICE recommend up to 6 cycles of IUI, but most studies have reported optimal outcome within the first 4 cycles.

⚬ There is no consensus on the role of simultaneous ovarian stimulation, but this should be considered in endometriosis when outcome is less favourable.

⚠ If >3 follicles develop the treatment cycle should be cancelled as there is a high rate of multiple pregnancies (>25%).

Egg donation
- May offer a chance of pregnancy for women previously considered to be irreversibly sterile.
- This includes women with:
  - ovarian failure (gonadal dysgenesis, premature, cancer patients secondary to surgery and chemo-radiotherapy or menopausal)
  - older women (>45 years)
  - those with repeated IVF failure.

Donor insemination
- Indicated in men
  - with azoospermia and failed surgical sperm recovery
  - at high risk of transmitting genetic disorders (eg. Huntington's disease)
  - at high risk of transmitting infections (HIV).
- Also used for women with no male partner.
- The success of ICSI has ↓ demand for DI.
- Insemination is usually intrauterine.
  - ± ovarian stimulation and 36–40 h after hCG administration.
- Success rates vary from 4% (aged 40–44) to 12% (<34 years).

Special concerns regarding donation of gametes

There are strict criteria for gamete donation, which is regulated by the HFEA.
- Ideally, donors should have no severe medical, psychiatric, or genetic disorders.
- Donors must be counselled.
- Donors must undergo a full infection screen.
- Donors may be known or anonymous to the recipient.
- Egg donors should ideally be <35 years old.
- Each donor can only be used in up to 10 families within the UK.

⚠ In April 2005 donor anonymity was lifted, meaning that when children born from the use of donor gametes reach the age of 18, they can contact the HFEA for identifying information on the donor.

▶ The supply of donor gametes in the UK is limited. The HFEA may authorize the procurement of gametes from abroad if the supplying clinic fulfils the same quality of standards as the UK.

Surrogacy

- IVF surrogacy:
  - the couple who want the child provide both sets of gametes
  - following IVF the embryos are transferred to the surrogate
  - this accounts for <0.1% of the total IVF cycles in the UK
  - indications include women who have congenital absence of the uterus (Rotikansky's syndrome), following hysterectomy, or with severe medical conditions incompatible with pregnancy.
- 'Natural surrogacy':
  - the surrogate is inseminated by the sperm of the male partner of the couple wanting the child.

⚠ Counselling and legal advice is necessary for all parties involved in the surrogacy.

Ovarian hyperstimulation syndrome (OHSS)

Ovarian hyperstimulation syndrome (OHSS) is a complication of ovulation induction or superovulation. Incidence is 0.5–10% and in 1/200 cases it is severe, requiring hospitalization. Vascular endothelial growth factor (VEGF) is central to underlying pathophysiology

- It is characterized by:
  - ovarian enlargement
  - shifting of fluid from the intravascular to the extravascular space.
- Fluid accumulates in the peritoneal and pleural spaces.
- There is intravascular fluid depletion, leading to:
  - haemoconcentration
  - hypercoaguability.
- Risk factors include:
  - polycystic ovaries
  - younger women with low BMI
  - previous OHSS.

Prevention

Management is focused on prediction and active prevention. This may involve low-dose gonadotrophins, cycle cancellation, 'coasting' during stimulation, or elective embryo cryopreservation for replacement in a further frozen–thawed cycle.

In vitro maturation may be used in women with polycystic ovaries, with high antral follicle counts collecting immature eggs, thus avoiding ovarian stimulation and the risk of OHSS.

Treatment

The treatment is supportive, with the aims of:

- Symptomatic relief.
- Prevention of haemoconcentration and thromboembolism.
- Maintenance of cardiorespiratory function.

Treatment should consist of:

- Daily assessment of:
  - hydration status (FBC, U&E, LFTs and albumin)
  - chest and respiratory function (pleural effusions)
  - ascites (girth measurement and weight)
  - legs (for evidence of thrombosis).
- Strict fluid balance with careful maintenance of intravascular volume.
- Thromboprophylaxis:
  - compression stockings
  - consider heparin.
- Paracentesis for symptomatic relief (± IV replacement albumin).
- Analgesia and antiemetics.

Sexual dysfunction: overview

Sexual health is a state of physical, emotional, mental, and social well-being in relation to sexuality, not merely the absence of disease or dysfunction. Sexual health necessitates the possibility of having pleasurable and safe sexual experiences, free of coercion, discrimination, and violence. Sexual rights must therefore be respected, protected and fulfilled.

The prevalence of female sexual dysfunction (FSD) is highly definition-dependent (whether dissatisfaction and disinterest constitute FSD is debated).

Rates up to 43% in women aged 18–59 compared to 31% in men. Increasing age is inversely proportional to sexually activity. 1/3 of all women over 60 may be sexually active (55% if married). Up to 50% of men will have some degree of erectile dysfunction, which rises to 67% by 70.

The menopause is associated with a deterioration of sexual function with one study suggesting an increase in FSD from 42–88% (45–55 year old).

Dyspareunia is common and may be present in up to 1/3 of women.

Normal sexual function

Masters and Johnson proposed 4 components of the sexual response: arousal/excitement, plateau, orgasm, and resolution (based on biological, predominantly male, responses). More recently, intimacy-based models include features of satisfaction, pleasure, and relationship context. Overall the 'normal' for female sexuality is not well characterized and currently female sexual dysfunction (FSD) is under construction.

Diagnosis

See the woman as she chooses to present herself, with or without a partner, and explore 'why now?' Many present when not in relationships, concerned about their sexual responses.

Presentation may be overt or covert—it is often useful to give the patient time to explore this and always think of the possibility of somatization of problems.

> **Vital questions in a psychosexual history**
> - Are you sexually active/ do you have a partner?
> - Do you have any difficulties?
> - Are they a problem for you?
> - Do you have pain associated with intercourse?

Examination

'The moment of truth' is a frequent occasion for disclosure of sexual problems manifesting as difficulties with examination, exposure, humiliation, or fantasies of disease or disgust.

Tips on handling consultations

- Be led by the patient.
- The patient is the expert—help her understand her behaviour.
- Reflect your thoughts and feelings.
- Try to understand relationship between the physical findings, such as prolapse, and the psychological reaction to them.
- Be aware of powerful subconscious defences in the patient, especially with lack of libido and desire disorders.

Consider discussing possible fantasies

- Feeling too small.
- Feeling too big.
- Feeling too loose.
- Vagina with teeth.
- Sharp penis.

📖 Institute of Psychosexual Medicine. www.ipm.org.uk

📖 British Association of Sexual & Marital Therapy. www.basrt.org.uk

📖 Vulval Pain Society. www.vulvalpainsociety.org.uk

📖 Mary Clegg—devices. www.maryclegg.com

Sexual dysfunction: classification of disorders

Desire disorder

Persistent or recurrent deficiency (or absence) of sexual fantasies/thoughts and/or desire for or receptivity to sexual activity, which causes personal distress (75% of women and 25% of men attending a psychosexual clinic).

The majority of women who have little or no desire are able to derive pleasure from sexual activity. Presentation itself indicates sufficient interest to be hopeful of cure.

Arousal disorder

Persistent or recurrent inability to attain or maintain sufficient sexual excitement, causing personal distress, which may be expressed as a lack of subjective excitement or genital (lubrication/swelling) or other somatic responses. Understanding the sequence of sexual events and the interplay of physical factors (pain, lubrication, environment) helps to deal with the root cause. Lack of sensation is a common presentation of secondary personal or relationship issues.

Orgasmic disorder

Persistent or recurrent difficulty, delay in, or absence of attaining orgasm following sufficient sexual stimulation and arousal, which causes personal distress.

7–10% of women never achieve orgasm with or without a partner. This may not be a concern. Those who can achieve orgasm with masturbation but not with a partner may need to explore their ability to let go or lose control. Up to 25% of women with lifelong anorgasmia have been sexually abused. Women with acquired orgasmic difficulties should explore hormonal status, concomitant medications and relationship issues. Up to 5% of women with anorgasmia will have an organic cause.

Sexual dysfunction secondary to a general medical condition

Endocrine disorders, psychiatric disorders and a number of medications will interfere with the sexual response cycle. Treatment of the condition or alteration of therapies may help but education and explanation may minimize the impact on sexual relationships.

Sexual pain disorders

Dyspareunia

- Dermatological disorders, e.g. psoriasis and lichen sclerosis, infections such as thrush and recurrent herpes, and atrophic vaginitis are treatable causes of superficial dyspareunia but may have significant psychological sequelae.
- Poor arousal may be the result or cause of sexual pain:
  - lubricants and topical anaesthetic gels may help break the cycle.
- Deep dyspareunia may be related to a number of medical conditions (endometriosis, PID, adhesions) determined by examination, ultrasound scan and if necessary laparascopy.

Vaginismus

- Difficulty of the woman to allow vaginal entry of a penis, finger, or object despite the wish to do so.
- This can involve pelvic floor and/or adductor thigh muscle spasm.
- Vaginismus should be regarded as a symptom or sign and not a diagnosis.
- It is generally secondary to another cause—physical, psychological, or both.
- Fear of pain and anticipation of difficulty evolves into avoidance behaviour.
- Check at examination for the presence of anatomical problems, e.g. vaginal septum.

Non-coital sexual pain disorders

- Vulval vestibulitis is the most common pain disorder, but frequently difficult to treat.
- Treatment of any skin condition, desensitization, and treatment with topical anaesthetics and lubricants is first line therapy in conjunction with an exploration of the psychosexual issues.
- Amitriptyline and gabapentin can be considered short term to interrupt the pain cycle.

Sexual dysfunction: treatment

Lifestyle
Address issues including those affecting body image and general well-being, reduction of stress, dealing with relationship/marital issues.

Education
- Teach people about their bodies and encourage exploration.
- Using 'bibliotherapy' for those needing 'permission' to look at erotic and sexual education material.
- Personal lubricants can be useful for those with arousal difficulties and atrophy (recommend oils or special preparations but be aware of mineral oil damage to condoms).

Hormonal treatments
- Oestrogen replacement in menopausal women may improve sexuality as well as symptoms of vaginal atrophy:
  - vaginal oestrogens can be used long term.
- Testosterone implants have been used successfully in those who have been oophorectomized and have hypoactive desire disorder (HSDD).
- Testosterone patches are also licensed in the UK.
- Tibolone is licensed for treatment of loss of desire in postmenopausal women.

Complementary therapies
No good evidence for Yohimbine, gingko, khat, or ginseng.

Behavioural therapy
Most sex therapists will use a combination of psychotherapeutic techniques and behavioural interventions. Sensate focus uses a programme of exercises building up in stages:
- Non-genital sensate focus
- Genital sensate focus
- Vaginal containment
- Vaginal containment with movement.

Devices for anorgasmia
- Clitoral stimulators.
- Vibrators.

Vaginal trainers or dilators
May be of use for women with vaginismus and are recommended for those having prolapse procedures and post radiotherapy.

Perineal injections
100 mg hydrocortisone, 10 mL 0.5% bupivicaine, and 1500 units hyaluronidase—may be of value for perineal injuries or for pain trigger points.

Surgery
Rarely necessary—may be for those with a rigid hymen, significant skin webs at the fourchette post surgery or childbirth, or septae.

Prognostic factors for the success of FSD interventions

- Motivation for treatment (especially in the male partner).
- Quality of the non-sexual relationship.

Sexual dysfunction: male disorders

If you have elicited a problem in a sexually active couple the difficulties of both partners should be gently sought.

Male sexual disorders

- Erectile dysfunction (ED)—most common.
- Desire disorders.
- Ejaculatory disorders.

Erectile dysfunction

Routine tests recommended are:

- Serum glucose.
- Lipids.
- Testosterone (early morning).
- Blood pressure.
- Pulse.
- Weight.
- Genitalia.
- Prostate.

⚠ New-onset erectile dysfunction may be a marker for cardiovascular disease.

Treatment options

- Phosphodiesterase inhibitors:
  - Sildenafil (Viagra®) and vardenafil ↑ erectile function in 60–70%
  - they act in 20–60 minutes and last for up to 8 hours.
- Tadalafil may be useful for premature ejaculation.
- Apomorphine:
  - dopamine agonist
  - less efficacious (40–50%).
- Androgens:
  - for men with hypogonadism.
- Intracavernous prostaglandin injections.
- Intraurethral prostaglandin pellets.
- Vacuum devices.
- Penile implants.

▶ It is important to remember the psychosexual aspects of sexual difficulties for both partners as well as concentrating on pharmacological treatments.

Sexual assault

Sexual assault: overview

Sexual offences and rape definitions vary from country to country.

Sexual Offences Act 2003 (UK)

- **Rape** is defined as non-consensual penetration of mouth, vagina, or anus by a penis.
- **Sexual assaults** are acts of sexual touching without consent. Sexual assault by penetration involves the insertion of object or body parts other than the penis into the vagina or anus (previously indecent assault).
- Children under 13 cannot legally consent to sexual activity and therefore do not need proof of consent. There is no defence in mistaken belief of age.

⚠ It is crucial that advice is sought (from the police or a sexual assault referral centre) **before** any examination is undertaken, to preserve possible evidence available.

Assessing a potential victim

It is important to establish:
- Whether a sexual act has occurred.
- Whether the victim gave consent when competent to give consent.
- Ability of the victim to give consent to forensic examination:
  - age, understanding, language, maturity, or intoxication.
- Need for interpreters for language difficulties.
- Need for 'appropriate adult' for anyone under age or with mental incapacity.

Presentation

Victims may present acutely but frequently there is delay which may be detrimental to evidence gathering. Acute on chronic presentation is also common, particularly with children.

Acute

Victims of acute sexual assault may report to the police directly, or to A&E, GU medicine, gynaecological, or psychiatric services with covert or overt symptoms. It is crucial to any criminal case that evidence is gathered appropriately and the chain of evidence maintained. 16–58% have genital injuries but a higher proportion (38–80%) have non-genital injuries.

⚠ Always consult with the police if there is any doubt about an individual's presentation.

Delayed

Can be with a number of symptoms (recent or historical). GU medicine, gynaecology, and psychiatry are frequent specialities for disclosure of sexual assault or abuse. As there is a significant increase in domestic violence and assault during pregnancy, antenatal services must include screening and referral facilities.

Sexual assault: facts and figures

- The lifetime risk of sexual assault is 1 in 4–6 for women.
- It is estimated that only 1 in 5 adult rapes is reported.
- 1 in 10 victims of sexual assault are men.
- 12% of assaults are by strangers.
- 45% are by acquaintances and 43% by intimate partners.
- 45% involve vaginal rape, 10% anal rape, 15% oral rape, and 25% digital penetration.
- The incidence of child sexual abuse is unknown + possibly only 1 in 20–50 assaults of children are known to supervising authorities.
- The prevalence is far higher than that reflected in numbers reported.

Sexual abuse in children

Concerns for children should be heightened in association with:
- Repeated A&E attendances.
- Poor parent/child interactions or behaviour.
- Child known to social services.
- Any injuries to child under 1 year.
- History of domestic abuse.
- Explanation inconsistent with injuries.
- Disclosure of abuse by child.
- Delay in presentation.

Sexual assault: history and examination

History
- **Consent** is taken before any forensic medical examination.
- **Confidentiality issues:** the victim may agree to only partial release of information and samples but is able to change this decision later; forensic samples can be stored for up to 30 years or 30 years after their 18th birthday.

Key history points
- Alleged assault and what happened since including eating, drinking, showering/bathing, passing urine, opening bowels, and douching.
- Basic medical, surgical, and psychiatric history.
- Medication—prescribed, over-the-counter, social, drugs of abuse.
- Gynaecological, obstetric, and sexual history.
- Last menstrual period, menstrual cycle, contraception.
- Police will also require details of meeting place and details of assault.

Examination
Timing of the examination and sampling should be noted. The presence of pre-existing conditions such as skin problems or markers of self harm must also be documented.

Key examination points
- Demeanour.
- Intoxication.
- Height/weight/BP/pulse/temperature.
- General findings.
- Injuries (record accurately with diagrams—photographs may be used (involvement of police photographer is favourable):
  - non-genital: none, bruising, petechiae, abrasions, lacerations, incisions, defence injuries
  - genital and anal: none, bruising, abrasions, lacerations, incisions, structure of hymen/remnants in those sexually active (or not)
  - oral: mucosa, teeth, tongue.
- Clothes may also be important for evidence.

Collecting evidence
- Evidence kits may be available in A&E departments or brought by the police/forensic examiner. If at all possible evidence by someone trained in this procedure, to ensure the highest standard.
- Evidential samples for sexual offences are likely to be: semen, saliva, vaginal samples, urine, blood, faeces, hair, fibres, vegetation, sanitary pads and/or tampons, toilet paper, clothes, and condoms.

Key samples for reported sexual assault
- Oral intercourse: mouth swab/saliva/mouth wash ± appropriate skin swab.
- Vaginal intercourse—swabs: vulval (×2), perineal (×2), low vaginal (×2), high vaginal (×1), endocervical (×1), from speculum (×1), lubricants ± pubic hair.
- Anal intercourse—swabs with proctoscope: perianal (×2), rectal (×2), anal (×2).
- Buccal swabs are taken for victim DNA.
- Double swabs = 1 dry + 1 wet (saline container).
- Skin samples collected within 48 hours, mouth 24–48 hours, anal 72 hours, and vaginal up to 7 days after the assault.

▶ Forensic examination at >7 days for women and >72 hours for men is unlikely to provide useful evidence.

Sexual assault: management

Principles

- Resuscitation/usual 'ABC' measures are of overriding importance.
- Consideration of collection of evidence.
- Prophylactic antibiotics.
- Post exposure prophylaxis for HIV.
- Emergency contraception.
- Hepatitis B vaccination.
- Analgesia.
- General advice and support.
- Follow-up including counselling.

Emergency contraception

This should be given if there has been any vaginal contact in women or menstruating girls, irrespective of stage of menstrual cycle. Current recommendations: levonorgestrel 1500 micrograms stat within 72 hours of sexual act or IUCD insertion with antibiotic cover within 5 days.

Sexually transmitted infections (STIs)

Risk is estimated at 4–56% depending on the local prevalence and degree of trauma. Consider prophylactic antibiotics particularly if the victim is unlikely to attend for follow-up: 1 g azithromycin + 500 mg ciprofloxacin (or follow local guidelines).

Psychological care

Those at immediate risk of self harm or suicide must be referred to on-call psychiatric services. Others may be referred to local counselling or support services as well as being given details of emergency out of hours contacts (see Websites and helplines, p. 593). Counselling should aim to contain the trauma of the experience and help the victim bear the 'unbearable'. Those with persistent symptoms after 6 months may have post-traumatic stress disorder and need referral to psychiatric services.

Child sexual abuse

It is difficult to know proportions of extrafamilial and intrafamilial sexual abuse because of under-reporting (possibly 2/3 to 1/3 respectively of reported abuse). Most children do not present acutely and may present because of Social Services or medical concerns regarding chronic physical illness/failure to thrive/neglect.

⚠Emergency contraception must be remembered in pubescent girls.

STIs diagnostic for child sexual abuse are:
- Gonorrhoea (if over 1 year).
- Syphilis and HIV (if congenital infection excluded).
- Chlamydia (if over 3 years).

HIV and sexual assault

Risk is dependent on the prevalence in the population and trauma of assault. The prescribing of postexposure prophylaxis (PEP) must be carefully balanced against the side effects and risks of taking them. Consider the higher risk factors: assailant HIV positive or in risk group, anal rape, trauma and bleeding, multiple assailants.

- **PEP:** currently 3 antiretroviral drugs taken ASAP (within 1 hour if possible) and within 72 hours. An HIV test is required at baseline and 6 months. Appropriate follow-up must be arranged because of the toxicity of these drugs. There are no studies of the efficacy of PEP after sexual exposure.

Risk of transmission of HIV with single exposure (higher if traumatic)
- Receptive vaginal intercourse: 1 in 600–2000.
- Receptive anal intercourse: 1 in 30–150.

📖 Rape Crisis Federation. www.rapecrisis.org.uk (local numbers available from website)

📖 Victim Support: for victims of all crimes including sexual assault. www.victimsupport.org.uk Tel. 0845 30 30 900

📖 The Havens: London Sexual Assault Referral Centres. www.thehavens.co.uk

📖 Samaritans. www.samaritans.org.uk Tel. 08457 90 90 90

📖 Brook: helpline and online enquiry service for the under-25s. www.brook.org.uk Tel. 020 7284 6040

📖 Rights of Women. www.rightsofwomen.org.uk Tel. 020 7251 6577

📖 Suzy Lamplugh Trust: for issues of personal safety. www.suzylamplugh.org.uk Tel. 020 8392 1839

Contraception

Combined oral contraceptive pill (COCP): overview

The COCP provides reliable, effective contraception with a failure rate of 0.2–0.3 per 100 woman-years. Modern COCPs all contain ethinylestradiol (20–35 micrograms) and are classified by the type of progestogen they contain.

Type of progestogen in the COCP

- **2nd generation:**
  - norethisterone
  - levonorgestrel.
- **3rd generation:**
  - desogestrel
  - gestodene (less androgenic)
  - norgestimate (metabolized to levonorgestrel).
- **Yasmin®** contains drospirenone (antiandrogenic and weak antidiuretic properties).
- **co-cyprindiol (Dianette®)** contains cyproterone acetate (antiandrogenic)
  - useful in the treatment of hirsutism and acne.

Mode of action

- Inhibition of ovulation (negative feedback on the hypothalamus + pituitary).
- Thickened cervical mucus preventing sperm penetration.
- Thin endometrium preventing implantation.

Side effects

- Breakthrough bleeding: may occur especially in the first 3 months:
  - missed pills, STIs and pregnancy should all be considered.
- Headache:
  - a ↓ dose of ethinylestradiol or change of progestagen may be tried.
- Weight gain:
  - there is no evidence of additional weight gain due to COCP use.

Contraindications to the COCP

- Pregnancy.
- Personal history of thromboembolic disease.
- Undiagnosed genital tract bleeding.
- Cardiovascular disorders.
- Migraine with aura.
- Oestrogen dependent tumours.
- Active hepatobiliary disease or liver tumours.
- Hypertension and diabetes.
- ≥ 35 years old who smoke (may use 1 year after cessation)
- BMI≥ 35.

Advantages of the COCP

- ↓ menstrual blood loss and pain.
- Menstrual cycle can be regulated and controlled.
- Decreased risks of benign ovarian tumours.
- ↓ incidence of PID.
- Improvement in skin condition in acne vulgaris.
- Possible ↓ symptoms—premenstrual syndrome + endometriosis.
- ↓ risks of colorectal cancer.
- ↓ ovarian cancer risk.
  - ≥50% during use and for >15 years after.

Disadvantages of the COCP

- ↑ risks of VTE, stroke, and cardiovascular disease (although absolute risk is very low).
- Small ↑ risk of breast cancer:
  - returns to the background risk 10 years after stopping.
- Very small association with ↑ risk of cervical cancer.

The pill and VTE

The absolute risk of VTE is:
- **Background risk:**
  - 5:100 000 women/year
- **2nd generation COCP:**
  - 10–15:100 000 women/year
- **3rd generation COCP:**
  - 25:100 000 women/year
- **Pregnancy**
  - 60:100 000 women/year

Current CSM advice regarding the COCP and VTE

▶ As long as women are well informed of the small increased risk of thrombosis associated with 3rd generation pills, and do not have any medical contraindications, it should be a matter of user preference and clinical judgement on which COCP is to be prescribed.

Combined oral contraceptive pill (COCP): regimes

'Pill-teach'

- Contraception is immediate if the woman starts the pills on day 1 of her cycle (the first day of her period).
- If her first pill is after day 2, other contraception needed for 7 days.
- Take the pill same time every day.
- One pill daily for 21 days followed by 7 pill-free days.
- If vomiting or diarrhoea use extra contraception from the onset of illness and continue it for the next 7 days.
- If taking antibiotics, use extra contraception during antibiotic usage and for the next 7 days.

Special circumstances

- Postpartum (not breastfeeding): start day 21 after delivery.
- Post termination: within 7 days of termination.
- Switching from other oral hormonal contraception: start immediately if using other contraception reliably.
- Switching from Implanon® or injectable progestogens: start at any time up to removal of Implanon or when injection is due.

Missed pills

⚠ Missed pills may lead to failed contraception. The risk of pregnancy is greatest at the beginning and the end of the pack.

Missed pill rules

- **Up to 2 pills, anywhere in pack** (or **one** if Loestrin 20®, Mercilon®, or Femodette®):
  - take the last pill missed as soon as possible.
  - take rest of the pack as usual.
  - leave the earlier missed pill.
  - no additional contraception needed.
- **3 or more** (**2** if taking Loestrin 20®, Mercilon®, or Femodette®):
  - take last pill you missed as soon as possible.
  - take rest of pack as usual.
  - leave any earlier missed pills.
  - use extra contraception for the next 7 days.
  - if unprotected sexual intercourse in the previous few days, consider emergency contraception (see p. 604).
- If **7 or more** pills are left in the pack after the missed pill:
  - finish the pack, have the usual 7-day break
- If **fewer than 7** pills are left in the pack:
  - finish the pack and begin new one straight away, missing out the pill-free break.

Progestogen-only pill (POP)

POPs currently marketed contain either levonorgestrel, norethisterone, or etynodiol acetate. The failure rate ranges from 0.3 to 4.0% per 100 woman-years and decreases with age.

▶ Cerazette®, a new POP (75 micrograms desogestrel), reliably blocks ovulation, increasing efficacy.

⚠ To be reliable, a POP must be taken at the same time every day.

Mode of action
- Thickened cervical mucus (4 hours after dose).
- Thin endometrium preventing implantation.
- Inhibition of ovulation (60% old POP, 97% Cerazette®).

Indications
Useful in conditions where COCP is contraindicated:
- During lactation—has no effect on quality or quantity of milk.
- Sickle cell disease.
- SLE and other autoimmune diseases.

Contraindications to the POP

- Pregnancy.
- Undiagnosed genital tract bleeding.
- Severe arterial disease.
- Active hepatic disease.
- History of recurrent follicular cysts.

Side effects
- Menstrual disturbance—regular, irregular, or even amenorrhoea.
- Headaches, nausea, mood swings, abdominal bloating, and breast tenderness—usually subside after a few months.

Drug interactions

▶ Broad spectrum antibiotics do not affect the efficacy of POP.

▶ Rifampicin and other enzyme-inducing drugs increase the metabolism of POP, leading to a reduction in efficacy.

How to take the POP

- Take the pill daily, at the same hour.
- If started on day 1 of the cycle no extra contraception is required.
- If started after day 5, extra contraception should be used for 48 hours.
- After miscarriage or TOP:
  - start on the day of the miscarriage or TOP.
- After delivery:
  - start on day 21 (whether breastfeeding or not).
- From COCP to POP:
  - if the first POP is taken the day after the last active COCP, no other contraception is needed.

Missed POP rules

- If >3 hours late or 27 hours since last dose:
  - take missed pill as soon as possible
  - take subsequent pill at the usual time
  - use extra contraception for the next 48 hours.
- If vomit within 2 hours of ingestion:
  - take another pill now
  - use extra contraception for the next 48 hours.

Other forms of contraception

Injectable progestogen Depo-provera® (MDPA) is advantageous for women who are unable or unwilling to take a pill. It contains 150 mg of medroxyprogesterone and is given 12-weekly.

▶ Very effective (failure rate <1 per 100 woman-years).

Side effects
- Menstrual disturbance (regular, irregular, or even amenorrhoea).
- Delayed conception (fertility may not return for 6–12 months).
- Weight gain (probably due to progestogen ↑ appetite).
- Bone loss (small risk of ↓ bone density with prolonged use).

Implanon® is a progestogen-only subdermal implant containing etonogestrel. Insertion and removal involve a small procedure under local anaesthetic (inserted into the arm). It lasts for 3 years.

▶ Highly effective (failure rate reported as <0.1 per 100 woman years)

Side effects
Menstrual disturbance.

Copper-bearing IUCD provide long-term reversible contraception. Insertion is usually easy and when inserted >40 years of age may be retained beyond the menopause.

▶ Very effective (failure rate of 0.6–0.8 per 100 woman-years)

Mode of action
- Foreign body reaction in the endometrium prevents implantation.
- Copper content may inhibit spermatozoa motility.

Complications
- Irregular PV bleeding, especially first 3–6 months.
- Risk of infection: screen for *Chlamydia* prior to insertion.
- IUD expulsion: most common in the first 3 months after insertion.
- Perforation: may be poor insertion technique or <4 weeks postpartum.
- Dysmenorrhoea.

Contraindications to copper-bearing IUCD

- Pregnancy.
- Undiagnosed genital tract bleeding.
- Active genital tract infection or PID.
- Uterine anomalies or fibroids distorting cavity.
- Copper allergy.

Timing of IUCD insertion
- Insert any time during cycle (as long as pregnancy excluded).
- Postpartum: safe to insert IUD from 4 weeks after delivery.
- Following TOP: insert within first 48 hours after termination.
- Switching from other contraception: any time as long as not pregnant.

Levonorgestrel-releasing system (Mirena IUS®)

The levonorgestrel-releasing system (LNG) has a T-shaped rod containing 52 mg levonorgestrel (20 micrograms released daily). It is a reversible, highly effective contraceptive with a failure rate of 0.18 per 100 woman-years.

⚠ Due to its progestogenic content, menstrual blood loss is decreased by >90%, and is as effective as endometrial ablation in the management of menorrhagia at 1 year.

Mode of action
- It acts on the endometrium, leading to endometrial atrophy and preventing implantation.
- Thickened cervical mucus inhibits sperm penetration.

▶ It is particularly useful when oestrogen is contraindicated.
- May be used in patients with a history of breast cancer:
  - no disease for 5 years and after consultation with breast surgeon.
- Breastfeeding:
  - can be inserted 4 or more weeks postpartum.

Side effects
- Irregular PV bleeding is common in the first 3–4 months:
  - amenorrhoea in up to 30% by 1 year.
- Hormonal symptoms: nausea, headache, breast tenderness, bloating.

📖 Faculty of Family Planning and Reproductive Health Care. www.ffprhc.org.uk

📖 Family Planning Association. www.fpa.org.uk

Emergency contraception (EC)

Emergency contraception is licensed for use to protect women from unwanted pregnancy following unprotected sexual intercourse (UPSI) or contraceptive failure.

The 2 main forms are:
- Oral emergency contraception—levonorgestrel (LNG EC).
- Copper intrauterine contraceptive device (IUCD EC).

Oral emergency contraception (LNG EC)
- Consists of a single oral dose of 1.5 mg of levonorgestrel:
  - if taken within 72 hours of unprotected coitus it is estimated to prevent 85% of expected pregnancies
  - it may be used up to 120 hours after, but efficacy is uncertain and it is not licensed for use after 72 hours.
- It may also be used more than once in a cycle if clinically indicated.
- It does not provide contraceptive cover for the remainder of the cycle, another method of contraception must be used.

Side effects
- Nausea is common after ingestion:
  - vomiting only affects 1%
  - if a woman vomits within 2 hours of ingestion, she should take a further dose as soon as possible.
- Erratic PV bleeding is common in the first 7 days following treatment.

Copper IUCD
- Intrauterine device acts as an emergency contraceptive by inhibiting fertilization by direct toxicity
  - Affects implantation by inducing an inflammatory reaction in the endometrium
  - The copper content may also inhibit sperm transport
- IUCD EC should to be inserted within 120 hours following UPSI.
- Failure rates are less than 1%.

The risks and complications for IUCD EC are similar to IUCD use in general. It can be removed after the next menstruation provided that no unprotected coitus has occurred since menstruation, or retained for ongoing contraception.

Female sterilization: preoperative considerations

Sterilization has become increasingly popular since the late 1960s and it is now the most commonly used method of contraception in women over 40 years of age.

History and examination

- This includes reasons for sterilization, menstrual history, current contraception, obstetric history, previous abdominal surgery, chronic medical conditions, and drug history.
- The patient's BMI should be noted and abdominal examination performed to look for scars from previous surgery or pelvic masses (previous surgery, endometriosis, PID, or fibroids may make the procedure technically difficult).

Counselling

It is important to establish that the woman is taking the decision of her own free will. Alternatives to the procedure must be discussed.

> *Alternative long-term methods of contraception*
> - Levonorgestrel (Mirena) IUS:
>   - failure rates comparable to sterilization
>   - lasts 5 years
>   - reversible
>   - useful in women with menorrhagia.
> - Vasectomy for the male partner:
>   - lower failure rates (1 in 2000 after 2 negative semen analyses)
>   - can be done under local anaesthesia with less procedure related risk.

- Must use effective contraception until her first period following sterilization (the commonest reason for failure is already being pregnant when the procedure is performed or in the same cycle!).
- Reassure that there is no increased risk of heavier periods in women >30 years of age (there is a small association with increased hysterectomy rates, but the reason is unclear).
- Laparoscopy and tubal occlusion with Filshie clips is usually the method of choice and must be explained including the operative risks.

▶ Counselling must be supported by printed information leaflets.

Consent for female sterilization

- Written informed consent must be taken from the patient prior to the procedure:
  - in case of doubt regarding mental capacity the case should be referred to court for judgement.
- The patient must fully understand that the procedure is intended to be permanent:
  - Success rates with reversal procedures are very small and are rarely provided by the NHS.
- Lifetime risk of failure with tubal occlusion is 1:200:
  - pregnancies can occur several years after the procedure
  - the longest follow-up data available for Filshie clips suggests a failure rate after 10 years of 2–3 per 1000 procedures.
- In case of failure there is an increased risk of ectopic pregnancy:
  - women must be advised to seek medical attention if they are pregnant or have abnormal pain and bleeding.
- There is a risk of injury to the blood vessels, bowel, and bladder with laparoscopic surgery:
  - women must be warned about the possibility of a laparotomy, particularly if they have had previous abdominal surgery.

Women at higher risk of regret

⚠ Care must be taken when considering sterilization for women from the following groups, as they are more likely to have regret and present requesting reversal:

- Under the age of 30 years:
  - current RCOG recommendation to avoid.
- Who do not have children
- Who decide during pregnancy
- Who have had recent relationship loss.

Female sterilization: the procedure

Preoperative—mandatory checklist

- Document last menstrual period.
- Check current contraception has been used to date.
- Pregnancy test must be performed (a negative test does not exclude the possibility of a luteal phase pregnancy).
- If **any doubt** exists about certainty of wishes or risk of pregnancy, the procedure should be abandoned.

Intraoperative

- Day case laparoscopic procedure is associated with quicker recovery rates and less morbidity than mini-laparotomy
- Usually general anaesthesia but local anaesthesia is an acceptable alternative.
- Laparascopic mechanical occlusion of the tubes by either Filshie clips or rings:
  - diathermy ↑ the risk of ectopic pregnancies and is less easy to reverse.
- When a mini-laparotomy is used, any effective surgical or mechanical method of tubal occlusion can be used (a modified Pomeroy procedure may be preferable for postpartum sterilization or at the time of Caesarean section due to lower failure rates).

Postoperative

- The patient must be informed about the method of occlusion used and any procedural complications.
- She must be advised to use effective contraception till her next menstrual period.

Special circumstances

- Tubal occlusion should ideally be performed after an appropriate interval following pregnancy.
- Sterilization postpartum or post-abortion carries a higher risk of regret and possibly increased failure rates.
- In cases of sterilization at the time of Caesarean section, counselling and consent should be taken at least 1 week before the procedure

Newer techniques

Hysteroscopic methods for sterilization are still under evaluation. Essure is the only form of hysteroscopic tubal occlusion licensed for use in the UK at present. It involves placing a metal micro-insert in the fallopian tubes under hysteroscopic guidance. This causes tubal blockage by subsequent fibrosis. A hysterosalpingogram is usually done 3 months after the operation to confirm tubal blockage.

Menopause

Menopause: overview

All women will go thorough the menopause and the average age is 52 years. The menopause is the cessation of the menstrual cycle and is caused by ovarian failure leading to oestrogen deficiency. Worldwide life expectancy is increasing and women live longer than men. A woman's average life expectancy at birth in the UK is currently 81 years and is estimated to reach 85 years by 2031. Thus UK women can expect more than 30 years of postmenopausal life. This population expansion will lead to an increasing importance of the health problems that affect postmenopausal women.

Definitions

- **Menopause** is the permanent cessation of menstruation that results from loss of ovarian follicular activity. Natural menopause is recognized to have occurred after 12 consecutive months of amenorrhoea for which no other obvious pathological or physiological cause is present.
- **Perimenopause** includes the period beginning with the first clinical, biological, and endocrinological features of the approaching menopause, such as vasomotor symptoms and menstrual irregularity, and ends 12 months after the last menstrual period.
- **Premenopause** is a term often used to refer either to the 1–2 years immediately before the menopause or to the whole of the reproductive period before the menopause. Currently, this term is recommended to be used in the latter sense.
- **Postmenopause** should be defined from the final menstrual period regardless of whether the menopause was induced or spontaneous.
- **Menopausal transition** is the period of time before the final menstrual period, when variability in the menstrual cycle usually is increased.
- **Climacteric** is the phase encompassing the transition from the reproductive state to the non-reproductive state. The menopause itself thus is a specific event that occurs during the climacteric, just as the menarche is a specific event that occurs during puberty.

Menopause: short-term consequences

Vasomotor symptoms

Hot flushes and night sweats are the commonest symptoms of the menopause, and, although they may begin before periods stop, the prevalence of flushes is highest in the first year after the final menstrual period. Although they usually are present for less than 5 years, some women will continue to flush into their 70s.

Sexual dysfunction

Changes in sexual behaviour and activity are common. The term **female sexual dysfunction** (FSD) is now used. The percentage of women with sexual dysfunction rises from 42% to 88% during the early to late menopausal transition. The underlying reasons for FSD are commonly multifactorial. For example, vaginal dryness, which results from declining levels of oestrogen, can cause dyspareunia. Low androgen levels have been implicated in low sexual desire though the evidence is conflicting. Non-hormonal factors, such as conflict between partners and life stress or depression are important contributors to a woman's level of interest in sexual activity. In addition, male sexual problems should not be overlooked.

Sexual problems are classified into various types:
- Loss of sexual desire.
- Loss of sexual arousal.
- Problems with orgasm.
- Sexual pain such as painful sex or dyspareunia.

Psychological symptoms

Psychological symptoms associated with the menopause include:
- Depressed mood.
- Anxiety.
- Irritability and mood swings.
- Lethargy and lack of energy.

However, most women do not experience major changes in mood at the menopause and psychological problems are likely to be associated with past problems and current life stresses.

Menopause: long-term consequences

Osteoporosis

Osteoporosis affects 1 in 3 women and 1 in 12 men. It is as 'a skeletal disorder characterized by compromised bone strength predisposing to an increased risk of fracture'. Bone strength reflects the integration of two main features: bone density and bone quality. Bone density is expressed as grams of mineral per area or volume and, in any given individual, is determined by peak bone mass and amount of bone loss. Bone quality refers to architecture, turnover, damage accumulation (for example, microfractures) and mineralization. A fracture occurs when a failure-inducing force, which may or may not involve trauma, is applied to osteoporotic bone. Thus, osteoporosis is a significant risk factor for fracture. Fractures are the clinical consequences of osteoporosis.

The most common sites of osteoporotic fractures are:
• Lower end of radius (wrist or Colles' fracture).
• Proximal femur (hip).
• Vertebrae.

Cardiovascular disease (CVD)

Myocardial infarction and stroke are the primary clinical endpoints. CVD is the most common cause of death in women over 60. Oophorectomized women are at 2–3-fold higher risk of coronary heart disease (CHD) than age-matched premenopausal women.

Urogenital atrophy

The lower urinary and genital tracts have a common embryological origin and are approximated closely in adult women. Oestrogen receptors and progesterone receptors are present in the vagina, urethra, bladder, and pelvic floor musculature. Oestrogen deficiency after menopause causes atrophic changes within the urogenital tract and is associated with urinary symptoms, such as frequency, urgency, nocturia, incontinence, and recurrent infection. These symptoms may coexist with those of vaginal atrophy, including dyspareunia, itching, burning, and dryness.

Table 20.1 Bone mineral density (BMD)

Description	Definition
Normal	A person has a BMD value between –1 SD and +1 SD of the young adult mean (T score –1 to +1)
Osteopenia	A person has a BMD reduced between –1 and –2.5 SD from the young adult mean (T score –1 to –2.5)
Osteoporosis	A person has a BMD reduced by equal to or more than –2.5 SD from the young adult mean (T score –2.5 or lower)

Table 20.2 Risk factors for osteoporosis

Risk factor	Example
Genetic	Family history of fracture (particularly a 1st-degree relative with hip fracture)
Constitutional	Low BMI Early menopause (<45 years of age)
Environmental	Cigarette smoking Alcohol abuse Low calcium intake Sedentary lifestyle
Drugs	Corticosteroids, >5 mg prednisolone or equivalent daily
Diseases	Rheumatoid arthritis Neuromuscular disease Chronic liver disease Malabsorption syndromes Hyperparathyroidism Hyperthyroidism Hypogonadism

Menopause: history taking and investigations

History

Symptoms, periods, and contraception
- Hot flushes and night sweats.
- Vaginal dryness.
- Other symptoms.
- Date of last menstrual period (could she be pregnant?).
- Frequency, heaviness and duration of periods.
- Contraception.

Gynaecological history
- Hysterectomy.
- Oophorectomy.

Past medical and surgical history
- Risk factors for osteoporosis.
- Confirmed deep vein thrombosis or pulmonary embolism.
- Risk factors for cardiovascular disease (e.g. smoking, hypertension, diabetes).
- Breast cancer, benign breast disease, and date last mammogram (if applicable).
- Does she have migraines?
- Current medications.
- Does she take alternative or complementary therapies?

Family history in close family members
- Breast, ovarian, or bowel cancer.
- Confirmed deep vein thrombosis or pulmonary embolism.
- Cardiovascular disease.
- Osteoporosis.

Investigations

- Follicle-stimulating hormone (FSH) only helpful if diagnosis is in doubt such as below age 40 and levels in menopausal range (>30 IU/L).
- Luteinizing hormone, oestradiol, progesterone are of no value in the diagnosis of ovarian failure.
- Thyroid function tests (free T4 and thyroid-stimulating hormone) as abnormalities of thyroid function can be confused with menopausal symptoms.
- Testosterone levels are of uncertain value.
- Bone mineral density (BMD) if significant risk factors for osteoporosis.

Premature menopause

Ideally, premature menopause should be defined as menopause that occurs at an age more than two standard deviations below the mean estimated for the reference population. The age of 40 years is used frequently as an arbitrary limit below which the menopause is said to be premature. It affects 1% of women younger than 40 years and 0.1% of those under 30 years. In most cases no cause is found.

Causes of premature ovarian failure

Primary
- Chromosome abnormalities.
- FSH receptor gene polymorphism and inhibin B mutation.
- Enzyme deficiencies.
- Autoimmune disease.

Secondary
- Chemotherapy and radiotherapy.
- Bilateral oophorectomy or surgical menopause.
- Hysterectomy without oophorectomy.
- Infection.

Presentation and assessment
- The most common presentation is secondary amenorrhoea or oligomenorrhoea (which may not necessarily be accompanied by hot flushes).
- Coexisting disease may be detected, particularly:
  - hypothyroidism
  - Addison's disease
  - diabetes mellitus
  - any chromosome abnormalities (especially those who have not achieved successful pregnancy).
- The diagnostic usefulness of ovarian biopsy outside the research setting has yet to be proved.

Consequences of premature menopause

- Women with untreated premature menopause (no oestrogen replacement) are at increased risk of osteoporosis and cardiovascular disease but at lower risk of breast malignancy.
- Premature menopause can lead to reduced peak bone mass (if <25 years old) or early bone loss thereafter.

⚠ Mean life expectancy in women with menopause before the age of 40 years is 2.0 years shorter than that in women with menopause after the age of 55 years.

Management issues in premature menopause

Fertility and contraception
- Reduced fertility.
- May require assisted conception.
- Need for contraception if no fertility goals.

▶ Women need oestrogen replacement until average age of natural menopause, which is usually regarded as 52.
- Hormone replacement therapy (HRT).
- Combined oral contraceptive pill (COCP).
- No evidence regarding use bisphosphonates, strontium ranelate, or raloxifene.
- No evidence regarding use of alternative and complementary therapies.

Hormone replacement therapy(HRT): overview

More than 50 hormone replacement therapy (HRT) preparations, which feature different strengths, combinations and routes of administration, are available. HRT can be given either systemically for hot flushes and osteoporosis or vaginally (or topically) for local symptoms such as vaginal dryness. In non-hysterectomized women HRT consists of an oestrogen combined with a progestogen.

Oestrogens

Oestrogens used in HRT include estradiol, estrone, and estriol, which, although chemically synthesized from soya beans or yams, are molecularly identical to the natural human hormone. Conjugated equine oestrogens containing about 50–65% estrone sulphate, with the remainder being equine oestrogens (mainly equilin sulphate) are also used.

Progestogens

The progestogens used in HRT are almost all synthetic and derived from plant sources. They are structurally different from progesterone. 17-hydroxyprogesterone and 19-nortestosterone derivatives are the progestogens used most commonly in HRT.

17-hydroxyprogesterone
- Dydrogesterone.
- Medroxyprogesterone acetate.

19-nortestosterone derivatives
- Norethisterone.
- Levonorgestrel.

Other hormones used at the menopause
- **Tibolone** is a synthetic steroid compound that itself is inert, but, on absorption, is converted to metabolites with oestrogenic, progestogenic, and androgenic actions. It is classified as HRT in the British National Formulary. It is used in postmenopausal women.
- **Testosterone** patches and implants may be used to improve libido.

Treatment of local symptoms

Some women do not wish to take, or cannot tolerate, systemic HRT and simply require relief of local symptoms, which are usually urogenital. Synthetic or conjugated equine oestrogens should be avoided, as they are well absorbed from the vagina. The options available are low-dose natural oestrogens, such as vaginal oestriol by cream or pessary or oestradiol by tablet or ring. Treatment is needed in the long term, if not lifelong, as symptoms return on cessation of treatment. With the recommended dose regimens, no adverse endometrial effects should be incurred, and a progestogen need not be added in non-hysterectomized women.

Types of systemic oestrogen-based HRT

- Oestrogen alone in hysterectomized women.
- Oestrogen plus progestogen in nonhysterectomized women.
  - oestrogen and cyclical progestogen in perimenopausal women
  - continuous combined oestrogen–progestogen ('no bleed' HRT) in postmenopausal women.
- Routes of administration of oestrogen:
  - oral
  - transdermal
  - subcutaneous
  - vaginal.
- Routes of administration of progestogen:
  - oral
  - transdermal
  - intrauterine (levonorgestrel).

Minimum bone-sparing doses of HRT

- Estradiol oral   1–2 mg
- Estradiol patch   25–50 micrograms
- Estradiol gel   1–5 g*
- Estradiol implant   50 mg every 6 months
- Conjugated equine oestrogens   0.3–0.625 mg daily

*Depends on preparation: lower doses may be effective.

Side effects of systemic HRT

- **Oestrogen-related:** fluid retention, bloating, breast tenderness or enlargement, nausea, headaches, leg cramps, and dyspepsia.*
- **Progestogen-related:** fluid retention, breast tenderness, headaches or migraine, mood swings, depression, acne, lower abdominal pain, and backache.*
- **Combined HRT:** irregular, breakthrough bleeding (may need investigation).
- **All types of HRT:** weight gain (but not proved in randomized trials).

* Changing dose, type, and route of administration (tablet to patch) may help.

Hormone replacement therapy(HRT): benefits

Two large studies, the randomized Women's Health Initiative (WHI) and the observational Million Women study (MWS) undertaken in women aged over 50 have resulted in controversy about the use of HRT. There are benefits and risks in its use, and some uncertainty concerning some claims made about HRT.

> **Benefits of HRT**
> - ↓ vasomotor symptoms.
> - ↓ urogenital symptoms and improved sexuality.
> - ↓ risk of osteoporosis.
> - ↓ risk of colorectal cancer.

Relief of vasomotor symptoms
- Oestrogen is effective in treating hot flushes:
  - improvement usually is noted within 4 weeks
  - maximum therapeutic response usually achieved by 3 months
  - should be continued for at least 1 year or symptoms often recur
  - the most common indication for a prescription of HRT
  - often is used for fewer than 5 years.
- Oestrogen is more effective than SSRIs or clonidine (largely ineffective).

Urogenital symptoms and sexuality
- Urogential symptoms respond well to oestrogen (which may be given vaginally or systemically).
- Improvement may take several months.
- Long-term treatment often is needed, as symptoms can recur.
- Urinary incontinence is not improved by systemic therapy.
- Sexuality may be improved with oestrogen alone, but it also may need the addition of testosterone especially in young oophorectomized women.

Osteoporosis
- HRT ↓ the risk of spine and hip and other osteoporotic fractures.
- Most epidemiological studies suggest that continuous and lifelong use is required for HRT to be an effective method of preventing fracture.
- The efficacy of alternatives such as bisphosphonates in perimenopausal or early postmenopausal women remains uncertain.
- HRT is significantly cheaper than alternative therapies, such as bisphosphonates, strontium ranelate, and parathyroid hormone.

Colorectal cancer
- HRT ↓ the risk of colorectal cancer by about 1/3.
- Little is known about the risk when treatment is stopped or in high risk populations.
- Currently, prevention of colonic cancer is not an indication for HRT.

Hormone replacement therapy (HRT): risks

Risks of HRT

- ↑ risk of breast cancer.
- ↑ risk of endometrial cancer with unopposed oestrogen.
- ↑ risk of venous thromboembolism (VTE).
- ↑ risk of gallbladder disease.

Endometrial cancer

- Unopposed oestrogen ↑ the risk of endometrial cancer.
  - the relative risk (RR) is 2.3
  - risk ↑ with prolonged use (RR 9.5 for ≥10 years)
  - risk remains ↑ for 5 or more years after stopping (RR 2.3).
- This risk is not eliminated completely with the addition of monthly sequential progestogen (especially if used for >5 years).
- No ↑ risk has been found with continuous combined HRT.

Venous thromboembolism (VTE)

⚠ HRT more than doubles the risk of VTE but the absolute risk remains small.

- For non-users, over a 5 year period, the incidence of VTE will be:
  - 3:1000 women aged 50–59 years
  - 8:1000 women aged 60–69 years.
- The number of additional VTE events in healthy women on HRT ≥5 years, is estimated to be:
  - 4:1000 women aged 50–59 years
  - 9:1000 women aged 60–69 years.
- The VTE is more likely in the first year of HRT.
- ↑ age, obesity and thrombophilia significantly ↑ risk of VTE.
- Using HRT after VTE has an ↑ risk of recurrence in the first year of use.
- Transdermal HRT may be associated with a lower risk than oral.

Gallbladder disease

- ☞ HRT appears to ↑ the risk of gallbladder disease but:
- The risk ↑ with age and obesity.
- Women who use HRT may have silent pre-existing disease.

Risk of breast cancer with HRT

- HRT confers a similar degree of risk to late natural menopause:
  - every year the menopause is naturally delayed, the risk ↑ by 2.8%
  - with HRT, the risk ↑ by 2.3% per year.
- The risk is dependent on duration of HRT.
- The effect is not sustained once HRT is stopped:
  - 5 years after stopping, the risk is the same as for women who have never had HRT.
- The risk of breast cancer with HRT is dependent on the regimen:
  - greatest with combined oestrogen–progestogen HRT
  - less with unopposed oestrogen (but ↑ risk of endometrial cancer)

⚠ Combined HRT probably accounts for an extra 3 breast cancers per 1000 women who start it at the age of 50 years and use it for 5 years.

☙ All risk estimates are based on starting HRT at 50; this effect is not seen in women who start it early for premature menopause (therefore duration of exposure to female sex hormones is probably relevant)

☙ The increase in risk of breast cancer found in nulliparous women, those with a high BMI, those who delay their first birth, and those who have a family history may be higher than that conferred by HRT.

Hormone replacement therapy (HRT): uncertainties

Uncertainties concerning HRT

- Cardiovascular disease.
- Dementia.
- Ovarian cancer.
- Quality of life.

Cardiovascular disease (CVD)

- The role of HRT in primary or secondary prevention is uncertain, and it should not be used primarily for this indication.
- The timing, dose, and possibly type of HRT, however, may be critical in determining cardiovascular effects:
  - women in the WHI who started HRT within 10 years of the menopause had a lower risk of coronary heart disease than women who started later.

Dementia and cognition

- Oestrogen may delay or ↓ the risk of Alzheimer's disease, but it does not seem to improve established disease.
- It is unclear if there is a critical age to start HRT or an optimal duration of treatment to prevent dementia.

Ovarian cancer

- There is ↑ risk in the very long term (>10 years) with oestrogen alone.
- This risk is not seen with continuous combined therapy.

✒ This issue is unresolved and requires further examination. Currently insufficient evidence is available to recommend alterations in HRT prescribing practice.

Quality of life

✒ Although some studies have shown improvement in both symptomatic and asymptomatic women, others have not. This area is difficult to evaluate because of the different measures used, varying levels of menopausal symptoms, a large placebo effect, and extrinsic factors that may alter women's responses.

Urogynaecology

Classification of urinary incontinence

Urinary incontinence is the complaint of any involuntary leakage of urine. It can result from a variety of different conditions and it is useful to classify them accordingly:

Stress urinary incontinence
The involuntary leakage of urine on effort or exertion, or on sneezing or coughing. It commonly arises as a result of urethral sphincter weakness.

Urge urinary incontinence
The involuntary leakage of urine accompanied by, or immediately preceded by, a strong desire to pass urine (void). Urge urinary incontinence can be a symptom of overactive bladder syndrome.

Mixed urinary incontinence
The involuntary leakage of urine associated both with urgency and with exertion, effort, sneezing, or coughing. Usually, one of these is predominant, i.e. either the symptoms of urge incontinence, or those of stress incontinence, are most bothersome.

Overflow incontinence
Occurs when the bladder becomes large and flaccid and has little or no detrusor tone or function. This is usually due to injury or insult, e.g. after surgery or postpartum. The condition is diagnosed when the urinary residual is more than 50% of bladder capacity. The bladder simply leaks when it becomes full.

Continuous urinary incontinence
The complaint of continuous leakage. Classically it is associated with a fistula or congenital abnormality, e.g. ectopic ureter.

Other types of incontinence
- Incontinence arising from urinary tract infections, medications, immobility, or cognitive impairment.
- Situational incontinence, e.g. giggle incontinence.

Urinary symptoms

- **Urinary incontinence** is the complaint of involuntary urinary leakage, which can be divided, broadly, into stress incontinence and urge incontinence.
- **Daytime frequency** is the number of times a women voids during her waking hours. There should normally be between 4 and 7 voids per day. Increased daytime frequency is when a woman perceives that she voids too often.
- **Nocturia** is the complaint of having to wake at night one or more times to void. Up to the age of 70 years, more than a single void is considered abnormal.
- **Nocturnal enuresis** is urinary incontinence occurring during sleep.
- **Urgency** is the sudden compelling desire to pass urine, which is difficult to defer. Urgency is most frequently secondary to detrusor overactivity, although inflammatory bladder conditions such as interstitial cystitis may also present with this.

- **Voiding difficulties** include:
  - hesitancy (difficulty in initiating micturition)
  - straining to void
  - slow or intermittent urinary stream.

These are all suggestive of urethral obstruction, an underactive detrusor muscle, or loss of coordination between detrusor construction and urethral relaxation. Intermittency is seen with neurological disease.

- **Postmicturition** symptoms include:
  - feeling of incomplete bladder emptying
  - terminal dribble (a prolonged final part of micturition)
  - postmicturitional dribble (the involuntary loss of urine immediately after passing urine).
- **Absent or reduced bladder sensation** is usually due to denervation caused by spinal cord injuries or pelvic surgery. It leads to infrequent micturition and a large-capacity bladder, and is often associated with overflow incontinence.
- **Bladder pain** is felt suprapubically or retropubically. Typically occurs with bladder filling and is relieved by emptying it. Pain is indicative of an intravesical pathology, such as interstitial cystitis or malignancy, and warrants further investigation.
- **Urethral pain** is felt in the urethra (the woman indicates this as the site of the discomfort).
- **Dysuria** is pain experienced in the bladder or urethra on passing urine. It is most frequently associated with urinary tract infections.
- **Haematuria** is the presence of blood in the urine. This can be microscopic or macroscopic (frank). It is always significant and always warrants further investigation.

Assessment of the lower urinary tract: history and examination

History
- The onset of urinary symptoms, their duration, and their severity should be recorded (the predominant bother symptom, e.g. urgency, urge incontinence, or stress incontinence, should be identified)
- Different underlying conditions can cause similar urinary symptoms history alone is often a poor predictor of pathophysiology.
- Check for coexisting medical conditions and optimize their treatment (the onset of diabetes significantly increases urine output and many pharmaceutical agents can alter bladder function).
- Enquire about colorectal symptoms and genitourinary prolapse.

Quality of life assessment
- Incontinence undoubtedly causes considerable distress.
- Disease-specific quality of life (QoL) questionnaires allow in-depth assessment of the impact-specific symptoms on a woman's life:
  - validated questionnaires are available from the International Consultation on Incontinence (🕮 www.iciq.net).

Frequency/volume chart
- The frequency/volume chart (Fig. 21.1) is a simple and practical method of obtaining objective quantification of fluid intake and voiding behaviour.
- Fluid intake, frequency, times of voiding, and leakage episodes (day and night) are recorded for at least 24 hours (typically 3 days).

Physical examination
General examination
- Weight (BMI), blood pressure, urinalysis.
- Check for signs of systemic disease.
- Mobility and mental state.
- Motivation and manual dexterity.
- Neurological examination, if there are any symptoms that point to a possible neurological cause.

Abdominal examination
- Exclude an abdominal or pelvic mass (⚠ including pregnancy).
- Exclude a full bladder (obstruction/retention).

Pelvic examination
- Condition of the vulval skin (any atrophy, erythema or oedema).
- Presence and degree of any concurrent uterovaginal prolapse.
- Assessment of urethral and bladder neck descent on straining.
- Assessment of pelvic floor muscle strength (graded 0 to 5 on a modified Oxford scale; see prolapse clinical assessment, p. 648)

Frequency/Volume Chart

Name: *Mrs Smith* Patient No. *1234567* Week commencing *26 Jan 2006*

Time	Date: 26.01.06 Day 1			Date: 27.01.06 Day 2			Date: 28.01.06 Day 3		
am	In	Out	Wet	In	Out	Wet	In	Out	Wet
1		300	X		500	X			
2		300	X						
3					600	X		700	X
4		350	X						
5									
6					600	X		600	X
7		500	X						
8				250	300			500	X
9	250	300		200			250		
10								300	
11							200		
12				200				100	
pm									
1	200	100			100				
2							200	300	
3									
4				200					
5	250	120						200	
6							200		
7				200	100				
8									
9		200			100				
10									
11		100			200		200	200	
12									
Total	650	2270		1050	2500		1050	2800	

Fig. 21.1 A 3-day frequency/volume chart showing severe nocturia

Information obtainable from a frequency/volume chart

- Functional bladder capacity.
- Volumetric summary of diurnal urinary frequency.
- Volumetric summary of nocturnal urinary frequency.
- Quantification of total fluid intake.
- Distribution of fluid intake throughout the day.
- Total voided volume and diurnal distribution of voiding.
- Evaluation of the severity of urinary incontinence.

Assessment of the lower urinary tract: investigations

Basic investigations

Urinalysis

- Reagent strip testing of urine for leucocyte esterase, nitrites, protein, blood, and glucose is a sensitive and cheap screening test.

Urine specimen

- Bacteriological analysis of a midstream urine specimen for microscopy, culture, and sensitivity is reserved for those with positive screening test.

Residual check

- A postvoid residual check should be carried out (either by ultrasound scan or by catheterization) to exclude incomplete bladder emptying.

Pad test

- This is a simple method of detecting and quantifying urinary leakage based on weight gain of absorbent pads during a set period of time.
- ▶ It is not helpful in determining the cause of urinary leakage.

Cystourethroscopy

- Allows visualization of all the lower urinary tract: urethra, bladder mucosa, trigone, and ureteric orifices.
- Can be performed using a rigid or flexible cystoscope, with or without anaesthesia.
- Bladder biopsies can be taken to obtain histological diagnosis and exclude malignancy.
- In cases of suspected interstitial cystitis a second-look cystoscopy should be performed after the initial bladder distension, to detect any glomerulations or petechial haemorrhages.

Indications for cystourethroscopy

- Recurrent UTIs.
- Haematuria.
- Bladder pain.
- Suspected urinary tract injury or fistula.
- To exclude bladder tumour or stones.
- If interstitial cystitis is suspected.

Assessment of the lower urinary tract: imaging

Imaging of the lower urinary tract is not justified as a routine investigation in all women presenting with urinary symptoms, but should instead be targeted at specific indications.

- **Ultrasonography,** widely used to:
  - exclude incomplete bladder emptying
  - check for congenital abnormalities, calculi, tumours
  - detect cortical scarring of the kidneys.
- **Plain abdominal radiograph** is useful for screening for a variety of conditions, including foreign bodies and calculi.
- **Intravenous urography** is indicated in women with neuropathic bladder, suspected congenital and acquired abnormalities e.g. utero-vaginal fistulae.
- **Micturating cystourethrography** is useful to demonstrate bladder and urethral fistulae, vesicoureteric reflux, and anatomical abnormalities of the lower urinary tract, such as urethral diverticulae.
- **Contrast CT** can detect and characterize solid renal masses as well as renal tract calculi, renal and perirenal infections, and associated complications.
- **MRI** remains predominantly a research investigative technique for incontinence and prolapse, because of its cost and availability. It is mainly used for characterization of renal or pelvic masses and tumour staging.

Conditions requiring imaging of urinary tract

- Recurrent UTIs.
- Haematuria.
- Urethral diverticula, which need to be differentiated from paravaginal cysts.
- Suspected ureteric injuries.
- Suspected urethral or vesical fistulae.
- Suspected malignancy or renal stones.

Assessment of the lower urinary tract: urodynamic investigations

Urodynamics

'Urodynamics' describes a combination of tests that look at the ability of the bladder to store and void urine. The tests include uroflowmetry, postvoid residual measurement, and cystometry. In addition, urethral pressure profilometry and videourodynamic investigations may be undertaken.

Uroflowmetry

- Simple, non-invasive investigation that can be used to screen for voiding difficulties. The patient voids in privacy on a commode incorporating a urinary flow meter, measures voided volume over time and plots it on a graph (Fig. 21.2).

Cystometry (Fig. 21.3)

- Involves measuring the pressure/volume relationship of the bladder during filling and voiding and is a useful test of bladder function.
- The bladder is filled with saline via a catheter, the first sensation of filling, first desire to void and any strong desire to void are recorded.
- Electronic subtraction of the intra-abdominal pressure from the intra-vesical enables the detrusor pressure to be calculated (Fig. 21.4).
- During filling the patient is asked to cough at regular intervals and to stand, in order to provoke the bladder.
- The presence of detrusor contractions and leakage through the urethra are noted.
- The woman is then asked to void at the end of the test, for pressure/flow analysis.

Video-urodynamics

- Combines fluoroscopic imaging of the bladder neck with cystometry, while filling the bladder with an iodine-based contrast medium.
- Enables detection of detrusor-sphincter dyssynergia, vesico-ureteric reflux or presence of abnormalities in the renal tract that are commonly seen in women with neurogenic bladder problems.

Ambulatory urodynamic monitoring

- A small recording device is worn and the information is later downloaded to a computer for analysis and review.
- The bladder is filled naturally and the woman should carry out her normal daily activities, including those that provoke symptoms.
- This approach is particularly useful for investigating detrusor overactivity when standard laboratory urodynamics have failed to replicate the symptoms experienced by the woman in her normal environment.

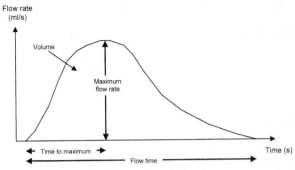

Fig. 21.2 Diagrammatic representation of normal urinary flow rate.
Voided volume: total volume expelled via the urethra, the area beneath the flow-time curve. Maximum flow rate: maximum measured value of the flow rate. Average flow rate: volume voided divided by the flow time. Flow time: the time over which measurable flow actually occurs.

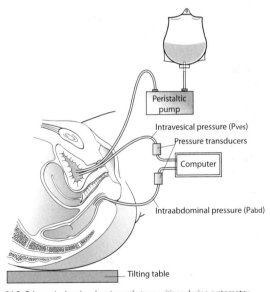

Fig. 21.3 Schematic drawing showing catheter positions during cystometry. Three catheters are required: the first in the bladder to fill it; the second in the bladder to measure vesical pressure; and the third in the rectum to measure abdominal pressure. Reproduced with permission from *Textbook of Female Urology and Urogynaecology*, 2001 by Cardozo L. and Staskin D., published by Taylor and Francis, London.

Stress urinary incontinence: overview

Definitions
- **Stress urinary incontinence (SUI)** is the complaint of involuntary leakage of urine on effort or exertion, or on sneezing or coughing.
- **Urodynamic stress urinary incontinence (USI)** is the involuntary leakage of urine during increased intra-abdominal pressure in the absence of detrusor contractions. Unlike SUI, it can only be diagnosed by urodynamic testing (Fig. 21.4).

Incidence
- The commonest urinary complaint for which women seek advice.
- 1 in 10 women will suffer from it at some point in their lives.
- 50% of incontinent women complain of pure stress incontinence.
- 30–40% of incontinent women have mixed symptoms of urge and stress incontinence.

Pathophysiology and aetiology
- SUI occurs when the intravesical pressure exceeds the closing pressure on the urethra.
- Childbirth is the most common causative factor, leading to denervation of the pelvic floor, usually during delivery.
- Oestrogen deficiency at the time of menopause leads to weakening of the pelvic support and thinning of the urothelium.
- Occasionally, weakness of the bladder neck can occur congenitally, or through trauma from radical pelvic surgery or irradiation.

Clinical features
- **Symptoms:** typically a woman will complain of leakage of urine when she coughs, sneezes, runs, jumps, or carries heavy loads. The leakage is usually a small, discrete amount, coinciding with the physical activity.
- **Signs:** prolapse of the urethra and anterior vaginal wall may be present. It may be possible to demonstrate stress incontinence by asking the woman to cough with a fairly full bladder.

Investigations
- **Midstream urine sample** should be taken to exclude infection or glycosuria
- **Frequency/volume chart:**
  - typically shows normal frequency and functional bladder capacity
  - slightly ↑ diurnal frequency may be observed, as women may void more frequently to prevent leakage.
- **Urodynamic studies** should be considered when surgery is indicated to:
  - confirm the diagnosis
  - check for any coexisting detrusor overactivity
  - check for voiding dysfunction.

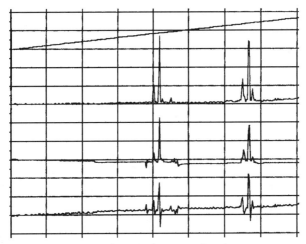

Fig. 21.4 Urodynamic trace showing urodynamic stress incontinence.
The upper trace shows intravesical pressure (P_{ves}) and the middle trace shows pressure within the abdomen (P_{abd}), both measured against time. The lower trace, obtained by subtracting intra-abdominal pressure fsrom intravesical pressure ($P_{det} = P_{ves} - P_{abd}$), shows the detrusor pressure. During the test there is no change in detrusor pressure, despite provocation with coughing, and leakage occurs only as a result of the momentary increase in intra-abdominal pressure caused by the coughing.

Stress urinary incontinence: conservative management

Stress urinary incontinence (SUI) interferes with a woman's quality of life but is not a life-threatening condition and therefore conservative measures should always be tried first. They include:

- **Lifestyle interventions:** weight reduction if BMI>30, smoking cessation, treatment of chronic cough and constipation.
- **Pelvic floor muscle training** for at least 3 months should be considered as the first line treatment:
  - physiotherapists usually individualize the programme, but 3 sets of 8–12 slow maximal contractions sustained for 6–8 seconds each per day is a common regimen
  - the exercises need to be continued long-term.
- **Biofeedback** refers to the use of a device to convert the effect of pelvic floor contraction into a visual or auditory signal to allow women objective assessment of improvement.
- **Electrical stimulation** can assist in production of muscle contractions in women who are unable to produce muscle contraction.
- **Vaginal cones** have been developed as a way of applying graded resistance against which the pelvic floor muscles contract.

Pharmacological management of SUI

- **Duloxetine** is the only drug licensed for the treatment of moderate to severe SUI.
- It is a serotonin and noradrenaline reuptake inhibitor (SNRI) that enhances urethral striated sphincter activity via a centrally mediated pathway.
- It is associated with significant and dose-dependent decreases in frequency of incontinence episodes.
- Nausea is the most frequently reported side effect (up to 25%).
- Other side effects (including dyspepsia, dry mouth, insomnia or drowsiness, and dizziness) can limit its use.

Indications for conservative treatment of stress urinary incontinence

- Mild or easily manageable symptoms.
- Family incomplete.
- Symptoms manifest during pregnancy.
- Surgery contraindicated by coexisting medical conditions.
- Surgery declined by patient.

Stress urinary incontinence: surgical management

Surgery may be considered when conservative measures have failed and the woman's quality of life is compromised. Before attempting surgical repair it is important to be clear about the underlying cause of the incontinence: USI may be successfully treated surgically but detrusor overactivity may be made worse, and the effects are largely irreversible.

Periurethral injections

- Injectable periurethral bulking agents have a lower immediate success rate (40–60%) and a long-term continued decline in continence.
- The procedure has low morbidity.
- The most commonly used periurethral bulking agents are:
  - glutaraldehyde cross-linked bovine collagen;
  - macroparticulate silicon particles) (Macroplastique®, Uroplasty Ltd).
- Injectables or bulking agents may be appropriate for:
  - frail, elderly, or unfit women
  - women who have had other multiple failed procedures.

Burch colposuspension

- Largely replaced by the TVT, now rarely performed.
- The retropubic space is entered through a low transverse suprapubic incision and two or three sutures placed between the paravaginal fascia and ipsilateral ileopectinal ligament (Cooper's ligament) at the level of bladder.
- Complications may include: haemorrhage; injuries to the bladder or ureter; voiding difficulties; de-novo detrusor overactivity; enterocele or rectocele formation.
- Overall, meta-analysis of published data suggests that that the efficacy of the Burch colposuspension as a primary procedure is 90% and as a repeat procedure is 83% (Table 21.1).

Laparoscopic colposuspension

- Efficacy and complications similar to those of the open procedure.
- The surgery is technically more demanding and requires considerable laparoscopic expertise.
- A quicker recovery time should be set against longer operating time and higher cost, due to the use of laparoscopic equipment and additional theatre time.

Table 21.1 Objective cure rate for first procedure and recurrent incontinence

Procedure	First procedure		Recurrent incontinence	
	Mean (%)	95% CI	Mean (%)	95% CI
Slings (TVT, TOT)	93.9	89.2–98.6	86.1	82.4–89.8
Burch colposuspension	89.8	87.6–92.1	82.5	76.3–88.7
Injectables	45.5	28.5–62.5	57.8	43.2–72.4

Tension-free vaginal tape (TVT)

▶ The most commonly performed surgical procedure for USI in the UK.
- A polypropylene tape is placed under mid-urethra via a small vaginal incision, using local, regional or general anaesthesia. (Fig. 21.5)
- Cystourethroscopy is carried out to ensure no damage to the bladder or urethra.
- The procedure is minimally invasive and most women return to normal activity within 2 weeks.
- Complications:
  - moderately high risk of bladder injuries 5–10%, but these do not seem to have long-term sequelae, if treated appropriately
  - bleeding in retropubic space, infection and voiding difficulties
  - tape erosion into the vagina and urethra has also been reported.
- The objective cure rate is 82–98% (mean 94%).

Transobturator tape (TOT)

- The polypropylene tape is passed via a transobturator foramen, through the transobturator and puborectalis muscles.
- The main difference from TVT is the retropubic space is not entered and the risk of bladder perforation is low.
- Early data suggests a success rate similar to that of TVT.

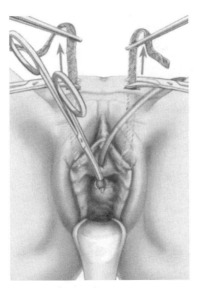

Fig.21.5 Insertion of tension-free vaginal tape.
The tape is placed in a U-shape under the urethra and the tension adjusted to prevent leakage as the woman coughs. Illustration reproduced by courtesy of ETHICON Women's Heatlth and Urology.

Overactive bladder syndrome (OAB): overview

Definition

- Overactive bladder syndrome (OAB) is a chronic condition, defined as urgency, with or without urge incontinence, usually with frequency or nocturia.
- It is used to imply probably underlying detrusor overactivity (DO) but this is a diagnosis made on urodynamic testing (Fig. 21.6).

Aetiology

- Idiopathic in most cases.
- Neurogenic DO is found in the presence of conditions such as multiple sclerosis, spina bifida, or upper motor neuron lesions.
- Secondary to pelvic or incontinence surgery.
- OAB due to outflow obstruction is uncommon in women.

Clinical features of OAB

- Symptoms of OAB include urinary frequency, urgency, urge incontinence, nocturia, and nocturnal enuresis.
- Provocative factors often trigger it, such as cold weather, opening the front door, or hearing running water.
- Bladder contractions may also be provoked by ↑ intra-abdominal pressure (coughing or sneezing), leading to complaint of stress incontinence, which may be misleading.
- Quality of life can be significantly impaired by the unpredictability and large volume of leakage.

Investigations

Urine culture

- Exclusion of infection is mandatory, as symptoms overlap those of UTI.

Frequency/volume chart

- Typical features are ↑ diurnal frequency associated with urgency and episodes of urge incontinence.
- Nocturia is a common feature of OAB.

Urodynamics

- Characterized by involuntary detrusor contractions during the filling phase of the micturition cycle, which may be spontaneous or provoked.
- Video-urodynamic testing is more appropriate in women with neurological diseases, to exclude vesicoureteric reflux or renal damage secondary to a persistent significant rise in intravesical pressure.

Diagnosis

- Urodynamic assessment is essential for the diagnosis of OAB in women with multiple and complex symptoms.
- Other factors, such as metabolic abnormalities (diabetes or hypercalcaemia), physical causes (prolapse or faecal impaction) or urinary pathology (UTI or interstitial cystitis), need to be excluded when a diagnosis of OAB is made.

Key points

- OAB is a common condition affecting around 1 in 6 women.
- The incidence of OAB increases with age.
- OAB is the second most common cause of urinary incontinence.
- OAB is the most common cause of incontinence in elderly women.
- Urodynamic assessment is required to make a diagnosis of DO.
- QoL is often severely affected by OAB symptoms.

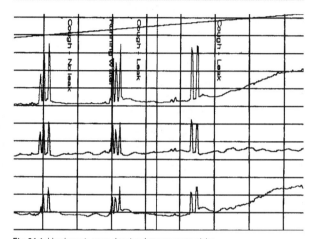

Fig. 21.6 Urodynamic trace showing detrusor overactivity.
The upper trace of intravesical pressure (P_{ves}) vs. time shows a sharp increase of
pressure within the bladder. The middle trace of pressure within the abdomen (P_{abd})
shows no similar increase. The lower trace, obtained by subtracting intra-abdominal
pressure from intravesical pressure ($P_{det} = P_{ves} - P_{abd}$), shows significant detrusor
overactivity.

Overactive bladder syndrome (OAB): management

Conservative management

It is wise to start with the simplest of conservative therapies and progress through to more radical treatments if necessary.

Behavioural therapy

- Advice to consume 1–1.5 L of liquids per day.
- Avoid caffeine-based drinks (tea, coffee, cola) and alcohol.
- Various drugs, such as diuretics and antipsychotics, alter bladder function and should be reviewed.

Bladder retraining

- The principles of bladder retraining are based on the ability to suppress urinary urge and extend the intervals between voidings.
- Reported cure rates using bladder retraining alone are 44–90%.

Hypnotherapy and acupuncture

- These can be successful in some cases.
- The relapse rate is very high.

Pharmacological interventions

Anticholinergic (antimuscarinic) drugs

- These remain the mainstay of pharmacotherapy, they block the parasympathetic nerves thereby relaxing the detrusor muscle.
- Patients should be advised about the side effects before starting treatment (some preparations may be better tolerated than others) (Table 21.2).
- The dosage may need to be titrated against efficacy and adverse effects.
- Adverse effects of anticholinergics may include:
  - dry mouth (up to 30%)
  - constipation, nausea, dyspepsia, and flatulence
  - blurred vision, dizziness, and insomnia
  - palpitation and arrhythmias.

Contraindications to anticholinergics

- Acute (narrow angle) glaucoma.
- Myasthenia gravis.
- Urinary retention or outflow obstruction.
- Severe ulcerative colitis.
- Gastrointestinal obstruction.

Antidepressants

- Imipramine has marked systematic anticholinergic effects.
- Its use is limited due to side effects.

Oestrogens

- In women with vaginal atrophy, intravaginal oestrogens may be tried.

Table 21.2 Anticholinergic drugs and their dosages

Drug	Delivery route	Adult dosage	Selectivity
Oxybutynin	(a) Oral	2.5–5 mg, 1–4 times/day	Selective, predominantly M1 and M3
	(b) Transdermal patch	1 patch, twice weekly (3.9 mg/24 hours)	
Propiverine	Oral only	15 mg, 2–4 times/day	Non-selective
Solifenacin	Oral only	5–10 mg daily	Selective, pre-dominantly M3
Tolterodine	Oral only	(a) 2 mg, twice daily (b) 4 mg, once daily (sustained release)	Non-selective
Trospium	Oral only	20 mg, twice daily	Non-selective
Darifenacin	Oral only	7.5 or 15 mg once daily (sustained release)	Selective, pre-dominantly M3

Surgical management and botulinium toxin A for OAB

- Surgery is reserved for those with debilitating symptoms and who have failed to benefit from medical and behavioural therapy.
- Procedures, such as bladder distention, sacral neuromodulation, detrusor myomectomy, and augmentation cystoplasty have limited efficacy and complication rates are high.
- Permanent urinary diversion is occasionally indicated in women with intractable incontinence.

Botulinium toxin A

- Botulinium toxin A blocks neuromuscular transmission, causing the muscle to become weak.
- Not yet licensed for use in OAB but is nevertheless being used increasingly in OAB refractory to anticholinergics, rather than resorting to the surgery.
- It is injected cystoscopically into the detrusor, usually under local anaesthetic
- It can cause urinary retention in 5–20% of cases, in which case intermittent self-catheterization may be required.
- Repeat injections are required every 6–12 months.
- The long-term effects of repeat injections are unknown and are the subject of ongoing research.

Anatomy of the pelvic floor

The pelvic floor consists of muscular and fascial structures that provide support to the pelvic viscera and the external openings of the vagina, urethra and rectum (Fig. 21.7). The uterus and vagina are suspended from the pelvic side walls by endopelvic fascial attachments that support the vagina at three levels.

Three levels of vaginal support (Fig. 21.7)

- **Level 1:** the cervix and upper third of the vagina are supported by the cardinal (transverse cervical) and uterosacral ligaments. These are attached to the cervix and suspend the uterus from the pelvic sidewall and sacrum respectively.
- **Level 2:** the mid portion of the vagina is attached by endofascial condensation (endopelvic fascia) laterally to the pelvic side walls.
- **Level 3:** the lower third of the vagina is supported by the levator ani muscles and the perineal body. The levator ani, together with its associated fascia, is termed the pelvic diaphragm.

The axis of the vagina is also important. It normally lies in a horizontal plane, flat on the levator muscles. This protects it during coughing and other activities that increase intra-abdominal pressure.

⚠ Damage occurring at the different levels of vaginal support causes different types of prolapse. It is therefore important to have an understanding of this anatomy.

Aetiology of prolapse

- **Pregnancy and vaginal delivery:** prolapse is uncommon in nulliparous women. Vaginal delivery may cause mechanical injuries and denervation of the pelvic floor. The risk is increased with large babies, prolonged second stage, and instrumental delivery (particularly forceps)
- **Congenital factors:** abnormal collagen metabolism, for example, in Ehlers–Danlos syndrome, can predispose to prolapse.
- **Menopause:** the incidence of prolapse increases with age. This may be due to the deterioration of collagenous connective tissue that occurs following oestrogen withdrawal.
- **Chronic predisposing factors:** prolapse is aggravated by any chronic increase in intra-abdominal pressure, resulting from factors such as obesity, chronic cough, constipation, heavy lifting, or pelvic mass.
- **Iatrogenic factors:** pelvic surgery may also influence the occurrence of prolapse:
  - hysterectomy is associated with subsequent vaginal vault prolapse, (particularly when the indication was prolapse)
  - continence procedures, although elevating the bladder neck, may lead to defects in other pelvic compartments (Burch colposuspension may predispose to rectocele and enterocele formation).

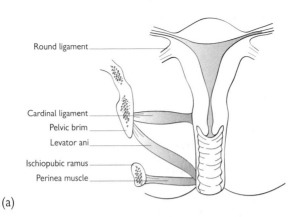

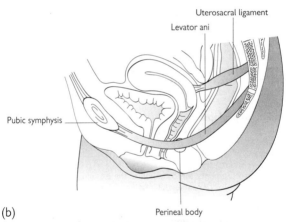

Fig. 21.7 (a) Coronal view of the pelvis, showing cardinal ligaments and levator ani. (b) Lateral view of the pelvis, showing the uterosacral ligaments and levator ani. Reproduced with permission from Impey L, *Obstetrics and Gynaecology*, Wiley-Blackwell Publishing, 1999.

Prolapse: classification

Definition

Prolapse is defined as protrusion of the uterus and/or vagina beyond normal anatomical confines. The bladder, urethra, rectum, and bowel are also often involved.

Incidence

The incidence of prolapse is difficult to define, as many women do not seek help and clinical examination does not necessarily correlate with symptoms. It is probably extremely common and is present in varying degrees in most older parous women.

Classification of prolapse

Types of uterovaginal prolapse are classified anatomically, according to the site of the defect and the pelvic viscera that are involved (Fig. 21.8).
- **Urethrocele** is prolapse of the lower anterior vaginal wall, involving the urethra only.
- **Cystocele** is prolapse of the upper anterior vaginal wall, involving the bladder. Often there is an associated prolapse of the urethra, in which case the term **cysto-urethrocele** is used.
- **Apical prolapse** is the term used to describe prolapse of the uterus, cervix, and upper vagina. If the uterus has been removed, the vault or top of the vagina, where the uterus used to be, can itself prolapse.
- **Enterocele** is prolapse of the upper posterior wall of the vagina. The resulting pouch usually contains loops of small bowel.
- **Rectocele** is prolapse of the lower posterior wall of the vagina, involving the anterior wall of the rectum.

Grading of prolapse

There are many grading systems. None is perfect, and some are complex and impractical. In 1996 the International Continence Society (ICS) Committee for Standardisation published its Pelvic Organ Prolapse (POP) quantitative scoring system.

For all measurements, the condition of the examination must be specified, i.e. position of the patient, at rest or straining and whether traction is employed.

Commonly used grading system for pelvic organ prolapse

0 No descent of pelvic organs during straining.
1 Leading surface of prolapse does not descend below 1 cm above the hymenal ring.
2 Leading edge of prolapse extends from 1 cm above to 1 cm below the hymenal ring.
3 Prolapse extends 1 cm or more below the hymenal ring but without complete vaginal eversion.
4 Vagina completely everted (complete procidentia).

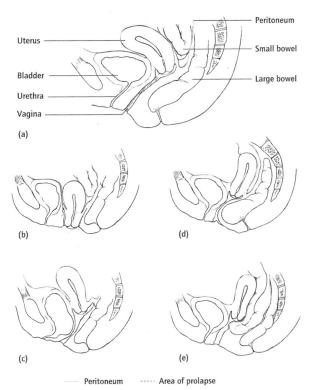

Peritoneum ----- Area of prolapse

Fig. 21.8 Types of prolapse. (a) normal pelvis, (b) uterine prolapse, (c) cystocele, (d) rectocele, (e) enterocele. Reproduced with permission from Impey L, *Obstetrics and Gynaecology*, Wiley-Blackwell Publishing, 1999.

Prolapse: clinical assessment

Symptoms

Symptoms are often absent, but the most commonly reported are:

- General:
  - dragging sensation, discomfort, and heaviness within the pelvis
  - feeling of 'a lump coming down'
  - dyspareunia or difficulty in inserting tampons
  - discomfort and backache.
- Cysto-urethrocele
  - urinary urgency and frequency
  - incomplete bladder emptying
  - urinary retention or reduced flow where the urethra is kinked by descent of the anterior vaginal wall.
- Rectocele
  - constipation
  - difficulty with defecation (may digitally reduce it to defecate).

Symptoms tend to become worse with prolonged standing and towards the end of the day. In case of grade 3 or 4 prolapse, there are may be mucosal ulceration and lichenification, resulting in vaginal bleeding and discharge.

Examination

- Exclude pelvic masses with a bimanual examination.
- Vaginal examination is best carried out with the woman in left lateral position, using a Sims speculum.
- The walls should be checked in turn for descent and atrophy.
- If absolutely necessary, a volsellum may be applied to the cervix so that traction will demonstrate the severity of uterine prolapse (this can cause marked discomfort and should be performed very gently).
- Sometimes, prolapse may only be demonstrated with the woman standing or straining.
- An assessment of pelvic floor muscle strength should be carried out (see box on p. 649).

Quality of life assessment

- Symptoms can affect quality of life, causing social, psychological, occupational, or sexual limitations to a woman's lifestyle.
- Self-completion questionnaires allow a comprehensive assessment of prolapse symptoms and their impact, such as the Vaginal Symptoms module of the International Consultation on Incontinence Questionnaire (ICIQ-VS); (☐ available at www.iciq.net.)

Investigations

- USS to exclude pelvic or abdominal masses (if suspected clinically).
- Urodynamics are required if urinary incontinence is present.
- ECG, CXR, FBC and U+E (if appropriate), to assess fitness for surgery.

Modified Oxford system for pelvic floor muscle strength

A system of grading using vaginal palpation of the pelvic floor muscles.
0 No contraction.
1 Flicker.
2 Weak.
3 Moderate.
4 Good (with lift).
5 Strong.

Prolapse: conservative management

Prevention of pelvic organ prolapse

- Reduction of prolonged labour.
- Reduction of trauma caused by instrumental delivery.
- Encouraging persistence with postnatal pelvic floor exercises.
- Weight reduction.
- Treatment of chronic constipation.
- Treatment of chronic cough (including smoking cessation).

Physiotherapy

Physiotherapy has a role in the management of mild prolapse in younger women, who find intravaginal devices unacceptable and are not yet willing to consider definitive surgical treatment.

- **Pelvic floor muscle exercises** (PFME) are most effective when taught under the direct supervision of a physiotherapist, these will improve the tone in young parous women but are unlikely to benefit older women with significant uterovaginal prolapse.
- **Biofeedback and vaginal cones** (see p. 636).

Intravaginal devices (pessaries)

Vaginal pessaries (Fig. 21.9) offer a further conservative line of therapy for women who decline surgery, who are unfit for surgery, or for whom surgery is contraindicated. They should be changed 6 monthly and topical oestrogen may be given to reduce the risk of vaginal erosion.

- The **ring pessary** is most commonly used and is available in a number of different sizes (52–129 mm), the ring is placed between the posterior aspect of the symphysis pubis and the posterior fornix of the vagina.
- The **shelf pessary** can be used when a correctly sized ring pessary will not sit in the vagina and/or where the perineum is deficient (it may be difficult to insert and remove, so its use is becoming less common).
- The **Hodge pessary** can be used to correct uterine retroversion. It is of classical interest but, in practice, is virtually never used now.
- **Cube and doughnut pessaries** are, very rarely, used for significant prolapse, when others are not retained.

Factors influencing management of prolapse

- Severity of symptoms.
- Extension of the signs (asymptomatic grade 1 prolapse does not require treatment).
- Age, parity and wish for further pregnancies.
- Patient's sexual activity.
- Presence of aggravating features such as smoking and obesity.
- Urinary symptoms.
- Other gynaecological problems such as menorrhagia.

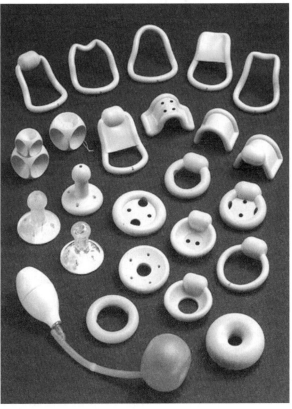

Fig.21.9 Types of pessary for uterovaginal prolapse: (a) ring pessary, (b) Gellhorn pessary, (c) Hodge pessary, (d) cube pessary, (e) doughnut pessary. Reproduced by courtesy of Milex Products Inc., Chicago © 2002

Prolapse: surgical management; anterior and posterior compartments

Surgery offers definitive treatment of prolapse. The choice of procedure depends on the patient and the type of prolapse that exists.

Anterior compartment defect

Anterior colporrhaphy (anterior repair)

- Appropriate for the repair of a cysto-urethrocele.
- A longitudinal incision is made on the anterior vaginal wall and the vaginal skin separated by dissection from the pubocervical fascia.
- Buttressing sutures are placed on the fascia.
- The surplus vaginal skin is excised and the skin is closed.
- The repair is traditionally performed under regional or general anaesthesia, but repair of a mild to moderate cystocele can also be performed under local anaesthesia, allowing early mobilization and discharge home.

Paravaginal repair

- Abdominal approach to correct an anterior defect.
- The retropubic space is opened through a Pfannenstiel incision and the bladder is swept medially, exposing the pelvic sidewall.
- The lateral sulcus of the vagina is elevated and re-attached to the pelvic sidewall using interrupted sutures.
- A cure rate of >95% has been reported (may also be done laparoscopically).

Posterior compartment defect

Posterior colpoperineorrhaphy (posterior repair)

- Appropriate for correction of a rectocele and deficient perineum.
- It involves the repair of a rectovaginal fascial defect and removal of excess vaginal skin:
  - care must be taken when removing redundant vaginal skin, as vaginal narrowing can result in dyspareunia.
- Perineoplasty is performed by placing deeper sutures into the perineal muscles, building up the perineal body to provide additional support.

Enterocele repair

- Similar to that of posterior colporrhaphy.
- The vaginal epithelium is dissected from the enterocele sac, which is closed with a purse-string suture.

Prolapse: surgical management; uterovaginal and vault

Uterovaginal (apical) prolapse

Vaginal hysterectomy

- May be combined with the above procedures in cases where there is significant uterine descent or menstrual problems.

Manchester repair (or Fothergill repair)

- Now rarely performed.
- Cervical amputation is followed by approximation and shortening of the cardinal ligaments anterior to the cervical stump.
- This is combined with an anterior and posterior colporrhaphy.

Sacrohysteropexy

- Can be performed if the patient wishes to preserve the uterus (Fig. 21.10).
- The uterus and cervix are attached to the sacrum using a bifurcated non-absorbable mesh.

Vaginal vault prolapse

Sacrospinous ligament fixation

- Involves suturing the vaginal vault to the sacrospinous ligaments, using a vaginal approach.
- Has a low immediate postoperative morbidity and success rate of 70–85%.

⚠ As the vaginal axis is changed by this procedure, there is a risk of postoperative dyspareunia.

Sacrocolpopexy

- The vault is attached to the sacrum using a non-absorbable mesh, can be performed either as an open procedure or laparoscopically.
- It has a higher success rate, of around 90%, and a better anatomical result than sacrospinous fixation.

⚠ Mesh erosion into the vagina, or rarely into the bladder or bowel, is a possible late complication.

Posterior intravaginal slingplasty

- Using 8 mm polypropylene tape, has been described as a minimally invasive procedure for treatment of vaginal vault prolapse.
- More studies are required to determine its safety and efficacy.

Recurrent urogenital prolapse

- Approximately 1/3 of all prolapse surgery is for recurrent defects.
- The vaginal epithelium may be scarred and atrophic:
  - making surgical correction technically more difficult
  - increasing the risk of damage to the bladder and bowel.
- The use of synthetic meshes is becoming increasingly common for repair of recurrent prolapse, as they may offer more support where the endopelvic fascia has proved to be deficient.

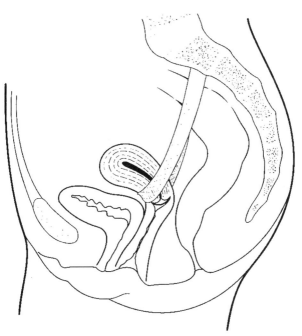

Fig. 21.10 Bifurcated mesh in position for sacrohysteropexy. Reproduced from Springer-Verlag London Ltd., *Female Pelvic Reconstructive Surgery*, 2002, p 187, Figure 13.10 Stanton and Zimmern. With kind permission of Springer Science and Business Media.

Benign and malignant gynaecological conditions

Benign neoplasms of the lower genital tract

Benign neoplasms are very common in the genital tract, most are innocent and easy to recognize.

Vulva

- **Bartholin's cyst:** arises from blocked Bartholin's duct in the lower third of the labia majora. It may present as a simple lump or an acute abscess after infection. Treatment: incision and marsupialization; send pus to microbiology if infected (some are due to gonococcal infection and may need treatment and referral to GUM for contact tracing).
- **Sebaceous cysts, boils, and carbuncles:** very common and if symptomatic should be treated by incision and drainage. They generally tend to recur.
- **Cysts of the canal of Nuck** (embryological remnants): appear in the anterior part of the vulva.
- **Mucinous cysts:** may arise from the minor vestibular glands.
- **Mesonephric cysts:** generally seen on the labia majora.
- **Endometriotic lesions:** especially on an episiotomy wound.
- **Lipomas and fibromas:** also common.
- **Condylomata acuminata** (HPV 6/11): sessile polypoidal mass on the vulva. Treatment: application of 80% trichloroacetic acid. Laser or electro diathermy under local anaesthesia is reserved for larger lesions.

Urethra

- **Urethral caruncle:** most common in postmenopausal women and children. Appears as a bright red, tender swelling at the posterior margin of the urethral meatus. May present with dysuria, bleeding, and dyspareunia. The treatment is excision using diathermy.
- **Prolapse of the urethra:** presents as a red lesion involving the entire circumference of the urethral meatal margin. It may be acute or chronic. Again, diathermy of the prolapsed mucosa is curative.

Vagina

- **Endometriotic deposits:** may present as small brown-black nodules.
- **Simple mesonephric (Gartner's) cysts and paramesonephric cysts:** usually appear in the fornices of the vagina. If symptomatic they should be marsupialized rather than excised.
- **Inclusion cysts:** can arise where the vaginal epithelium is embedded under the surface during a perineal surgery. Treatment is warranted only when patients are symptomatic.

Cervix

- **Cervical polyps (adenoma):** common and due to overgrowth of the endocervical mucosa. Sometimes arise in the endometruim (pedunculated) and protrude from the cervix. These are very rarely malignant (1:6000). However, they should be removed and a hysteroscopy to rule out further polyps should be considered if symptoms warrant it.
- **Nabothian cysts:** mucous-retention cysts caused by blockage of endocervical mucous glands. Treatment is not required.

Benign neoplasms of the uterus

Uterine fibroids

These are the most common benign tumours arising from the myometrium of the uterus. Also called **leiomyomata**, these tumours are composed primarily of smooth muscles but may contain fibrous tissue. Present in 20–40% of women in the reproductive age group, it has a higher incidence in Afro-Caribbean women and those with a family history of fibroids. Many women are asymptomatic but may present with: dysmenorrhoea, menorrhagia, pressure symptoms (especially frequency), and pelvic pain. Infertility may be associated and, in <10% cases, caused solely by the fibroids. In pregnancy they can cause pain from degeneration, abnormal lie, and obstruction if cervical, and difficulty in Caesarean section. The association with miscarriage is as yet unproven.

> *Types of uterine fibroids*
> * **Submucous:** >50% projection into the endometrial cavity.
> * **Intramural:** located within the myometrium.
> * **Subserous:** >50% of the fibroid mass extends outside the uterine contours.
> * **Cervical:** relatively uncommon and can cause surgical difficulty due to the proximity to the bladder and the ureters.
> * **Pedunculated:** mobile and prone to torsion.
> * **Parasitic:** have become detached from the uterus and attached to other structures.

Diagnosis

Clinical examination (hard, irregular uterine mass) may be sufficient. Transvaginal or abdominal ultrasound can differentiate the types and dimensions of the fibroids. Rarely MRI may be needed when the scan is inconclusive.

Endometrial polyps (adenoma)

These are focal overgrowth of the endometrium and are malignant in <1%. They are more common in women >40, but may occur at any age. Treatment is usually resection during hysteroscopy and the polyp should be sent for histological assessment.

Treatment options for uterine fibroids

- No treatment may be necessary if minimal symptoms.
- GnRH analogues shrink fibroids but should only be used for this purpose prior to surgery.
- **Myomectomy:** open, laparoscopic, or hysteroscopic depending upon location (especially when wish to preserve fertility and when the fibroids are distinctly isolated on scan—fibroids often recur).
- **Hysterectomy:** women who have either completed their family or are over 45 years—guaranteed cure of fibroids.
- **Uterine artery embolization:** uterine artery is catheterized generally using the unilateral approach; polyvinyl alcohol powder or gelatin sponge is used as the embolic material (minimally invasive procedure with avoidance of a general anaesthetic).

Benign neoplasms of the fallopian tube

Hydrosalpinx, pyosalpinx, and tubo-ovarian masses following pelvic inflammatory disease or endometriotic adhesions may present as a benign mass in the pelvis. The diagnosis is essentially by ultrasound and laparoscopy. Most tumours of the fallopian tubes are malignant, although they are rare.

Benign ovarian tumours: diagnosis

Ovarian cysts are extremely common, and frequently physiological, due to follicular cyst (≤3 cm) and corpus luteal cyst (≤5 cm) formation during the menstrual cycle. In a woman who is having periods, a cyst of <5 cm should not cause concern (or referral) unless there are other suspicious features or she is symptomatic (e.g. pain). A re-scan in 6 weeks is recommended (when she will be at another point in her cycle) to see if the cyst has resolved. Small cysts are also frequently seen in postmenopausal women (up to 14%) on transvaginal ultrasound.

Ultrasound features and the tumour marker CA125 are used to determine the risk of malignancy index (RMI). This is useful for identifying patients with a high risk of cancer who should be referred to a cancer centre for treatment (sensitivity 87.4%, PPV 86.8% in recent series) (see Table 22.1).

Presentation of benign ovarian tumour

- Asymptomatic.
- Chronic pain:
  - dull ache
  - pressure on other organs (urinary frequency or bowel disturbance)
  - dyspareunia (endometrioma)
  - cyclical pain (endometrioma).
- Acute pain:
  - bleeding (into the cyst or intra-abdominal)
  - torsion
  - rupture.
- Abnormal uterine bleeding.
- Hormonal effects.

History and investigation

History

Menstrual history (LMP, cycle length, menorrhagia); pain (site, nature, radiation; typically down leg, duration, precipitating factors); bowel/bladder function; abdominal distension; medical and family history.

Examination

- **Systemic:** pulse; BP; anaemia; temperature.
- **Abdominal:** mass arising from pelvis; tenderness; signs of peritonism; upper abdominal masses or ascites suggest cyst less likely to be benign.
- **Pelvic:** PV discharge/bleeding; cervical excitation; adnexal mass or tenderness (mobile or fixed, smooth or nodular, size).

Haematological tests

- FBC.
- Tumour markers:
  - CA125
  - consider other tumour markers especially in a young woman a with solid mass: AFP, hCG, LDH, inhibin, and oestradiol.

Imaging

- Abdominal/pelvic USS—presence and appearance of pelvic mass and ascites.

Risk of malignancy index

$RMI = U \times M \times CA125$

- U = ultrasound score (0, 1, or 3).
- M = menopausal status (1 = premenopausal, 3 = postmenopausal)
- CA125 = serum CA125 level (U/L)

Ultrasound scoring system

- 1 point for each of the following features on USS:
  - multilocular cyst
  - evidence of solid areas
  - evidence of metastases
  - ascites
  - bilateral lesions.
- Final U score:
  - 0 if no features
  - 1 if 1 feature
  - 3 if 2 or more features.

Table 22.1 RMI score and ovarian cancer risk

Risk	RMI score	Risk of cancer
Low	<25	<3%
Moderate	25–250	20%
High	>250	75%

Data from: Davies AP, Jacobs I, Woolas R, et al. The adnexal mass: benign or malignant? Evaluation of a risk of malignancy index. *Br J Obstet Gynaecol* 1993;**100**(10): 927–31.

Non-gynaecological causes of pelvic masses

Other benign masses due to non-gynaecological conditions in the pelvis should always be borne in mind as a differential diagnosis:

- Bladder tumours
- Intestinal tumours
- Diverticular disease
- Inflammatory bowel disease.

Benign ovarian tumours: histology

Histology

It is difficult to know the true incidences of benign ovarian tumours, as most will be functional cysts and are not removed, hence ratios of functional/benign/malignant tumours are highly dependent on the age and selection of the population studied.

Non-neoplastic
- Functional:
  - **follicular cysts** (normally <3 cm)
  - **corpus luteal cysts** (normally <5 cm (may show signs of haemorrhage into cyst or cause haemoperitoneum).
- Pathological:
  - **ovarian endometriotic cyst** (filled with old altered blood, 'chocolate cyst', see 🔲 p. 556)
  - **polycystic ovarian syndrome** (generally bulky ovaries with multiple small follicles, fibrotic capsule and smooth surface, 'ring of pearls sign on TVUSS)
  - **theca leutin cysts** (multiple ovarian cysts, occur in conditions with ↑hCG, e.g. hydatidiform molar pregnancy—resolve if ↑hCG levels fall)
  - **ovarian oedema** (secondary to ovarian torsion, the ovary is enlarged and boggy—exclude germ cell tumour in young woman).

Benign neoplastic
- Epithelial tumours:
  - **serous cystadenoma** (usually unilocular and 20–30% are bilateral, may have septations)
  - **mucinous cystadenoma** (often multiloculated, but usually unilateral (5% bilateral)– can get extremely large, >150 kg)
  - **Brenner tumours** (1–2% of ovarian tumours, unilateral and have solid grey, white, or yellow appearance to cut surface, fibrous elements and transitional epithelium).
- Benign germ cell tumours:
  - **mature teratoma or dermoid cyst** (10% are bilateral, 90% occur in women in reproductive age group, usually full of sebaceous material and hair, but often contain hair, teeth, skin, cartilage, fat, or bone; can cause chemical peritonitis if contents spill).
- Sex-cord stromal tumours (see 🔲 p. 700):
  - **fibroma** (commonest stromal tumour, up to 40% present with Meig's syndrome, ascites and pleural effusion)
  - **Sertoli–Leydig cell tumour** (1% of ovarian tumours; produce androgens and present with virilization)
  - **thecoma** (produce oestrogens—present with abnormal vaginal bleeding)
  - **lipoma**.

Benign ovarian tumours: management

Most cysts presenting acutely will present with lower abdominal pain, but without signs of peritonism or systemic upset. Manage conservatively with analgesia, as most will resolve spontaneously. However, if the woman presents with an acute abdomen and/or signs of systemic upset, due to ovarian torsion, rupture or haemorrhage of a cyst, urgent diagnostic laparoscopy or laparotomy may be required. In these cases, blood should be sent for tumour markers at the time of surgery, as if the cyst is not benign, this will aid follow-up.

Adolescent women

Manage as for premenopausal women. Germ cell tumours are more common in this age group (up to 20% in some series), especially in those presenting with ovarian torsion. Aim for conservative surgery (cystectomy if possible) to diagnose, but preserve fertility.

Premenopausal women

Malignant tumours are rare in this age group (0.4–9:100 000). Aim is to exclude malignancy and preserve fertility. Re-scan in 6 weeks. If cyst is persistent then either monitor with USS and CA125 (e.g. 3 months and 6 months (~50% <5 cm will resolve, less with larger cysts). Calculate RMI.

Management of low-risk cysts
- Transvaginal cyst aspiration can be performed under USS guidance, but has no advantage over expectant management.
- If cyst still persistent or >5 cm then consider laparoscopic cystectomy.
  - if cyst <5 cm and simple: cyst fenestration and wall biopsy for histology is acceptable
  - if cyst >5 cm or is a dermoid then aim to prevent spillage of contents, e.g. cystectomy and removal of cyst in an 'endobag'
  - if suspicious findings at laparoscopy, abandon procedure (take peritoneal biopsy for diagnosis) and refer to a cancer centre for a full staging laparotomy.

⚠ Do not use a morcellator and try not to spill cyst contents.
- If a dermoid cyst, this can cause a chemical peritonitis.
- If cyst ruptured and contents spill out this can disseminate an otherwise early ovarian cancer (although rare in this age group).

Postmenopausal women

Low RMI (<25) Simple, <5 cm cyst and normal CA125; follow up for 1 year with USS and CA125 every 4 months. If no change then discontinue monitoring. If change and RMI still low or women requests removal, laparoscopic oophorectomy (usually bilateral) is appropriate.

Moderate RMI (25–250) Oophorectomy (usually bilateral) in a cancer centre is recommended. It may be acceptable to perform this laparoscopically in some cases. If malignancy found then full staging laparotomy will be needed.

High RMI (>250) Refer to a cancer centre for a full staging laparotomy.

📖 Ovarian cysts in postmenopausal women RCOG guideline no. 34 (2003) ww.rcog.org.uk

Vulval dermatoses: lichen sclerosus

Skin conditions of the vulva can cause distressing symptoms and be difficult to diagnose and manage. Irritation leads to scratching and excoriation, which may make the appearance clinically difficult to differentiate, especially when added to changes seen following secondary infection or use of topical creams.

Vulval dermatoses refers to a range of benign skin conditions, which generally cause white thickening of the vulval skin: lichen sclerosus; lichen planus; vulval dermatitis; vulval psoriasis.

Lichen sclerosus

- Chronic inflammatory condition (lymphocyte mediated).
- May be hereditary (association with HLA-DQ7).
- Usually confined to anogenital area.
- More common in women.
- Incidence estimated as 1:300–1:1000 women.
- Normally in perimenopausal women, but can occur in young girls (2/3 improve at puberty—may be misdiagnosed as signs of abuse).
- Associated with other autoimmune diseases:
  - e.g. thyroid disease; diabetes; vitiligo; pernicious anaemia
  - 20–34% have association with autoimmune disease
  - up to 74% have autoantibodies.

See Fig. 22.1.

Clinical presentation of lichen sclerosus
- Burning pain or itch, occasionally asymptomatic.
- Figure of 8 appearance around vulva and anus.
- White, shiny, wrinkly, atrophic appearance 'like tissue paper':
  - may have white patches, purpura or telangesctasia
  - hyperkeratosis and lichenification if chronic scratching
  - over time can develop loss and fusion of labia minora, narrowing of introitus, resulting in problems with intercourse and micturation.

⚠ Long-term risk of vulval squamous cell carcinoma (4–6%), so need long-term observation, follow-up and biopsy of suspicious lesions.

A wide range of useful patient information leaflets is available on the Internet:

📖 www.bad.org.uk

📖 www.lichensclerosus.org

📖 www.prodigy.nhs.uk/patient_information/pils/lichen_sclerosus.htm

Management of lichen sclerosus

- Biopsy for diagnosis (ideally before starting steroids).
- Biopsy suspicious lesions (risk of vulval cancer).
- FBC, thyroid function tests, glucose, serum iron, autoimmune antibodies, intrinsic factor and B_{12}.
- Potent corticosteroids—clobetasol propionate 0.05% b.d. initially once a night for 4 weeks, alternate nights for 4 weeks, twice weekly for 4 weeks, then use 'as required' for flares; the shiny appearance will remain.
- Follow-up at 3 months to check response.
- Annual review with GP and advice re contacting urgently if ulcers, bleeding or suspicious lesions.

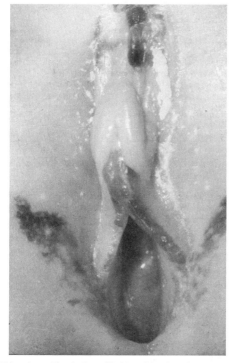

Fig. 22.1 Lichen sclerosus. Note the fusion of the labia and the vulva, and symmetrical white lesions with marked atrophy and spots of haemorrhage. Reproduced from Mackie, R. *Clinical dermatology*, 5th edn, OUP, 2003. By permission of Oxford University Press.

Other vulval dermatoses

Vulval dermatitis
- Dermatitis or eczema.
- If scratched so that thickening of skin → lichen simplex chronicus.
- Association with other atopic illnesses (asthma, hay fever, or eczema).
- Common irritants:
  - soaps, shower gels, condoms, deodorants, creams
  - often diagnosed as candidiasis; topical creams can be additional irritant.

Clinical presentation of vulval dermatitis
- Itch—burning and pain secondary to scratching.
- Erythema ± scaling of skin.
- No loss or fusion of labia.

Management
- Avoid irritant and apply general vaginal care (see text box p. 669).
- Low vaginal swabs for secondary infection (e.g. *Candida*).
- Severe disease—treat with steroid cream—clobetasol propionate or betamethasone valerate, if less severe. Use twice daily initially; reduce to daily, then twice weekly, as improves.
- Consider sedating anti-histamine (e.g. chlorphenamine 4 mg) at night to prevent scratching.

Lichen planus
- Rare condition.

Clinical presentation of lichen planus
- Purplish papules and plaques—can have white streaks on top— 'Wickham's striae'. May involve mouth too.
- May cause painful, red, ulcerated areas around introitus. Occasionally can cause severe desquamative vaginitis.
- Cause itch, pain, postcoital bleeding or discharge.

Management
- As for lichen sclerosus, including follow up, as also have an increased risk of developing vulval cancer.
- Biopsy; potent steroids; good vulval skin care; local anaesthetic gel.

Vulval psoriasis

Clinical presentation of vulval psoriasis
- Classically well-defined erythematous patches, may have scaling on pubic area, but not necessarily on vulval skin.

Management
- Good vulval skin care; bland emollients; mild topical steroids.
- Other psoriatic medications often too harsh for vulval skin.

Vulval skin care

- Keep area clean but avoid soap:
  - use soap substitutes; soap-free shower gels; bath oil; just water
  - salt baths *may* help.
- Don't soak in hot bath.
- Allow air circulation to avoid sweating:
  - loose underwear and bed clothes; avoid jeans, etc.
- Cotton next to skin:
  - avoid synthetics (esp. nylon) and wool (intrinsically itchy!).
- Avoid vaginal lubricants:
  - may be irritating;
  - can use saliva or oil (vegetable, olive, almond)—avoid perfumed oil.

⚠ Oils weaken condoms!

📖 www.prodigy.nhs.uk/patient_information/pils/lichen_planus.htm

📖 www.bad.org.uk

Idiopathic vulval itch and pain

Pruritis vulvae
- Common (1 in 10 women).
- Persistent itch, often worse at night and may disturb sleep.

Management
- Identify cause and treat appropriately
  - may need swabs; skin scrapings; skin biopsy; U&E; LFTs.
- General vulval skin care and bland emollients.
- Short course of weak steroid cream (hydrocortisone 1–2 weeks).
- Sedating antihistamine at night (e.g. chlorphenamine 4 mg) (break itch/scratch/itch cycle).

  www.prodigy.nhs.uk/patient_information/pils/pruritus_vulvae_itchy_vulva.htm

Vulvodynia/vestibulodynia
These are dysaesthesia, which involve pain in the vulva or around the introitus in the absence of a specific cause.
- Burning, stinging or raw discomfort.
- Typically worse when sitting down.
- May occur as sequelae to inflammatory vulval condition, e.g. lichen sclerosus.
- Neuropathic pain.

Management
- Investigate and exclude other causes.
- General vulval skin care.
- Topical local anaesthetic gel.
- Amitriptyline; start on low dose (10 mg) at night and increase as tolerated/required—reduce gradually after 3 months.
- Antiepileptics (used rarely and with specialist referral—e.g. chronic pain service):
  - gabapentin and pregabalin.

  www.bad.org.uk

  www.vulvalpainsociety.org/

Ulcers
- Aphthous ulcers.
- Infectious:
  - **herpes simplex virus:** multiple, extremely painful ulcers
  - **syphilis primary chancre:** painless unless infected
  - **tropical** (chancroid; granuloma inguinale; lymphogranuloma venerium).
- Inflammatory/autoimmune:
  - Crohn's disease
  - Behçet's disease (causes orogenital ulcers and ophthalmic inflammation; uncommon in women, HLA-B51 association).

Causes of pruritis vulvae
- Infection:
  - candidiasis
  - threadworms
  - *Phthirus pubis* (genital lice)
  - *Sarcoptes scabiei* (scabies, from Latin 'to itch').
- Vulval dermatoses:
  - lichen sclerosus
  - vulval dermatitis
  - lichen planus
  - vulval psoriasis.
- Vulval intraepithelial neoplasia or vulval carcinoma.
- Urinary incontinence.
- Systemic conditions:
  - liver failure
  - uraemia.
- Medication.
- Pregnancy/menopause.
- Idiopathic.

Guidelines for the NHS Cervical Screen NHSCSP Publication No. 20. April 2004 www.cancer-screening.nhs.uk

Cancer screening in gynaecology: overview

The intention of screening is early identification of a disease, prompt referral for diagnostic tests, and appropriate intervention and management. A screening test does not necessarily diagnose a condition or disease but may reduce the associated incidence, mortality, and morbidity.

> ## WHO principles of screening (1968)
>
> - The condition should be an important public health problem.
> - An effective intervention should be available.
> - Clear, recognizable early stage and known natural history of condition.
> - There should be a suitable screening test available.
> - The test should be acceptable to the population.
> - Benefits of the test should outweigh the risks.
> - There should be an agreed policy on who to treat.
> - The total cost of finding a case should be economically balanced.

Sensitivity, specificity, positive and negative predictive values

- **Sensitivity:** the ability of the screening test to detect the disease—acceptable sensitivity detects most disease.
- **Specificity:** the ability of the screening test not to identify those who do not have the condition—acceptable specificity excludes most without the disease.
- **Positive predictive value (PPV):** the proportion with a positive test result who have the disease.
- **Negative predictive value (NPV):** the proportion with a negative test result who do not have the disease.

Ovarian and endometrial cancer screening

Ovarian carcinoma presents with advanced disease in nearly 75% of cases and therefore necessitates a reliable screening test. Cancers of the ovary are less well studied than other gynaecological malignancies and only a few aetiological factors have been identified.

The main predisposing factors to epithelial cancer of the ovary are:
• Nulliparity.
• Non-use of oral contraceptives (RR 0.40 if used for >36 months).
• Family history.
There is lack of robust evidence for other factors such as age at menarche, menopause, and first childbirth.

Genetic factors

If a first-degree relative develops ovarian cancer aged <50 the risk increases by 6–10-fold. If 2 or more close relatives were affected, the lifetime risk rises to 40%. Possibly 1% of families in the UK may belong to a very high risk group. This familial risk is associated with a mutation of the *BRCA1* gene on chromosome 17, but other loci may also be involved. *BRCA1* and *BRCA2* have been identified in almost all families with both breast and ovarian cancer and in 40% of families with breast cancer alone.

⚠ Genetic advice to women with one of these genes should be given by a clinical geneticist.

▶ Women with a family history of ovarian cancers in one first-degree relative should be reassured. Although their risk of ovarian cancer is increased the absolute risk remains small (lifetime risk of 2–5% vs 1% in the general population).

▶ Oopherectomy should not be used as a primary prophylactic procedure but may be considered in women who have a strong family history and have completed their family. The risk of other peritoneal cancers cannot be ruled out in these women.

Endometrial cancer screening

Ultrasound assessment of endometrial thickness and sampling of the endometrium have been described, but there is no evidence to use these as screening methods in clinical practice. Endometrial cancer tends to present early with aberrant bleeding and as such has a good prognosis, so screening is unlikely to be beneficial in the general population.

Ovarian cancer screening

The efficacy of screening for ovarian cancer is not proven. The results from a large UK Collaborative Trial of Ovarian Cancer Screening (UKCTOCS) are awaited. Currently, any screening offered to women, should be as part of a clinical trial.

- Pelvic TVS can identify ovarian cysts. In a young woman most of these will be physiological, but features suggestive of malignancy are large size of cyst, internal septa, solid areas, and increased blood flow on Doppler examination. Operator expertise is extremely important in the screening process.
- CA125 is a glycoprotein shed by 85% of epithelial tumours. Normal levels are 30–65 IU/L, but false positives are commonly seen in other malignancies (liver, pancreas), endometriosis, PID, and early pregnancy. Sensitivity is improved using serial measurements and the trends. Up to 50% of stage 1 tumours will present with a CA125 level of <30 IU/L.
- Both ultrasound examination and CA125 estimation can give rise to a false positive result in nearly 2–3% of postmenopausal women. The use of the two tests together reduces the chance of false positives.

📖 www.ukctocs.org.uk/

Cervical cancer:pathology and screening

Cervical intraepithelial neoplasia (CIN) is widely regarded as a necessary precursor lesion for carcinoma of the cervix. CIN is a histological diagnosis and needs persistent cervical infection with human papillomavirus (HPV) to develop. There are about 15 oncogenic subtypes of HPV, the most common being types 16, 18, 31, and 33.

> **Risk factors for CIN**
>
> - Persistent HPV infection.
> - Multiple partners increases the risk of exposure to HPV infection.
> - Smoking as a promoter.
> - Immunocompromise, e.g. HIV, immunosuppressive agents.
> - Use of the combined oral contraceptive pill (COCP) has an association, probably due to non-barrier method and exposure to HPV.

Normal and abnormal physiology of transformation zone

The endocervix is composed of a thin secretory glandular epithelium; the ectocervix consists of a stronger stratified squamous epithelium. The two are in continuity and meet at the squamolumar junction. Under the influence of oestrogen the glandular epithelium is pushed out onto the ectocervix and in response to low pH undergoes physiological squamous metaplasia—the **transformation zone** (TZ). The TZ is usually ectocervical in women of reproductive age but tends to become endocervical in postmenopausal women.

As an area of high mitotic activity the TZ is vulnerable to HPV-driven neoplastic change, if persistent. (i.e. not eradicated). Most work suggests an average of 8–10 years from acquisition to development of cancer. Cervical cancer is therefore, in theory, a completely preventable disease.

Screening for cervical premalignancy

The NHS Cervical Screening Programme (NHSCSP) has been systematic since the 1980s and has since been shown a 50% reduction in mortality from cervical cancer. Regular cervical screening reduces the risk of death from cervical carcinoma by 75% (but does not eliminate it).

Screening is based on the natural course of cervical cancer where CIN (dysplasia) precedes overt malignancy and is a progressive condition. However, in reality CIN may also revert back to normal. Routine screening carries a 50–70% sensitivity to detect CIN III.

> **Current UK criteria for cervical screening**
>
> - Sexually active women 25–64.
> - 3-yearly 25—50, if normal 5-yearly till 64.
>
> ▶ 3-yearly screening identifies more than 95% of abnormalities tested by annual screening and is cost-effective.

Table 22.2 Management of abnormal smears

Papanicoulaou class	Histology	Management
Normal	0.1% CIN II–III	Repeat smear in 3 years
Inflammatory	6% CIN II–III	Repeat in 6 months (colposcopy after 3 consecutive)
Borderline nuclear changes	20–30% CIN II–III	Repeat in 6 months (colposcopy after 3 consecutive)
Mild dyskaryosis	30% CIN II–III	Colposcopy
Moderate dyskaryosis	50–75% CIN II–III	Colposcopy
Severe dyskaryosis	80–90% CINII–III	Colposcopy
Invasion suspected	50% invasion	Urgent colposcopy
Abnormal glandular cells	Adenocarcinoma of the cervix	Urgent colposcopy

📖 Guidelines for the NHS Cervical Screen NHSCP Publication No. 20. April 2004. www.cancer-screening.nhs.uk

Cervical cancer: cytology, colposcopy, and histology

Cervical cytology

The primary screening tool for cervical malignancy. Until recently the standard was a smear of cells from the transformation zone obtained with a wooden spatula. However, failure to adequately sample the lesion and failure by cyto-screeners to detect cytological abnormalities can lead to increase in false negative results. NICE now recommends liquid-based cytology for the cytological preparation of cervical cells—cleaner preparation, easier to read, inadequate cytology cut by 80% and more cost-effective.

> *Cytological markers seen with abnormal smears:*
> - Increased nuclear/cytoplasmic ratio.
> - Shape of the nucleus (poikilocytosis—abnormal shape).
> - Density of the nucleus (koilocytosis—abnormal density).
> - Inflammation, infection, and mitoses.

Dyskaryosis is a cytological term. False positive and false negative rates are 10–15% and 5–15% respectively. Due to these problems with sensitivity and specificity, abnormal cytology is further assessed by colposcopy.

Colposcopy

Involves the magnified (6–40×) visualization of the transformation zone after application of 5% acetic acid (preferentially taken up by neoplastic cells) or Lugol's iodine (not taken up by glycogen-deficient neoplastic cells). Upon identification of colposcopic abnormalities either:
- Directed punch biopsy to gain histological confirmation, or
- Definitive treatment ('see and treat').

> *Adequate colposcopic assessment requires:*
> - Visualization of the entire transformation zone.
> - Any lesion identified must be completely seen (esp. upper extent).
>
> Problem areas: postmenopause, post-treatment, and postpartum.

Histology

CIN is a histological diagnosis and is characterized by loss of differentiation and maturation from the basal layer of the squamous epithelium upwards.
- Bottom 1/3 = CIN I.
- Bottom 2/3 = CIN II.
- Full thickness = CIN III.
- Mitotic figures are present throughout the epithelium in all grades.

Referral criteria for colposcopy

- Any single smear showing mild, moderate, or severe dyskaryosis.
- Any smear suggestive of malignancy.
- Any smear suggestive of glandular abnormality.
- 3 consecutive borderline smears.
- 3 consecutive inadequate smears.
- Keratinizing cells (?underlying CIN).
- Postcoital bleeding
- Abnormal-looking cervix.

Colposcopic appearances of CIN

- Aceto-white epithelium (AWE).
- Vascular abnormalities, esp. mosaic and punctuation.
- Bizarre or grossly abnormal vessels are suggestive of micro-invasive carcinoma.

Management of cervical intraepithelial neoplasia (CIN)

CIN can be managed conservatively, by excision, by destruction, or rarely by hysterectomy. Management depends upon the grade of CIN and patient preference but excision is the preferred treatment modality. This is usually by large loop excision of the transformation zone (LLETZ).

Benefits of LLETZ

- Easy and safe.
- Usually possible with local anaesthetic.
- Tissue available for histology and assessment of excision margins.

Low grade CIN (CIN I)

Will spontaneously regress in at least 50–60% within 2 years. Malignant potential is very low but still up to 10× greater than women with normal cytology. Management options are:

- Conservative monitoring with colposcopy and cytology 6 monthly.
- LLETZ.

High grade CIN (>CIN I)

Will progress to cancer in up to 3–5% (CIN II) and 20–30% (CIN III) within 10 years. Spontaneous regression will occur less often.

- Definitive treatment with LLETZ is necessary.

Follow-up and management after LLETZ

Complete excision

- **Low grade:** follow-up cytology 6, 12, 24 months then return to normal screening.
- **High grade:** follow-up cytology at 6 and 12 months then annually for 10 years before return to normal screening.

Involved endocervical margins

- Colposcopy and cytology (with endocervical sampling) at 6 months.
- Repeat LLETZ if abnormal cytology and/or incomplete colposcopy, especially with high grade histology.

Involved ectocervical margins

- Colposcopy and cytology at 6 months (less likely to need repeat LLETZ as colposcopy usually complete).

📖 www.bsccp.org.uk/docs/public/pdf/nhscsp20.pdf

Complications of LLETZ

Short term:
- Haemorrhage.
- Infection.
- Vaso-vagal reaction.
- Anxiety (disproportionately high in colposcopy clinic attenders).

Long term:
- Cervical stenosis (dysmenorrhoea and/or difficulty in follow-up),
- Possible cervical incompetence (evidence suggests a small association, though absolute risk very low).

Management of cGIN and HPV

Dysplasia originating primarily in the glandular epithelium is known as cGIN. It is divided into low and high grade: the latter is a full-thickness abnormality. It can coexist with CIN or stand alone and is mainly associated with HPV 18. It poses difficulties in management because:

- The endocervical epithelium extends beyond view (up to 10% of cGIN lesions will have higher 'skip' lesions).
- The natural history is less well understood than squamous CIN.
- Typical colposcopic appearances and current management strategies are not widely agreed.
- Follow-up is difficult and the only known guaranteed 'cure' is hyster-ectomy.
- The incidence of adenocarcinoma appears to be rising compared to squamous cell carcinoma.

Management of cGIN

All glandular cytological abnormalities should be referred for colposcopy.

Colposcopy ± hysteroscopy may need to be performed. Endocervical curet-tage has a very low yield and is no longer recommended. In the presence of colposcopic abnormalities or high grade cytology a LLETZ with deep 'top hat' or cold knife cone biopsy is recommended. Hysterectomy may be required after completion of family or if colposcopic assessment is incom-plete with repeated cytological abnormality.

Prevention and the role of HPV typing and vaccination

HPV is a necessity for the development of CIN and cancer. HPV testing for high risk serotypes (hr HPV) has been evaluated and shown to be useful for:

- Triage of borderline and mild abnormalities to either colposcopy or cytological surveillance.
- Follow-up of high grade abnormalities after treatment.
- Management of HPV 18 positivity as a marker for cGIN.

It is unlikely that HPV testing can ever replace cytology, and it is not used in routine practice as an adjunct because it is not cost-effective. HPV vaccines have recently shown very promising results. They utilize the type-specific HPV-like particles (HPV-LPs). The two commercially available vaccines induce excellent antibody production against 4 and 6 HPV types respectively and in trials have been shown to reliably prevent CIN (types 16 +18 commonly) and anogenital warts (types 6 + 11).

HPV vaccines—what we know:

- They reliably induce excellent type specific antibody titres vs HPV.
- There is good trial evidence for reliable prevention of CIN (and presumably therefore ultimately cancer) and anogenital warts.
- Due to absolute type specificity they will not prevent all cancers—there are 15 hr-HPVs (current vaccines target 2 + 4 hr-HPVs only).
- The long-term antibody response is not yet known, although current limited data suggest it is likely to be good—?further vaccination required.
- They will need to be widely used in young girls before sexual debut to be most effective—this is a difficult area.
- They offer no protection once HPV-infected.
- Cost-effectiveness is still unknown and will take decades to determine, including whether they truly prevent cervical carcinoma.

CIN, VAIN, VIN + PAIN

The presence of any form of intraepithelial abnormality of the lower genital tract is a marker for a 'field change'. The vagina (VAIN), vulva (VIN), and perianal area (PAIN) are all at risk in the presence of CIN and vice versa. When the cervical appearances are normal with abnormal cytology the abnormal cells may be derived from elsewhere—they should be examined at colposcopy.

Gynaecological cancer: a multidisciplinary approach

Optimal treatment of the gynaecological cancer patient is provided by coordination of care within a multidisciplinary team (MDT). This team is made up of a range of doctors, nurses, and allied professionals with an interest in treating gynaecological cancer patients and should, at a minimum, consist of: gynaecological oncologist (surgeon); clinical oncologist; medical oncologist; radiologist; histopathologist; colposcopist; gynaecological cancer nurse specialist (CNS); and multidisciplinary team coordinator. Ideally, because of the complex nature of gynaecological cancer patients, their treatments and the complications they may encounter, teams should also include or have ready access to a: palliative care team; dietician; fertility specialist; lymphoedema specialist; lower gastrointestinal surgeon; urological surgeon; stoma therapy nurse; psychologist; and psychosexual counsellor.

The role of the team is to provide the following areas of care:
- Diagnosis, staging, primary surgical and adjuvant treatment, and coordination of follow-up care.
- Psychological preparation for anti-cancer treatment and follow-up.
  - Psychosexual support is a vital aspect, since many of the treatments can have major impacts on sexual functioning, either physically or psychologically, and may deprive women of their sense of femininity.
- Information on diagnosis, treatment plans, likely side effects, and follow-up plans.
- Access to financial, social, and psychological support:
  - Often required as patients may be young and have either young or elderly dependants, for whom they may be either the financial provider or primary carer.
- Advice on future fertility and treatments available.
- Aiding rehabilitation and preventing complications, e.g. provision of dilators following pelvic radiotherapy.
- Support with issues of survivorship.
- Appropriate and timely transition from active care to palliative care.
- Recruitment to clinical trials.
- Training of junior doctors and nurses.
- Audit of practice.

The CNS is often the central point of contact for the patient and ideally is trained to fulfil a supportive, advisory, advocacy role, in addition to being experienced in caring for women with complex medical issues and treatments.

Provision of appropriate care within a MDT has been shown to improve not just outcomes in terms of life-expectancy and cure rates, but also benefits patients' functional, cosmetic and psychological well-being.

📖 National Cancer Guidance Steering Group, Department of Health. *Improving outcomes in gynaecological cancers—guidance for commissioners: the manual.* London: NHS Executive, 1999. www.dh.gov.uk/en/publicationsandstatistics

Sources of information for patients

Excellent patient advice and information leaflets are available from:

📖 Cancer Backup. www.cancerbackup.org.uk

📖 Cancer Research UK. www.cancerresearchuk.org

📖 Ovacome, an ovarian cancer support network. www.ovacome.org.uk

📖 www.dipex.org (very useful website that uses patient experiences of disease to help patients and their carers).

Cervical cancer: aetiology and presentation

Cervical cancer is the second most common cancer in women worldwide (83% occur in developing countries), but mortality is declining in the UK due to the success of the cervical screening programme, introduced in the 1980s (decreased from 4000 to <1000 deaths/year)—one of the few screening tests which meets the WHO criteria for effectiveness (see p. 672). There are dual peaks in incidence (30–39 year age group and over 70s). The UK national screening programme is changing the spectrum of disease—↑ proportion of microscopic disease and adenocarcinomas.

Aetiology

The overwhelming majority of cervical cancer is associated with persistent infection with high-risk human papilloma virus (HPV) subtypes (mainly HPV 16 and 18). The natural history is well known; untreated high grade CIN leads to cervical cancer in 20–30% of women over 10 years.

> *Risk factors for cervical cancer*
> - Exposure to HPV:
>   - early 1st sexual experience
>   - multiple partners
>   - non-barrier contraceptive.
> - Combined oral contraceptive and high parity may have direct hormonal effect, but difficult to show independent role from indirect effect on sexual behaviour.
> - Smoking: strong dose/response effect—reduces viral clearance.
> - Immunosuppression: HIV and transplant patients especially.

Presentation

- Cervical smear demonstrating ?invasion (but not 100% reliable, so if suspect cancer clinically need colposcopy and biopsy).
- Incidental at treatment for pre-invasive disease (CIN).
- Postcoital bleeding (PCB).
- Postmenopausal bleeding (cervical cancer present in <1% of women with PMB).
- Rarer presentations (often suggestive of advanced disease):
  - heavy bleeding PV
  - ureteric obstruction
  - weight loss
  - bowel disturbance
  - fistula (vesicovaginal most common).

Histology of cervical cancers

- Squamous cell carcinoma (85–90%).
- Adenocarcinoma (10–15%).
- Neuroendocrine tumour (<1%):
    - originates from argyrophil cells in the cervix
    - may present with carcinoid syndrome (very rare)
    - median survival <2 years.
- Clear cell carcinoma (<1%):
    - <25 years 2° to DES exposure in utero (not now given)
    - > 45 years not associated with DES
    - treat as per adenocarcinoma, but prognosis worse.
- Glassy cell carcinoma (<<1%):
    - median age 35 years
    - presents with bleeding—often normal smear history
    - similar prognosis to adenocarcinoma.
- Sarcoma botryoides of the cervix (<<1%):
    - type of embryonal rhabdomyosarcoma;
    - median age ~14 years (range 5 months -45 years);
    - local excision (conservative surgery if possible) ± chemotherapy.
- Lymphoma of cervix (0.06%):
    - no need for surgical excision
    - responds well to combination chemotherapy.

Cervical cancer: diagnosis

Investigation

History
PCB; abnormal menstruation; PMB; PV discharge; risk factors; parity; fertility wishes.

Examination
- **Vaginal and bimanual examination:** roughened hard cervix, ± loss of fornices and fixed cervix if there is extension of disease.
- **Colposcopy:** irregular cervical surface, abnormal vessels, dense aceto-white changes.

Histology
Take a punch biopsy or small loop biopsy at colposcopy.

⚠ Do not try to treat with LLETZ if cancer is suspected—it may bleed +++, which is not ideal if done under LA in a colposcopy clinic!

Further investigations if cancer confirmed on biopsy
- U&E, LFTs, FBC.
- CXR (staging and pre-op assessment).
- MRI scan (can be very accurate at staging and examining for suspicious lymph nodes (LN), although staging still based on clinical examination **not** MRI or histology) and has largely replaced IVU, which was previously used to assess for hydronephrosis for staging (see Table 22.3).
- Examination under anaesthetic (EUA):
  - bimanual vaginal examination, cystoscopy, hysteroscopy, fractional curettings (try to take from endocervix, then uterine cavity) and PV/PR examination ± sigmoidoscopy
  - less often performed now as MRI is good and many tumours are microscopic, but it still has important role in Ib1 tumours when considering surgery.

Table 22.3 FIGO staging of cervical cancer

Stage			Extent of disease	5-year survival*
0			Cervical intraepithelial neoplasia (CIN)	
I			Limited to cervix	
	Ia		microscopic disease	> 95%
		Ia1	microscopic disease: invasion ≤ 3 mm; width ≤ 7 mm	
		Ia2	microscopic disease: invasion ≤ 5 mm; width ≤ 7 mm	
	Ib		macroscopic disease or microscopic disease > 5 mm depth and/or > 7 mm width	
		Ib1	<4 cm in diameter	~90%
		Ib2	>4 cm in diameter	~80–85%
II			*Extended beyond cervix (uterus/parametria/vagina), but not out to pelvic side wall, or lower 1/3 vagina*	~75–78%
	IIa		No obvious parametrial involvement	
	IIb		Obvious parametrial involvement	
III			*Extension to pelvic side wall and/or lower 1/3 vagina*	~47–50%
	IIIa		Lower 1/3 vagina involved	
	IIIb		Extension to pelvic side wall (includes all cases with hydronephrosis)	
IV			*Extension beyond true pelvis or involvement of bladder/bowel mucosa*	~20–30%
	IVa		Extension to adjacent organs	
	IVb		Distant metastases	

Data from Shepherd JH. Revised FIGO staging for gynaecological cancer. *BJOG* 1989; 96(8): 889-92 and Benedet JL et al. Carcinoma of the cervix uteri. *Int J Gynaecol Obstet* 2003; 83 suppl 1: 41-78.

Cervical cancer: treatment

Management depends on stage and age. Age is not an independent adverse prognostic factor, but is associated with ↑ stage at presentation. RCTs show that for Ib disease Wertheim's hysterectomy and radiotherapy have equivalent survival. However, if +ve LN on histology, will need radiotherapy as well, which ↑ morbidity and mortality. Aim is to perform pelvic lymphadenectomy, check for LN involvement (either frozen section at time of hysterectomy or paraffin section in a two-stage procedure -?laparoscopic lymphadenectomy) and proceed with Wertheim's hysterectomy only if LN –ve.

Role of laparoscopic surgery

Increasingly laparoscopic surgery is used in cervical cancer treatment. Pelvic lymphadenectomy can be performed laparoscopically, and this may be done as a separate procedure to the Wertheim's hysterectomy, to allow for formal paraffin-embedded histology of the LN, rather than frozen section. Wertheim's hysterectomy can also be performed laparoscopically.

Fertility-sparing surgery

In young women who are keen to preserve their fertility, fertility-sparing surgery (e.g. radical trachelectomy) is an option for early stage disease (stage 1a2 and early stage 1b1) if LN are proven to be negative following lymphadenectomy. This a vaginal procedure and involves the removal of cervix and paracervical tissue, to the level of the internal os with the introduction of a cerclage suture at the level of the internal os.

☛ The procedure is still 'experimental' and not proven to be as safe as conventional treatment, but case series demonstrate successful pregnancies can be achieved, although ↑ risk of late miscarriage, PPROM, and preterm delivery.

> ### Treatment options for cervical cancer according to stage
>
> - **Stage Ia1:**
>   - local excision or TAH (risk of +ve LN <1%).
> - **Stage Ia2-Ib1:**
>   - lymphadenectomy + Wertheim's hysterectomy if –ve LN (~5% +ve LN).
> - **Stage Ib2 and early IIa:**
>   - radiotherapy (?combination chemoradiotherapy)
>   - consider lymphadenectomy and Wertheim's hysterectomy in very selected LN –ve cases.
> - **>Stage Ib2**
>   - radiotherapy (?combination chemoradiotherapy).

Complications of treatment

- Wertheim's hysterectomy and lymphadenectomy:
  - bleeding
  - infection
  - DVT/PE
  - ureteric fistula
  - bladder dysfunction
  - lymphoedema
  - lymphocysts.
- Radiotherapy:
  - acute bowel and bladder dysfunction (tenesmus, mucositis, bleeding)
  - 5% late bowel and bladder dysfunction (ulceration, strictures, bleeding, fistula formation)
  - vaginal stenosis, shortening, and dryness.

Ovarian cancer: aetiology

Ovarian cancer is the leading cause of death from gynaecological malignancy in the UK, with around 6500 new cases per year. The ovary is a collection of several different cell types, each of which can have neoplastic development. However, 90% are epithelial ovarian cancers (EOC) and are commonly referred to as ovarian cancer (and will be below unless otherwise stated). Peak incidence of ovarian cancer is in women aged 75–84 years.

Aetiology

Believed to be due to irritation of ovarian surface epithelium by damage during ovulation.

- ↑ risk if multiple ovulations and ↓ risk if ovulation suppressed:
  - nulliparity ↑ risk
  - early menarche and/or late menopause ↑ risk;
  - combined oral contraceptive pill ↓risk (RR 0.5)
  - pregnancy ↓ risk.

BRCA mutations

BRCA1 and BRCA2 gene products involved in repair of damaged DNA. Mutations lead to ↑ risk of ovarian and breast cancer (see Table 22.4).

HNPCC (Lynch II syndrome)

Identified in families with strong history of colorectal, uterine, and ovarian cancer.

- Rarer than BRCA1 and BRCA2 mutations.
- Lifetime risk of ovarian cancer ~12%.
- If prophylactic surgery then consider hysterectomy in addition to BSO.

> ### Refer for clinical genetics counselling if:
>
> - Two primary cancers (breast and/or ovary) in one 1st or 2nd degree relative
> - Three 1st and 2nd degree relatives with any of the following cancers:
>   - breast
>   - ovary
>   - colorectal
>   - stomach
>   - endometrial.
> - Two 1st or 2nd degree relatives, one with ovarian cancer at any age, **and one** with breast cancer under 50.
> - Two 1st or 2nd degree relatives with ovarian cancer at any age.

Screening of genetically high-risk individuals

Need a blood sample from a consenting affected relative (often a problem as may have died). Mutations may occur anywhere within the BRCA1 and BRCA2 genes, so the entire sequence of the BRCA genes should be screened. However, a deletion may not be found, in which case patient is still at moderately high risk.

Management if BRCA mutation is identified:

- Surveillance with repeated CA125/ TVUSS (UKFOCSS trial ongoing).
- Prophylactic surgery:
  - bilateral oophrectomy and salpingectomy (BSO)
  - evidence that many tumours actually arise from the **fallopian tubes,** so remove as much tube as possible
  - counsel re risk of finding occult tumour at time of surgery
  - screen with CA125 and USS within 2 months prior to surgery (to ensure no evidence of cancer prior to prophylactic surgery, in which case a full staging laparotomy would be required rather than laparoscopic BSO)
  - can still develop primary peritoneal cancer post-surgery, so risk of cancer not reduced to zero
  - ↓ breast cancer risk following oophorectomy if premenopausal, even on combined HRT
- Theoretically ↓ risk of breast cancer further if only oestrogen HRT required (but would need hysterectomy).
- Hysterectomy only recommended if required for other reasons (fibroids, menorrhagia, etc.).

Table 22.4 Ovarian cancer risk in *BRCA1* and *BRCA2* positive women

Cumulative risk by age	BRCA1	BRCA2
30	0%	0%
40	3%	2%
50	21%	2%
60	40%	6%
70	46%	12%

Data from King MC et al. Breast and ovarian cancer risks due to inherited mutations in BRCA1 & BRCA2. *Science* 2003; 302(5645): 643–6.

Ovarian cancer: presentation and investigation

Presentation

Women present with a range of vague, common symptoms which may be misinterpreted as other conditions, e.g. irritable bowel syndrome, diverticular disease, or 'middle-aged spread'. ~50% of women will present to a specialty other than gynaecology. Combination of these symptoms should increase suspicion. 75% of women will present once disease has spread to the abdomen (FIGO stage III—see Table 22.5, p. 697).

- **Common symptoms include:** abdominal distension (often described as bloating, but persistent); increased girth; urinary symptoms; change in bowel habit; abnormal vaginal bleeding; detection of pelvic mass.

Investigation

History

Symptoms; risk factors; co-morbidities; family history (if strong, consider referral for genetic screening).

Clinical examination

Pelvic/abdominal mass (fixed/mobile); ascites; omental mass (common site for metastasis, may involve whole omentum—'omental cake'); pleural effusion; supraclavicular lymph nodes.

Haematological tests

- FBC, U&E, LFTs—esp. albumin.
- Tumour markers:
  - **CA125:** ↑ in 80% of epithelial cancers. Risk of malignancy index (RMI) useful for identifying patients at high risk of cancer and who should be referred to a cancer centre for treatment (sensitivity 87.4%, PPV 86.8% in recent series) (see 📖 p. 663)
  - **CEA:** raised in colorectal cancers, normal in ovarian cancer
  - **CA19.9:** may be raised in mucinous tumours, which are more likely to have normal CA125 (also raised in pancreatic and breast cancer)
  - tumour markers for rarer ovarian tumours if appropriate: AFP, hCG, LDH, inhibin, and oestradiol.

Imaging

- Abdominal/pelvic USS: presence of pelvic mass and ascites.
- CXR: pleural effusion or lung metastases (for staging and pre-op work up)
- CT abdo/pelvis: omental caking, peritoneal implants, liver metastases and para-aortic LN.

Management of ascites and pleural effusion

Diagnosis
- Ascitic or pleural fluid should be sampled and sent for:
  - histology
  - microbiology
  - biochemistry (U&E).

▶ Send as much fluid as possible as it may be relatively acellular.

Symptom control
- Drainage of massive tense ascites or a pleural effusion pre-operatively.
- For ascitic drainage use a small suprapubic catheter (e.g. Bonanno), use aseptic technique, and instil LA into skin and through abdominal wall.

▶ Consider USS guidance, especially if bowel metastases are suspected or previous abdominal surgery.

⚠ Albumin may ↓ precipitously following ascitic drainage. Suggest dietitian referral and use of high-protein supplements to avoid problems with hypoalbuminaemia and severe generalized oedema.

Ovarian cancer: treatment

Surgery

Current standard care for patients with a high RMI is for a staging laparotomy to be performed through a midline incision. Ideally this should be performed at a cancer centre by a gynaecological oncologist, as studies have demonstrated that this ↑ prognosis. The laparotomy should aim to remove as much tumour as possible—ideally with no macroscopic tumour remaining. Achievement of optimal debulking is a positive prognostic factor.

A full surgical staging laparotomy consists of:

- Laparotomy.
- Hysterectomy.
- Bilateral salpingo-oophrectomy.
- Omentectomy.
- Lymph node sampling (pelvic and para-aortic).
- Peritoneal biopsies.
- Pelvic washings/ascitic sampling.

See Table 22.5.

☞ There is no evidence to support routine 'second-look surgery' to see if there is still tumour present after chemotherapy.

☞ There is no consensus on the use of interval debulking surgery (IDS) (following 3 cycles of chemotherapy), if 1° surgery does not achieve optimal debulking.

Mucinous cystadenocarcinomas may present with **pseudomyxoma peritonei**—a thick, jelly-like ascites with mucinous tumour deposits throughout the abdominal cavity. Frequently these may arise from a primary tumour of the appendix and an appendicetomy is recommended as part of the debulking surgery for diagnosis.

Two specialist centres for pseudomyxoma peritoneii exist in the UK, at Manchester and Basingstoke. Optimal treatment requires extensive abdominal surgery (Sugarbaker technique) and intraperitoneal chemotherapy.

Table 22.5 FIGO staging of ovarian cancer

Stage	Extent of disease	5-year survival
I	*Limited to ovaries*	75–90%
Ia	One ovary	
Ib	Both ovaries	
Ic	Ruptured capsule, tumour on ovarian surface or positive peritoneal washings/ascites	
II	*Limited to pelvis*	45–60%
IIa	Uterus or tubes	
IIb	Other pelvic structures	
IIc	Positive peritoneal washings/ascites	
III	*Limited to abdomen*	30–40%
IIIa	Microscopic metastases	
IIIb	Macroscopic metastases <2 cm	
IIIc	Macroscopic metastases >2 cm	
IV	*Distant metastases outside abdominal cavity*	<20%

Data from Shepherd JH. Revised FIGO staging for gynaecological cancer. *BJOG* 1989;96(8): 889–92 and Engel J et al. Moderate progress for ovarian cancer in the last 20 years: prolongation of survival, but no improvement in the cure rate. *Eur J Cancer* 2002; 38(18): 2435-45.

Ovarian cancer:chemotherapy and follow-up

Adjuvant chemotherapy

Adjuvant chemotherapy (following surgery) is recommended for all patients other than those with low risk early stage disease (stage Ia–b low grade disease). For advanced disease (stage II and greater) RCTs have demonstrated that platinum agents are superior and that carboplatin ≈ cisplatin in terms of prognosis, but has ↓ side effects.

▶ Normal regimen is 6 cycles of carboplatin ± paclitaxel every 3 weeks.

✒ There is conflicting evidence that paclitaxel gives additional survival benefit, although it certainly increases side effects (uniformly causing alopecia as well as ↑ side effects caused by platinum agents). Current NICE guidance is that the decision to use paclitaxel in addition to platinum agents should be left up to the 'individual woman and her doctor'.

✒ Recent trials have suggested that intraperitoneal (i.p.) chemotherapy may improve survival (improved regional pharmacokinetics), although at the cost of increased side effects (many related to the i.p. catheter).

Investigations before starting chemotherapy

• Baseline CT scan (to assess response).
• Creatinine clearance, or
• ^{51}CrEDTA (to assess renal function).

▶ Assessment of renal function is needed to determine platinum agent dosing.

Neoadjuvant chemotherapy

Neoadjuvant chemotherapy (chemotherapy before surgery) is currently recommended only for women with cytologically or histologically proven ovarian adenocarcinoma, who are unfit for surgical treatment. The role of neoadjuvant chemotherapy is being investigated for use in all women with advanced ovarian cancer (stage 3c or more) in 2 ongoing RCTs.

Follow-up

Patients are monitored using clinical examination and tumour markers, where previously raised (every 3 months for 1st year, every 4 months 2nd year, then, if no recurrence, every 6 months for up to 5 years).

✒ There is currently debate about whether maintenance therapy improves outcome and when chemotherapy should be commenced following a rise in tumour markers. These issues are being assessed in RCTs, as is the choice of chemotherapy agents to be used for relapsed disease. Various novel agents are being investigated in clinical trials, including antibodies against vascular endothelial growth factor (VEGF) (bevacizumab) and epidermal growth factor receptor (EGFR) (cetuximab), in addition to tyrosine kinase inhibitors (gefitinib).

Rare ovarian tumours: germ cell

Germ cell tumours account for <5% of ovarian tumours and can arise anywhere down the tract of the embryological genital ridge, along which the primordial germ cells migrate from the yolk sac, although most occur in the ovaries. The degree of differentiation of the primordial germ cell affects the type of cancer produced: undifferentiated germ cells cause dysgerminomas; cells which have undergone initial differentiation can undergo embryonal or extraembryonal differentiation, to produce choriocarcinoma/endodermal sinus tumours (yolk sac) or teratomas respectively. Germ cell tumours most commonly occur in young women and account for 70% of ovarian tumours in the under 20s; when ~30% of these are malignant.

Dermoid cyst

- Common benign ovarian tumour.
- Often bilateral (10%).
- Commonly contain sebaceous material; sometimes hair and teeth.

Dysgerminoma

- Commonest malignant germ cell tumour.
- Female equivalent of a seminoma.
- 80% present at stage I and so treat with conservative surgery.
- Can be bilateral (10–20%) and require close follow up of the conserved ovary.
- Common in XY karyotypically abnormal gonads, e.g. X0/XY Turner's syndrome mosaic, and prophylactic removal should be recommended.

Dysgerminomas may require chemotherapy if more advanced. Combination chemotherapy regimens include: bleomycin, etoposide, and cisplatin (BEP); vinblastin, bleomycin, and cisplatin (VBP); and cisplatin, vincristine, methotrexate, bleomycin, actinomycin, cyclophosphamide, and etoposide (POMB/ACE).

⚠ Aim is to conserve fertility if appropriate in young women but ↑ risk of secondary malignancies following chemotherapy.

Immature teratomas

- Present most commonly in girls 10–20 years.
- Conservative surgery and chemotherapy unless stage Ia (BEP regimen).

Endodermal sinus tumours (previously yolk sac tumours)

- Median age 18 years at presentation.
- Raised AFP levels.
- Conservative surgery and chemotherapy (BEP or POMB/ACE).
- 2-year median survival 60–70%.

Choriocarcinoma of ovary and embryonal carcinoma

- Presentation in women <20 years.
- Raised hCG levels (choriocarcinoma) or hCG and AFP (embryonal carcinoma).
- Treat as other germ cell tumours.

Rare ovarian tumours: other

Sex-cord stromal tumours (~5%)

Granulosa cell tumour
- Solid ovarian tumours, which commonly produce oestrogens.
- Peak incidences in young girls and postmenopausal women.
- Present with postmenopausal bleeding (PMB), menstrual problems, or precocious pseudopuberty, depending on age.
- May be associated with concurrent endometrial cancer (2° to unopposed oestrogens).
- Often have raised inhibin (produced by granulosa cells to cause negative feedback on FSH levels from pituitary gland) and oestradiol levels—used as tumour markers for monitoring recurrence.
- Treat with surgery (conservative surgery in young woman, i.e. remove affected ovary, biopsy omentum and LN ± biopsy other ovary) as most (~80%) present at stage I and so fertility can be preserved.
- Often recur, which may be many years later and may require repeated surgical debulking.

Sertoli–Leydig cell tumour
- Produce androgens.
- Present with hirsuitism, amenorrhoea, and virilization (male pattern baldness, clitoromegaly, deepening voice, hairiness, oily skin, etc.).
- Normally benign tumours—treat surgically.

Fibroma
- Benign solid tumour.
- May present with ascites and pleural effusion (R > L)—Meig's syndrome.

Tubal carcinoma
- Present similarly to ovarian cancer (and may often be misdiagnosed as ovarian cancer and probably not as rare as previously thought).
- Normally serous cystadenocarcinoma.

See Table 22.6.

Table 22.6 Ovarian cancer: histological subtypes

Epithelial (85–90%)	Sex cord–stromal (5%)	Germ cell (5%)
Serous cystadenocarcinoma (75%)	*Granulosa-stromal cell tumours*	Dysgerminoma
Mucinous cystadenocarcinoma	Granulosa cell	*Embryonal carcinoma*
Endometrioid adenocarcinoma	Thecoma	Immature teratoma
Clear cell	Fibroma	Mature teratoma
Undifferentiated	*Androblastomas*	Stuma ovarii
	Sertoli cell	Carcinoid
	Sertoli–Leydig cell	Endodermal sinus tumour (yolk sac)
	Leydig cell	Choriocarcinoma

~5% of ovarian tumours are 2° tumours: endometrium; cervix; fallopian tube; Krukenburg tumours (breast, stomach, colon); lymphoma; melanoma; carcinoid.

Data from Gredmarek T et al. Histopathological findings in women with postmenopausal bleeding *BJOG* 1995; 102(2); 133–6.

Borderline ovarian tumours

Borderline ovarian tumours arise from the ovarian surface epithelium. They are not benign tumours, and are staged as for ovarian cancer. They were previously known as 'tumours of low malignant potential' and account for ~15% of ovarian epithelial cancers, although more common in younger women.

Borderline tumours are:
- Often confined to ovary.
- Occur in premenopausal women:
  - even in girls and teenagers.
- Can have metastatic implants:
  - these may be non-invasive or invasive.
- Associated with a much better prognosis than epithelial ovarian cancer.
- Difficult to diagnose histologically.
- Of predominately serous histology.
- CA125 may be elevated and if so can be a useful tumour marker for recurrence.

There are no trials to suggest that women with borderline tumours without invasive implants benefit from chemotherapy. Surgery is the recommended treatment. In young women a conservative surgical approach is valid, with the aim of preserving fertility (i.e. unilateral oophrectomy with appropriate staging biopsies). In stage I disease an RCT found that conservative treatment was safe; relapse rate was 8% over 2–18 years. They may relapse at a very late stage, after the traditional 5-year follow-up, and can occur anything up to 25 years after initial presentation.

Endometrial hyperplasia

Endometrial hyperplasia is a premalignant condition, which can pre-dispose to, or be associated with, endometrial carcinoma. It is characterized by the overgrowth of endometrial cells and is caused by excess unopposed oestrogens, either endogenous or exogenous, similar to endometrial cancer, with which it shares a common aetiology (see Risk factors for endometrial cancer, p. 706).

Presentation

Endometrial hyperplasia was commonly diagnosed on endometrial biopsies of women investigated for infertility. However, these are not routinely performed, and it is now most commonly diagnosed in women over 40 years old with irregular menstruation or in those with postmenopausal bleeding.

Histology

Endometrial sampling or formal endometrial curettage is necessary for diagnosis. Degree of hyperplasia (simple or complex) depends on the glandular:stromal ratio (much less stroma in complex hyperplasia). Atypia describes the appearance of the individual glandular cells (increased nuclear:cytoplasmic ratio—similar to CIN). Back-to-back atypical glandular cells (i.e. no stromal component) = endometrial carcinoma.

Management of endometrial hyperplasia

Depends on age of patient, histology, symptoms, and desire for retaining fertility.

Endometrial hyperplasia (no atypia)
- Exclude treatable causes of unopposed oestrogens:
  - oestrogen-only HRT
  - oestrogen-secreting tumour (e.g. granulosa cell tumour of ovary).
- Treat with progestogens, e.g.:
  - continuous oral progestogens daily for 3–6 months: 5 mg norethisterone (premenopausal); 10 mg medroxyprogesterone acetate (MPA) (perimenopausal); 20 mg MPA (postmenopausal)
  - levonorgestrel intrauterine device if postmenopausal.
- Risk of progression to cancer:
  - simple hyperplasia ~1%
  - complex hyperplasia 3.5%.
- Re-biopsy only if abnormal bleeding continues.

Classification of endometrial hyperplasia

- Endometrial hyperplasia
  - simple
  - complex (adenomatous).
- Atypical endometrial hyperplasia.

Atypical endometrial hyperplasia

⚠ 46% of women with atypical hyperplasia will have a concurrent adenocarcinoma and if not concurrent, there is a very high risk the woman will develop adenocarcinoma.

▶ Counsel about high risk of developing endometrial carcinoma.

▶ Unless fertility if desired or unacceptably high operative risk, recommend TAH (+ BSO if >45 years).

⚠ If conservative treatment, then treat with high-dose progestogens, e.g. MPA 100 mg daily. Re-biopsy every 3–6 months until progression or regression, and continue with long-term surveillance.

Endometrial cancer: aetiology and histology

Endometrial cancer, predominantly affects post-menopausal women (91% of cases in >50 year olds). Worldwide differences in prevalence reflect differences in risk factors (22:100 000 in N. America cf. 3.5/100 000 in Africa), and incidence is rising with increasingly 'Western' lifestyles.

Aetiology

Presence of unopposed oestrogen (i.e. no protective effect of progesterone), whether endogenous or exogenous.

- Endogenous:
  - peripheral conversion in adipose tissue of androstenedione to oestrone
  - oestrogen-producing tumour (granulosa cell tumour)
  - polycystic ovarian syndrome or anovulatory cycles at menarche or during climacteric period (lack of progesterone as no luteal phase).
- Exogenous:
  - Oestrogen-only HRT
  - tamoxifen (oestrogen agonist in endometrial tissue).

Risk factors

- Obesity and conditions predisposing or associated with obesity (including type II diabetes mellitus, hypothyroidism, hypertension).
- Reduced endogenous progesterone production:
  - nulliparity (pregnancy associated with high progesterone levels);
  - PCOS (anovulatory cycles—no corpus luteum, ∴ no progesterone)
  - early menarche/late menopause (anovulatory cycles).
- Genetic predisposition:
  - HNPCC (Lynch II syndrome) with high risk of colorectal, endometrial, and ovarian tumours (40–60% lifetime risk of endometrial cancer; inherited as autosomal dominant condition; inherited mutation in one copy of a mismatch repair gene)
- Breast cancer (shared lifestyle risk factors and tamoxifen usage).

Protective factors

- Parity (high progesterone dose in pregnancy).
- Combined oral contraceptive pill (RR ~ 0.5) (progesterone effect and lack of cycling of hormones).

Histology

Endometrial cancer arises from the endometrial lining. The major prognostic indicators in endometrial cancer are their grade of differentiation and FIGO stage of disease. These factors guide use of adjuvant treatment.

⚠ Endometrial hyperplasia with atypia (but not without) is a premalignant condition and may have coincidental cancer in at least 50% of women.

Histological types of endometrial cancer

Adenocarcinoma:
- Endometriod adenocarcinoma 87%
- Adenosquamous carcinoma* 6%
- Clear cell or papillary serous carcinoma* 6%
- Mixed mesodermal Mullerian tumours (MMMT)* 1%

* high risk of advanced disease at presentation and recurrence—all G3.

Grading

- Well differentiated (G1)
- Moderately differentiated (G2)
- Poorly differentiated or high risk cell type (G3)

Endometrial cancer: presentation and investigation

Presentation

Most commonly presents with postmenopausal bleeding (PMB). Younger women present with menstrual disturbance (heavy or irregular periods). 1% are picked up on routine cervical smear tests.

⚠ 1 in 10 women with PMB will have endometrial cancer or atypical hyperplasia (Table 22.7).

▶ Endometrial sampling required for women >40 years with abnormal menstrual symptoms.

⚠ PV discharge and pyometra may occur instead of bleeding—have a ↑ index of suspicion in postmenopausal women with ↑ PV discharge (50% of postmenopausal women with pyometra have underlying carcinoma).

Investigation

History

Presenting symptoms; menstrual history; parity; co-morbidities; drug history (COCP, HRT, tamoxifen, antihypertensives, oral hypoglycaemics); family history.

Examination

- Rule out other causes of bleeding (vulval, vaginal and cervical pathology) with vulval, vaginal, and speculum examination.
- Bimanual examination: uterine size, mobility, adnexal masses.

Haematological investigations

- FBC, U&E, LFTs.

Imaging investigations

- Transvaginal USS (TVUSS):
  - < 4 mm endometrial thickness/echo (ET) ≈ very low risk of endometrial pathology in postmenopausal women (96% NPV)—no requirement for endometrial sampling.
- MRI pelvis: in experienced hands very good at determining local extent of tumour and presence of grossly involved pelvic lymph nodes.
- CXR (staging).

Endometrial biopsy

Perform endometrial sampling if ET ≥4 mm or persistent bleeding in woman with ET <4 mm (in which case consider formal hysteroscopy).

- Blind outpatient sampling (e.g. pipelle, vabra).
- Hysteroscopy: under LA as outpatient or GA as inpatient.

Table 22.7 Histopathology findings in women with PMB

Histological diagnosis	%
Atrophy	49.9
Proliferatory/secretory	5.5
Benign polyps	9.2
Hyperplasia	
No atypia	27.8
Atypical hyperplasia	5.5
Adenocarcinoma	8.1
Not diagnostic	14.2
Other disorders	3.3

Endometrial cancer: treatment

Treatment

Surgery

Total abdominal hysterectomy and bilateral salpingo-oophrectomy (TAH & BSO) and pelvic washings. This can be performed via a transverse or midline incision. Increasingly, laparoscopic hysterectomy is gaining popularity and should give similar results to open TAH, although no trials have compared the outcomes of women with endometrial cancer.

Pelvic lyphadenectomy

Role in low-grade early disease is controversial (and is debated fiercely across the Atlantic divide!). Preliminary results of the ASTEC RCT (Women with stage Ib G2 and G3 endometrial carcinoma. Randomization arms for pelvic lymphadenectomy **and** radiotherapy) suggest no survival advantage in early disease (see Table 22.8).

Adjuvant radiotherapy

Adjuvant radiotherapy reserved for women with stage Ib G3 disease, or stage Ic or greater disease with any grade of tumour.

> **PORTEC trial**
> This trial compared adjuvant radiotherapy vs no adjuvant radiotherapy in women with early endometrial adenocarcinoma who were still at risk of recurrence: G1 with deep myometrial invasion (>50%; stage Ic); G2 with any myometrial invasion (stage Ib or Ic); and G3 with superficial invasion (stage Ib).
> • Radiotherapy reduced pelvic recurrences but gave no survival advantage to women with stage Ib endometrial cancer and intermediate risk histology (G2).
> • This was because pelvic recurrences were amenable to radiotherapy in previously non-irradiated patients.

The role of radiotherapy in early disease was also examined in the ASTEC RCT (Stage Ib G2 and G3 endometrial carcinoma. Randomization arms for pelvic lymphadenectomy and radiotherapy)—results awaited.

Hormonal

• High dose progesterone used for advanced and recurrent disease.
• Largely aiming for palliation of symptoms (bleeding)—no survival advantage demonstrated.

Table 22.8 FIGO staging of endometrial cancer

Stage	Extent of disease	5-year survival*
I	*Tumour limited to uterine body*	*85%*
Ia	Limited to endometrium	
Ib	< 1/2 myometrial depth invaded	
Ic	> 1/2 myometrial depth invaded	
II	*Tumour limited to uterine body and cervix*	*75%*
IIa	Endocervical invasion only	
IIb	Invasion into cervical stroma	
III	*Extension to uterine serosa, peritoneal cavity and/or lymph nodes*	*45%*
IIIa	Extension to uterine serosa, adnexae, or positive peritoneal fluid (ascites or washings)	
IIIb	Extension to vagina	
IIIc	Pelvic or para-aortic lymph nodes involved	
IV	*Extension beyond true pelvis and/or involvement of bladder/bowel mucosa*	*25%*
IVa	Extension to adjacent organs	
IVb	Distant metastases or positive inguinal lymph nodes	

* Amant F, Moerman P, Neven P, et al. (2005) Endometrial cancer. *The Lancet* **366**(9484),491–505.

Data from Shepherd JH. Revised FIGO staging for gynaecological cancers. *BJOG* 1989: 96(8); 389–92.

Rare uterine malignancies

Uterine sarcomas

Uterine sarcomas are very rare, accounting for 3–5% of uterine cancers and have an incidence of 2:100 000 women. Abnormal bleeding is the most common presenting feature; other symptoms include pain and a pelvic mass. Polypoid masses may protrude through the cervical os.

⚠ Uterine corpus sarcomas account for 3–5% of all uterine cancers, but cause 26% of the mortality.

> **Types of uterine sarcomas**
>
> - Leiomyosarcoma (46%).
> - Endometrial stromal sarcoma (12%).
> - Carcinosarcoma (27%).
> - Not specified/others (15%).

The peak incidence for leiomyosarcoma and endometrial stromal sarcoma is 50–64 years of age. Peak incidence for carcinosarcoma is older, at 65–79 years. Age, stage, and tumour type are important prognostic factors.
- The 5-year survival figures are:
  - leiomyosarcoma, stage I 65%, stage IV 0%
  - carcinosarcoma, stage I 62%, stage IV 17%
  - endometrial stromal sarcoma, stage I 85%, stage IV 37%.

▶ There was no improvement in survival for stage I and II uterine sarcoma with postoperative chemotherapy.

Vulval intraepithelial neoplasia (VIN)

VIN can occur in any age group, but is more common in postmenopausal women. There has been an ↑ in incidence of VIN (×2 or ×3 over 30 years), especially in younger women, probably reflecting changes in sexual practice as well as ↑ recognition. The natural history of VIN is not as well understood as CIN, but ~80% of women with untreated VIN will progress to vulval cancer over several years. VIN is difficult to treat and frustrating to patient and doctor.

Aetiology

VIN is a dysplastic lesion of the squamous epithelium. As with its cervical counterpart, CIN, it is associated with persistent infection with HPV in >90% of cases, especially HPV 16. HPV infection may cause multifocal disease, and patients with VIN should be carefully screened for CIN. Smoking is also associated with development of VIN.

Histology

The histological staging and features of VIN are the same as for CIN: VIN I ≈ loss of differentiation in the lower 1/3 of the epidermis; VIN II ≈ loss of differentiation in the lower 2/3 of the epidermis; VIN III ≈ loss of differentiation in the entire epidermis but with an intact basement membrane. However, a newer classification system now uses VIN to refer to previous VIN II–III, whereas VIN I is now thought to be non-specific inflammatory changes and is not premalignant.

Presentation and investigation

Symptoms are primarily those of itch, but include pain and ulceration; over 20% may be asymptomatic. Lesions may be raised and warty or flat and erythematous and are frequently found at multiple sites on the vulva (~50%). Diagnosis is made by punch or excision biopsy. Since HPV causes multifocal disease, patients require regular cervical smears.

Paget's disease of the vulva

- Non-mammary adenocarcinoma in situ:
  - In breast Paget's disease is normally associated with underlying malignancy; whereas only 10–12% with vulval Paget's disease have an invasive adenocarcinoma component, and another ~8% have an underlying adenocarcinoma (e.g. colorectal).
- Postmenopausal women.
- Presents with itching and vulval soreness.
- Eczematous or raised and velvety appearance—may weep serous fluid.
- Extent of disease spreads well beyond clinical lesion—difficult to excise completely.
- May be associated with rectal adenocarcinoma, especially if Paget's in perianal area.
- Treat with surgical excision and exclude underlying malignancy.
- Can recur and if does so is normally another adenocarcinoma in situ.

Vulval intraepithelial neoplasia (VIN): management

Although small, painful lesions can be excised, it must be remembered that there is normally a field change, and so it is difficult to completely excise the VIN, and recurrence rate is ↑, even after radical vulvectomy. The aim of treatment is therefore to minimize symptoms and side effects of disease and to exclude development of vulval cancer.

Surveillance
Careful follow-up of patients with VIN is required and suspicious lesions should be biopsied.

Surgery
Excision of painful/irritating lesions can be performed, but skinning vulvectomy or laser ablation is rarely recommended, due to the high recurrence rate (40–70%) and poor functional outcome. Development of pain is associated with ↑ risk of vulval cancer.

Immunotherapy
Imiquimod, an immune modifier, has been shown to help clearance of genital warts. Stimulates monocytes and macrophages; these secrete cytokines which result in T-helper cell coordination of a cell-mediated immune response. Apply cream 2–3× weekly. ~30% response rate, most will relapse. Treatment limited by side effects—soreness and burning.

Vaccination
Vaccinia virus encoding HPV genes under investigation.

Chemotherapy
❧ Patients can be treated with topical 5-fluorouracil (5-FU). This is usually ineffective and badly tolerated.

Vulval cancer: aetiology and investigation

Vulval carcinomas are uncommon, but approximately 90% are squamous cell carcinomas and ~5% are 1° vulval melanomas, with basal cell, Bartholin's gland carcinoma, and rarely sarcomas, accounting for the rest. Most occur in older women (median age at presentation 74 years), although younger women are at risk, especially those with multifocal VIN.

Aetiology

Vulval squamous carcinomas (vulval cancer) commonly arise on a background of lichen sclerosus or VIN.

Presentation

Vulval cancers commonly present with a lump, pain, irritation, or bleeding. There may be an obvious ulcer present. Elderly women in particular may delay presentation due to embarrassment. Referral to secondary care may also be delayed if there is not an adequately high index of suspicion.

Investigation

History

Vulval symptoms, treatments (prescribed or self), past medical history, and performance status (see Table 22.9).

Clinical examination

Palpable groin lymph nodes (LN), size and location of lesion, general medical condition. May be too painful for examination unless under GA, so if obvious tumour, do this at time of biopsy.

Haematological investigations

- FCS, U&E, LFTs.

Imaging investigations

- CXR (staging and preoperative).
- As yet no role of imaging groins for LN (see later)

Anaesthetic review

Patients with vulval cancer are often very elderly and may be quite frail. Involve an anaesthetist at an early stage in the pre-op work-up. Remember that regional anaesthetic may be a preferred option in some patients.

Histology

All suspicious vulval lesions should be biopsied. Small lesions can be excised and larger lesions should have a wedge biopsy taken, including the edge of the lesion if possible (in ulcerated lesions, it may be difficult to get a diagnosis from the sloughed tissue central to the lesion).

Table 22.9 ECOG performance status

Grade	Performance criteria
0	Fully active
1	Reduced physical activity, but ambulatory and able to perform light work, e.g. light housework, office work
2	Ambulatory and capable of all self-care, but unable to carry out work activities. Up and about more than 50% of waking hours
3	Limited self-care, confined to bed or chair more than 50% of waking hours
4	Totally confined to bed or chair cannot carry out any self-care

Reproduced from Oken, M.M., et al. Toxicity and response criteria of the Eastern Cooperative Oncology Group. *Am J Clin Oncol* 5:649–655, 1982. Reproduced with permission from Lippincott, Williams and Wilkins.

Vulval cancer: treatment

Surgery

Surgery is the mainstay of treatment in vulval cancer, both for curative intent and also for palliation.

- All patients with disease > 1 mm invasion should have groin lymphadenectomy performed.
- Lateral disease can have an ipsilateral LN dissection.
  - if +ve LN, bilateral groin LN dissection is required.
- Central disease requires bilateral groin LN dissections.

The importance of lymphadenectomy was recognized in the 1940s by Way and Taussig, who developed the 'butterfly' incision en-bloc dissection, which removed the entire vulva and inguinal LNs with all connecting tissue. These wounds frequently broke down and took many months to heal by secondary intent. The triple incision vulvectomy, with separate groin incisions, was subsequently developed to reduce morbidity. Current treatment aims for wide local excision (ideally margins > 1 cm) of the vulval lesion and LN dissection through separate incisions along the inguinal ligament. Occasionally plastic surgical reconstruction is required.

⚠ Groin recurrence is very difficult to treat and carries a very ↑ mortality.

Complications

- Wound breakdown and infection.
- Lymphocysts.
- Lymphoedema.
- DVT/PE.

Radiotherapy ± chemotherapy

- Can be used before surgery to shrink primary to reduced morbidity of surgery (e.g. if urethra or anus involved).
- Is used after surgery if positive groin LNs, to prevent regional recurrence. External beam radiotherapy given to treat potentially +ve pelvic LN.
- Can combine with chemotherapy (5-FU and mitomycin C).

☛ Should not be used as an alternative to groin dissection (RCT halted early as 5/26 had groin recurrences, cf. none in surgical arm).

Sentinel lymph node biopsy

Morbidity ↑ from groin LN dissection. The theory is that there is a single LN which primarily drains the tumour. If this is identified and is negative, patient can be spared full groin dissection. Identify sentinel LN with blue dye and radiolabelled tracer. Currently under RCT investigation for safety. See Table 22.10.

Vulval/vaginal melanoma
- Staged, like other melanomas, rather than vulval cancer:
  - Breslow depth and American Joint Committee on Cancer (AJCC) staging (2002).
- Most common site lower anterior vaginal wall (so easy to miss on speculum examination).
- Very poor prognosis—5-year survival 13–19%.

Table 22.10– FIGO staging of vulval cancer

Stage	Extent of disease	5-year survival*
0	Intraepithelial neoplasia (VIN)	
I	Tumour limited to vulva or perineum <2 cm diameter (negative lymph nodes)	98%
Ia	<1 mm depth of invasion	
Ib	>1 mm depth of invasion	
II	Tumour limited to vulva or perineum >2 cm diameter (negative lymph nodes)	85%
III	Tumour spread to vagina, urethra, anus, and/or lymph nodes	74%
IV	Tumour spread beyond vulva and immediately adjacent areas	31%
IVa	Tumour spread to upper urethra, bladder, bowel, pelvic bones, and/or bilateral inguinal lymph nodes	
IVb	Distant metastases and/or positive pelvic lymph nodes	

* Homesley, HD, et al. (1991) Assessment of current International Federation of Gynecology and Obstetrics staging of vulvar carcinoma relative to prognostic factors for survival (a Gynecologic Oncology Group study). *Am J Obstet Gynecol.* **164**(4):997–1003.

Data from Shepherd JH. Revised FIGO staging for gynaecological cancers. *BJOG* 1989: 96(8); 889–92.

Vaginal cancer

All primary vaginal carcinomas are rare and account for only 1% of gynaecological malignancies. Most vaginal tumours are metastases from either above (cervical or uterine) or below (vulval). Of the remaining true vaginal tumours, most are squamous cell carcinomas and are present in elderly women. Many will have a previous history of intraepithelial neoplasia or invasive carcinoma of the vulva, vagina, or cervix. Other predisposing factors include pelvic radiotherapy and long-term inflammation due to a vaginal pessary or procidentia.

Vaginal clear cell adenocarcinoma

Occur in younger women and are strongly associated with diethylstilbestrol (DES) exposure *in utero*. DES was administered to several million pregnant women at risk of miscarriage or premature delivery between 1940 and 1971. The critical time for exposure was in the first 20 weeks of pregnancy.

Vaginal clear cell adenocarcinoma in DES-exposed women
- Probably only of historical significance.
- Appear after 14 years of age; peak incidence of 19 years.
- R.R. of developing clear cell adenocarcinoma is 40.7 (95% CI, 13.1–126.2).
- Cumulative incidence rate is only 1.5 per 1000 DES-exposed women.

Vaginal clear cell adenocarcinoma in women not exposed to DES
- Peak incidence 50–60 years.

⚠ The DES-exposed cohort is only just reaching this age, so the total effect of DES exposure is not yet known.

Treatment of vaginal clear cell adenocarcinoma
Aim to preserve reproductive function in (often) young women. Stage I tumours treated with wide local excision. In more advanced stage disease, 1° radiotherapy is indicated. See Table 22.11.

Embryonal rhabdomyosarcoma (sarcoma botryoides)
- Rare tumour with a multicystic grape-like form (sarcoma botryoides).
- Derived from rhabdomyoblasts.
- Presents in infancy (girls <3 years).
- Cervical rhabdomyosarcoma can occur in teenagers and uterine rhabdomyosarcoma has been described in postmenopausal women.
- Presents with a grape-like mass arising from the vagina; can present with vaginal bleeding or a single polyp.
- Treatment—preserve fertility and vaginal function.
  - smaller tumours excised followed by combination chemotherapy (vincristine, dactinomycin, and cyclophosphamide)
  - neoadjuvant chemotherapy given for larger tumours, to reduce their size prior to surgery.
- Survival rates of 90% can be achieved:
  - refer to centres with expertise—may need reconstructive surgery.

Table 22.11 FIGO staging of vaginal cancer

Stage	Extent of disease	5-year survival*
0	Intraepithelial neoplasia (VAIN)	95%
I	Tumour limited to vaginal wall	~67%
II	Tumour limited to vagina and sub-vaginal tissue, but not extending to pelvic side wall	<39%
III	Tumour spread to pelvic side wall	~33%
IV	Tumour spread beyond true pelvis and/or into bladder/bowel mucosa	<19%
IVa	Tumour spread to bladder/bowel or directly invading beyond true pelvis	
IVb	Distant metastases	

*Beller U et al. Carcinoma of the vagina. *Int J Gynaecol Obstet* 2003; 83 Suppl 1:27–39.

Data from Shepherd JH. Revised FIGO staging for gynaecological cancers. *BJOG* 1989: 96(8); 889–92.

Gestational trophoblastic disease (GTD): hydatidiform mole

Gestational trophoblastic disease (GTD) covers a spectrum of diseases caused by overgrowth of the placenta. This includes hyatidiform mole, choriocarcinoma, invasive mole, placental site trophoblastic tumour.

- **Incidence:** 0.6–2.3 per 1000 pregnancies.
- **Background:** 50% cases follow hyatidiform mole, 25% a normal pregnancy, and 25% a miscarriage or ectopic pregnancy.

Hyatidiform mole

Can be subdivided into complete and partial mole based on genetic and histological features.

Complete mole

- Consists of diffuse hydropic villi with trophoblastic hyperplasia.
- This is diploid, derived from sperm duplicating its own chromosome following fertilization of an 'empty' ovum. This is mostly 46XX with no evidence of fetal tissue.

Partial mole

- Consists of hydropic and normal villi.
- This is triploid (69XXX, XXY,XYY) with one maternal and two paternal haploid sets. Most cases occur following two sperms fertilizing an ovum, and a fetus may be present.

Diagnosis

Symptoms and signs (with approximate frequency)

- Irregular first-trimester vaginal bleeding (>90%).
- Uterus large for dates (25%).
- Pain from large theca lutein cysts (20%) resulting from ovarian hyper-stimulation by high hCG levels.
- Vaginal passage of vesicles containing products of conception (10%).
- Exaggerated pregnancy symptoms:
  - hyperemesis (10%)
  - hyperthyroidism (5%)
  - early preeclampsia (5%).

▶ Serum hCG is excessively high with complete moles, but levels may be within the normal range for partial moles.

Risk factors for hyatidiform mole

- **Age:** extremes of reproductive life (>40 years and <15 years of age) in complete moles, not partial moles.
- **Ethnicity:** ×2 higher in east Asia, particularly Korea and Japan.
- **Previous molar pregnancy:** ×10 higher risk of developing future molar pregnancy.

USS findings (see Fig. 22.2)

Complete mole

- 'Snowstorm' appearance of mixed echogenecity, representing hydropic villi and intrauterine haemorrhage.
- Large theca lutein cysts.

Partial mole

- Fetus may be viable, with signs of early growth restriction or structural abnormalities.

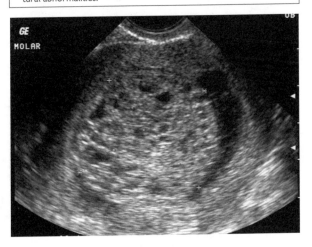

Fig. 22.2 Ultrasound of hydatidiform mole

Hydatidiform mole: management

Management

- **Complete mole:** Surgical evacuation is advisable and should be performed by an experienced surgeon as risks of uterine perforation and haemorrhage are significant. Oxytocin may be required to reduce the risk of haemorrhage, but its use is associated with a theoretical risk of tissue dissemination leading to metastatic disease to the lungs or brain.
- **Partial mole:** surgical evacuation is preferable but medical evacuation can be used.
- Histological examination of products of conception is essential to confirm diagnosis.

Treatment of persistent GTD

Risk of requiring chemotherapy is 15% after a complete mole and 0.5% after a partial mole.

Indications for chemotherapy

- Serum hCG levels >20 000 IU/L at 4 weeks after uterine evacuation
- Static or rising hCG after uterine evacuation in absence of new pregnancy.
- Persistent symptoms, e.g uterine bleeding and/or abdominal pain.
- Evidence of metastases.
- Histological diagnosis of choriocarcinoma.

Prognosis

- With effective registration and treatment programme, cure rate is high (98–100%) with low chemotherapy rates (5–8%).
- Recurrence rate is low (1/55).
- Women should be advised not to conceive until hCG level has been normal for 6 months.
- hCG levels should be checked 6 and 10 weeks after each subsequent pregnancy.

Contraception and HRT

- Barrier contraception should be used until serum hCG is normal.
- The COCP and HRT are safe to use after hCG levels have returned to normal.

📖 www.hmole-chorio.org.uk

📖 Sheffield Trophoblastic Tumour Screening and Treatment Centre.

www.sheffield.ac.uk/~co/troph

📖 The management of gestational trophoblastic neoplasia. RCOG Guidelines No.38.

Specialist follow up for molar pregnancy

In the UK, all women with any molar pregnancy should be registered at one of the three specialist centres (Sheffield, Dundee, London). The protocol for follow-up varies amongst the specialist centres. At Charing Cross Hospital (London), follow-up with hCG ranges from 6 months to 2 years after uterine evacuation.

- Serum hCG should be checked fortnightly until levels are normal (<4 IU/L).
- Following this, urine hCG is requested at 4 weekly intervals until 1 year post evacuation and then every 3 months in the second year of follow-up.
- If hCG normalizes within 8 weeks, follow-up will be limited to 6 months.
- Patients who do not have normal hCG values within 8 weeks of evacuation should have the 2-year follow-up.

Gestational trophoblastic disease: choriocarcinoma

This is a highly malignant tumour consisting of syncytio- and cytotrophoblast with myometrial invasion. Local spread and vascular metastases to the lung are common. 50% of the cases are preceded by hyatidiform mole, 40% by normal pregnancy, 5% by miscarriage or ectopic pregnancy, and 5% are non-gestational in origin.

Incidence

1 in 30 000 pregnancies in western countries and 1 in 11000 in east Asia.

Diagnosis

Signs and symptoms
- Vaginal bleeding.
- Abdominal or vaginal swelling.
- Amenorrhoea.
- Dypnoea and haemotypsis (secondary to lung metastases).
- Intra-abdominal haemorrhage (due to uterine perforation by tumour tissue).
- Less common sites for metastases include brain, kidney, liver, or spleen; these present with symptoms related to their site

Investigations
- USS.
- Serum hCG.
- CXR ('cannonball' or 'snowstorm' appearance).
- CT of chest and abdomen.

Treatment

The chemotherapy regime used is determined by a prognostic scoring system which is based on:
- Age of patient and type of antecedent pregnancy.
- Extent of tumour burden (hCG level, number, site and size of tumour, site of metastases).
- Interval from antecedent pregnancy.
- Response to previous chemotherapy.

Prognosis
- Overall survival rate is >90%.
- Poorer prognosis is associated with patient aged >40 years, antecedent pregnancy being term pregnancy, time interval from antecedent pregnancy to chemotherapy >4 months, large tumour burden, and poor response to previous chemotherapy.
- Subsequent fertility does not appear to be impaired by chemotherapy with no increased risk of fetal abnormalities.

Chemotherapy for GTD

- Low risk patients:
  - methotrexate and folinic acid (well tolerated with main side effects of mucositis and pleuritic chest pain).
- Medium risk patients:
  - drugs in sequence, including methotrexate and etoposide.
- High risk patients:
  - intensive weekly schedule of EMA (etoposide, methotrexate, and dactinomycin) alternating with CO (cyclophosphamide and vincristine)
  - salvage surgery may be required (craniotomy, pleurotomy, hysterectomy).

Principles of chemotherapy

Chemotherapy, together with radiotherapy and surgery, is used in the treatment of gynaecological cancers for control (and in some cases cure) of these diseases or palliation of their symptoms.

The cell cycle

- Chemotherapeutic agents interfere with cell division by acting on a specific phase of the cell cycle (see 📖 p. 729) (e.g. taxanes active against cells in G2/M) or non-specifically (e.g. alkylating agents exert their effects throughout the cell cycle).
- One of the characteristics of cancer cells is uncontrolled proliferation. As chemotherapy has a propensity for actively proliferating cells, they are more vulnerable than normal cells. However, they do act on normal cells so side effects are not unusual (see 📖 p. 730).

Practical aspects

- Before embarking on chemotherapy, and indeed any other form of therapy, the intent of treatment (i.e. curative or palliative) for each patient should be discussed within the MDT and clearly explained to the patient.
- It is important to weigh up the potential risks and anticipated benefits so that optimal survival and quality of life may be achieved. Factors to consider are:
  - Disease-related
    - type and stage of cancer
    - response to previous treatment
  - Patient-related
    - performance status (PS; the general condition of the patient); in general, chemotherapy is not indicated if PS>2
    - concurrent medical problems
    - nutritional status
    - patient's wishes.
- Chemotherapy is generally delivered on an outpatient basis.
  - Each course of systemic treatment is composed of 6 cycles, depending on response assessed after the 3rd one.
  - Each cycle lasts 21–28 days.
  - The gap between consecutive cycles enables damaged 'normal' cells to repair and regenerate.
- Response to treatment is assessed by:
  - Changes in evaluable disease on CT/MRI scans (RECIST criteria)
  - Trends in tumour markers (e.g. CA 125 levels for ovarian cancer)
  - Symptoms
  - Signs.

Phases of the cell cycle

- G0   Resting phase.
- G1   RNA and protein synthesis.
- S   DNA synthesis.
- G2   Protein synthesis, mitotic spindle formation.
- M   Mitosis.

ECOG performance status

- Grade 0 Asymptomatic, fully active.
- Grade 1 Restricted in strenuous activity by symptoms but fully ambulatory.
- Grade 2 Symptomatic, able to self care but not work, in bed <50% of the day.
- Grade 3 Symptomatic, in bed >50% of the day.
- Grade 4 Confined to bed or chair, unable to self-care.
- Grade 5 dead.

RECIST criteria

- Stands for 'Response Evaluation Criteria In Solid Tumours'
- Complete response:
  - disappearance of all lesions with no evidence of new lesions on 2 occasions of at least 4 weeks apart.
- Partial response:
  - ≥30% decrease in the sum of the longest diameters of the lesions.
- Stable disease:
- Progression:
  - ≥20% increase in the sum of the longest diameters of the lesions or presence of new lesions.

Some classes of cytotoxic agents

- Antimetabolites:
  - interfere with DNA and RNA synthesis
  - e.g. 5-FU, gemcitabine, methotrexate.
- Alkylating agents:
  - form covalent bonds with DNA bases
  - e.g. cyclophosphamide, ifosfamide.
- Intercalating agents:
  - bind to DNA, thus inhibiting its replication
  - e.g. cisplatin, carboplatin (most widely used in gynaecological cancer).
- Antitumour antibiotics:
  - complex mechanism of action leading to inhibition of DNA synthesis
  - e.g. bleomycin, doxorubicin, etoposide.
- Drugs against spindle microtubules:
  - prevent mitosis
  - e.g. paclitaxel, vincristine.

Side effects of chemotherapy: haematological and gastrointestinal

Chemotherapy is associated with a range of side effects due to its action on normal cells as well as cancer cells. The pattern of toxicity varies between drugs as well as between individual patients. Most side effects are self-limiting, but recognizing and seeking ways to prevent and manage them, whenever possible, is important to enable maintenance of a good quality of life.

Haematological

Bone marrow suppression leads to a gradual fall in blood count, which eventually recovers. The *nadir* (period of lowest count) occurs around 7–14 days after chemotherapy.
- **Neutropenic sepsis:** potentially fatal, urgent action required:
  - neutropenia = neutrophil count $\leq 1.0 \times 10^9$/L
  - must have a high level of suspicion in any patient having chemotherapy presenting with a temperature of ≥ 38 °C and feeling unwell
  - take FBC, cultures—blood, urine, etc., start intravenous broad-spectrum antibiotics as per hospital protocol (e.g. tazocin and gentamicin), and inform an oncologist
  - prophylaxis with GCSF (granulocyte colony stimulating factor) and oral antibiotics such as ciprofloxacin may be appropriate if there have been previous episodes of neutropenic sepsis.
- **Anaemia** (Hb ≤ 11 g/dL):
  - may be seen after several cycles of chemotherapy
  - treatment depends on severity and includes blood transfusion, iron tablets, erythropoietin.
- **Thrombocytopaenia** (platelet count ≤ 100):
  - rarely problematic with chemotherapy used for gynaecological cancers
  - avoid invasive procedures.

Gastrointestinal

Gastrointestinal side effects are due to loss of epithelial cells.
- **Nausea and vomiting:**
  - can be prevented in most cases with effective anti-emetics (e.g. domperidone, metoclopramide, and/or 5-HT3 antagonists).
- **Mucositis:**
  - resolves spontaneously with epithelial healing
  - helpful measures are good mouth care, use of local anaesthetic agents, treatment of oral candidiasis
  - commonly occurs with methotrexate and 5-FU.
- **Constipation:**
  - attention to diet and fluid intake
  - short-term use of laxatives.
- **Diarrhoea:**
  - exclude infection/constipation
  - control with codeine phosphate, loperamide, and rehydration.

Side effects of chemotherapy: other

Alopecia
- Taxanes (e.g. paclitaxel), doxorubicin, and etoposide commonly cause temporary hair loss.
- Carboplatin and cisplatin are not usually associated with this side effect.
- Has a psychological impact on some women. Individual preference for wigs, scarves, or hats.

Neurological
These are dose-related side effects that slowly subside on dose reduction or on stopping the offending drug.
- **Peripheral neuropathy:**
  - usually sensory changes such as numbness and tingling
  - commonly seen with paclitaxel and cisplatin.
- **Tinnitus:**
  - associated with cisplatin.

Constitutional
These symptoms tend to have cumulative effects as treatment progresses, but resolve on its cessation.
- **Lethargy**
- **Anorexia.**

Reproductive function
- **Fetal abnormality:**
  - most chemotherapeutic agents are teratogenic and should be avoided during the 1st trimester. Some agents may be used after 12 weeks if necessary—data is generally reassuring but limited
  - contraception is necessary until a period of time has elapsed following completion of treatment.
- **Ovarian failure:**
  - more likely to be caused by alkylating agents than other chemotherapy
  - permanent ovarian failure in premenopausal patients results in early menopause and infertility
  - young women with premature menopause are predisposed to osteoporosis, cardiovascular disease, and postmenopausal symptoms; hormone replacement therapy can be used without evidence of increase risk of cancer recurrence, except in endometrioid ovarian cancer and endometrial cancer which are oestrogen-dependent diseases
  - cryopreservation of embryos and ovarian tissue is possible for women who wish to preserve their fertility options prior to chemotherapy.

Chemotherapy for gynaecological cancer

General points

- Chemotherapy has a narrow therapeutic index; close monitoring whilst on treatment is essential.
- Before the start of each cycle of treatment, blood tests (FBC, U&E, LFT) are taken, patient's performance status and side effects are assessed.
- Chemotherapy when used alone has a palliative rather than curative role, except for choriocarcinoma which is highly chemosensitive.
- Response rate is better when chemotherapy is used in combination with surgery or radiotherapy, this may be given:
  - neoadjuvantly: **before** definitive treatment (i.e. surgery or radiotherapy) to reduce tumour bulk
  - adjuvantly: **after** definitive treatment to reduce the risk of recurrence.

The future

Standard chemotherapy agents do not differentiate between cancer cells and normal cells. Side effects are common because these agents damage DNA of potentially all cells. It is known that cancer cells have certain characteristics that enable them to continue to proliferate. Much attention has been focused on exploiting the differences between normal and cancer cells in order to develop targeted therapy.

- Targeted therapy is defined as a drug that acts on a defined target or biological pathway that is present on the cancer cells only, because normal cells are relatively unaffected, side effects are likely to be less problematic.
- Targeted agents that have shown some response in ovarian cancer are:
  - bevacizumab: a VEGF inhibitor. VEGF is needed for blood vessel formation (angiogenesis); successful angiogenesis will enable the tumour to be supplied with oxygen and nutrients for its continued growth
  - pertuzumab: a HER2 (human epidermal growth factor receptor 2) dimerization inhibitor; overproduction of HER2 by cancer cells leads to further uncontrolled growth.

Common chemotherapy regimens for gynaecological cancers

- Ovarian cancer:
  - sensitive to platinum-based regimens, response rate ~70%
  - carboplatin ± paclitaxel (may be used neoadjuvantly, adjuvantly, or palliatively)
  - >50% of patients will relapse and require further treatment, if >6 months have elapsed since initial chemotherapy, tumour more likely to be sensitive to carboplatin therefore it is often given again
  - intraperitoneal chemotherapy (instillation of agents such as cisplatin directly into the peritoneal cavity) has shown clinical benefit (not widely available, as special facilities required for its administration).
- Endometrial cancer:
  - chemotherapy has a limited role, reserved for recurrent or metastatic disease
  - carboplatin ± paclitaxel
  - doxorubicin and cisplatin
- Cervical cancer:
  - cisplatin combined with radiotherapy has been shown to reduce risk of relapse for those undergoing radiotherapy after surgery
  - cisplatin and methotrexate may be used for metastatic disease but the response rate is low.
- Vulval cancer:
  - 5-FU ± cisplatin is used in combination with radiotherapy for patients unfit for surgery
  - 5-FU and cisplatin may be used as sole therapy for symptom control in metastatic disease
- Trophoblastic tumour:
  - chemotherapy alone may be curative
  - bleomycin-containing regimen used
  - treatment given at specialist centres.

Radiotherapy: principles

Radiotherapy, unlike chemotherapy, is local and not systemic treatment. It may be used with curative and palliative intent in some gynaecological cancers.

Radiobiology

- Radiotherapy kills cells by the use of ionizing radiation:
  - X-rays
  - gamma-rays
  - beta-particles.
- Radiation can lead to breakage of DNA directly or indirectly via production of free radicals.
- Sensitivity of any cell to radiation depends on
  - cell type (for example, cells of the small bowel have low tolerance to radiation)
  - cell cycle (cells in G0, resting, phase are relatively resistant, whereas cells in G1 and G2 phases are sensitive)
  - microenvironment (cells in areas of low oxygen are radioresistant).
- Many cells are able to repair a certain amount of DNA damage but cancer cells do this less effectively, thus a significantly higher proportion will be destroyed.
- The total dose of radiotherapy that can be given to one area is limited by the tolerance of the surrounding normal tissue of that area.

Delivery of radiotherapy

Radiation may be given by external beam therapy and/or brachytherapy.
- External beam therapy:
  - radiation is distant from the patient
  - delivered from a linear accelerator
  - use of conformal radiotherapy (i.e. shaping the radiation beam to shape of tumour) encompasses less normal tissue within the field therefore reduces side effects.
- Brachytherapy:
  - placement of radioactive source directly within or around the tumour site (e.g. intravaginal/intrauterine brachytherapy for cervical cancer)
  - advantage: higher radiation dose to the tumour, lower exposure to normal tissue
- Side effects may be reduced by giving radiotherapy in divided doses so that normal tissues can recover.

Radiotherapy: side effects

The side effects of radiotherapy depend on the site being irradiated. In gynaecological cancers this is the pelvis, therefore tissues in this area are prone to damage. Problems may become apparent during and immediately after treatment (early effects) or occur months or years later (late effects).

Early side effects

- Due to damage of rapidly dividing cells such as the mucosa. Usually self-limiting.
- Skin:
  - erythema
  - moist desquamation
  - management: aqueous cream, hydrocortisone cream.
- Mouth/bowel
  - mucositis: treat with mouthwash, analgesia, nystatin if thrush present
  - nausea (less so vomiting): antiemetics for prophylaxis or treatment
  - diarrhoea: exclude infection, treat with loperamide or codeine phosphate.
- Bladder:
  - cystitis causing frequency and dysuria
  - management: exclude infection, ensure adequate fluid intake, oxybutynin may help.
- Tiredness:
  - treat anaemia if present
  - rest.
- Bone marrow suppression.

Radiotherapy: gynaecological cancers

Management of gynaecological cancers is multimodal in nature, combining surgery, chemotherapy, and radiotherapy. Surgery is the mainstay of treatment whenever possible. The choice of treatment depends on the type of cancer, the extent of disease, and the patient's fitness and wishes.

Cervical cancer
- Early disease (stage Ib):
  - radiotherapy as effective as radical hysterectomy (cure rate ~80%)
  - for those who have had surgery, radiotherapy may be given afterwards (adjuvant treatment) to reduce the risk of pelvic recurrence.
- Locally advanced disease (stage II—IVa):
  - adjuvant use of external beam radiotherapy and brachytherapy ± chemotherapy
- Recurrent disease:
  - localized recurrence may be treated by surgical resection or radiotherapy.
- Distant metastatic disease (stage IVb):
  - best supportive care, palliative radiotherapy or palliative chemotherapy.

Endometrial cancer
- Early disease (stage I):
  - if patient unfit for surgery, radiotherapy used as primary treatment
  - if fit for surgery, brachytherapy ± external beam therapy to the pelvis adjuvantly, especially if high risk features present (e.g. poorly differentiated tumour, deep myometrial involvement).
- Locally advanced disease (stage II—IIIc):
  - postoperative (adjuvant) radiotherapy.
- Recurrent disease:
  - as for cervical cancer.

Vulval cancer
- Early disease:
  - primary radiotherapy if unfit for surgery.
- Locally advanced disease:
  - radiotherapy to the pelvis after surgery if lymph nodes found to be involved
  - radiotherapy in combination with chemotherapy being evaluated to shrink extensive disease before surgery.
- Recurrent disease:
  - radiotherapy may be possible if the maximum dose has not been exceeded.

Ovarian cancer
- No evidence to support the use of radiotherapy in the primary or adjuvant setting.
- Radiotherapy may have a role in the palliation of localized symptoms.

Radiotherapy for symptom palliation

- Radiotherapy is used to control some symptoms caused by metastatic disease. Examples are:
  - pain from bone / brain metastases
  - bleeding from fungating tumour.

Pain and its management

Most patients with advanced cancer experience moderate to severe pain that can be attributed directly to the cancer.

Type of pain
- Somatic (e.g. bone pain).
- Visceral (e.g. liver capsular pain).
- Neuropathic (e.g. lumbosacral plexus involvement, often described as burning, sharp).

Assessment
- Ask questions about pain (SOCRATES) to assess its nature and distinguish whether acute or chronic.
- Measurement of pain may be done using scales; for example, by asking the patient to score her pain out of 10.
- Consider psychological factors which might contribute to or exacerbate pain, such as anxiety and depression.

Methods for the management of pain
- Non-pharmacological:
  - relaxation/message
  - acupuncture
  - TENS (transcutaneous electrical nerve stimulation)
  - radiotherapy
  - nerve block.
- Pharmacological:
  - use analgesia according to WHO ladder
  - increase dose of analgesia at each step to its maximum; if pain is still not controlled, move up the ladder
  - give regularly
  - anticonvulsants (gabapentin) ± antidepressants (amitriptyline) for neuropathic pain
  - corticosteroids for pressure due to metastases
  - bisphosphonates for bone pain due to metastases

▶ Remember to **assess and re-assess** frequently to maintain good pain control.

Side effects of opioids
- Commonly:
  - nausea
  - constipation
  - sedation.
- Inform patient of potential problems.
- Give antiemetics and laxatives.

⚠ Do not allow concerns about potential dependence prevent you from prescribing adequate amounts of opiates.

'SOCRATES'

- **S**ite
- **O**nset
- **C**haracter
- **R**adiation
- **A**ssociations
- **T**iming
- **E**xacerbating/relieving factors
- **S**everity

WHO analgesic ladder

Step 1: non-opioid (e.g. paracetamol, NSAIDs).
Step 2: weak opioid (e.g. codeine) + non-opioid.
Step 3: strong opioid (e.g. morphine) + non-opioid.

Symptoms of advanced gynaecological cancer

Gastrointestinal symptoms

Nausea and vomiting
- Causes:
  - ascites
  - metabolic (e.g. ↑ Ca^{2+})
  - brain metastases
  - constipation
  - bowel obstruction
  - medication.
- Treat cause, if possible:
  - radiotherapy and corticosteroids for brain metastases
  - paracentesis for ascites
  - hydration and bisphosphonates for hypercalcaemia.
- Antiemetics.

Constipation
- Causes:
  - ↓ fluid intake
  - lethargy
  - metabolic (e.g. ↑ Ca^{2+})
  - immobility
  - bowel obstruction
  - medication (esp. opioids).
- Treat cause, if possible.
- Laxatives.

(Subacute) bowel obstruction
- Caused by tumour seedling within the peritoneum.
- Exclude constipation with AXR.
- Best to manage conservatively; however, if patient is reasonably fit and there is only one area of obstruction, surgery may be an option.

Other symptoms
- Vaginal discharge and bleeding:
  - may be infective, therefore give metronidazole
  - tranexamic acid ± embolization for bleeding.
- Fistulae:
  - difficult to manage, limited role for surgery.
- Fatigue:
  - dexamethasone may give a sense of well-being.
- Anorexia and cachexia:
  - caused by the secretion of proinflammatory cytokines
  - dexamethasone or megestrol / medroxyprogesterone may improve appetite
  - total parental nutrition is rarely indicated.
- Dyspnoea:
  - causes: pleural effusion, cachexia, lymphangitis, anaemia, lung metastases, pulmonary embolism
  - suspect pulmonary embolism if acute onset of shortness of breath.

Principles of palliative care

The World Health Organization (WHO) defines palliative care as the 'active, holistic care of patients with advanced, progressive illness'.

Good communication and rapport with the patient (and her family) are essential to facilitate frank discussion of prognosis and formulate a plan of care that is most suited to her.

Goals of palliative care

- To achieve optimal symptom relief.
- To promote the best quality of life.

In order to palliate effectively, it is necessary to individualize each patient's care and take her wishes into account. Aspects to explore include:

- Physical symptoms.
- Psychological symptoms.
- Social issues.
- Spiritual issues.

Multidisciplinary approach

- Symptoms may be controlled by pharmacological or non-pharmacological means.
- The expertise of different specialties may be needed depending on the nature of the patient's problems, e.g. advice from dietitians about nutrition, from clinical oncologists about radiotherapy for bone pain, from surgeons about feasibility of resection for bowel obstruction.
- Palliative care is delivered at home, in a hospice, or in hospital.

Terminal care

- Aim for a peaceful and dignified death.
- Maintain comfort, psycho-social-spiritual support.
- Avoid unnecessary/uncomfortable procedures.
- Review medication. Most can be stopped, but continue the following:
  - analgesics
  - antiemetics
  - anxiolytics
  - anticonvulsants.

Miscellaneous gynaecology

Imaging: pregnancy, postmenopausal bleeding, and menstrual disorders

Gynaecological practice has changed enormously over the last 20–30 years principally due to improvements in pelvic imaging, particularly ultrasound (USS).

Early pregnancy

USS is the imaging modality of choice for early pregnancy allowing assessment of pregnancy location, viability and gestational age. Table 15.1 summarizes the main diagnostic criteria used.

- In a normal intrauterine pregnancy, a gestational sac should be visible from 5 weeks gestation and fetal heart pulsations visible from 6 weeks using transvaginal ultrasound (TVS).
- In the first trimester accurate dating is performed by measuring the crown-rump length (optimum time is 8–12 weeks gestation).
- It should be possible to see up to 90% of ectopic pregnancies on TVS.
- Other pathology may also be discovered e.g. ovarian cysts.

Post-menopausal bleeding (PMB)

Approximately 10% of women with PMB will have endometrial cancer. A TVS examination with measurement of endometrial thickness (ET) can discriminate between women at high and low risk.
- Using a cut-off of an ET of 4 mm:
  - 96% of endometrial carcinomas can be identified using TVS (high negative predictive value).
  - Up to 55% of women with no disease will also have a positive result (lower positive predictive value).

Other methods for assessing the endometrium

- Saline infusion sonography (infusion of saline into uterine cavity during scanning) allows assessment focal endometrial lesions (agreement between saline infusion sonography and hysteroscopy is excellent).
- MRI may be indicated in the presence of fibroids.

Menstrual disorders

Imaging methods can be used to diagnose anatomical abnormalities such as endometrial polyps, fibroids or adenomyosis. Other causes of bleeding disturbance such as hormonal dysfunction, hormonal treatment, and infections cannot be reliably established using imaging methods.
- TVS and saline infusion sonography allow assessment of endometrial pathology such as polyps and submucous fibroids.
- USS and MRI have a similar ability to diagnose uterine fibroids, but MRI is superior to USS in determining the exact location, especially when there is a large uterus with more than 4 fibroids.

Imaging: pain and subfertility

Pelvic pain

Acute pelvic pain
USS is the diagnostic imaging method of choice. The following can reliably be diagnosed on TVS: ovarian cysts, some sequelae of PID (including pyosalpinx and tubo-ovarian abscess) and fibroid degeneration. Colour Doppler may aid in adnexal torsion but the diagnosis is usually made on clinical findings.

Chronic pelvic pain
USS may help to diagnose endometriosis, adenomyosis, or adhesions.
- Endometriosis may be diagnosed on TVS by the finding of characteristic cysts (endometriomas) on the ovary and occasionally by the visualization of endometriotic nodules elsewhere in the pelvis such as the rectovaginal septum, although these may be better visualized with MRI or rectal USS.
- Adenomyosis is associated with a thickening of the myometrium with areas of both ↓ and ↑ echogenicity.
- There are few published data on the diagnostic accuracy of imaging methods to assess pelvic adhesions. However, poor definition of pelvic structures on TVS has been shown to predict adhesions at laparoscopy (3-D USS in combination with serum Ca-125 levels has also been shown to be helpful).
- 'Soft markers' including the presence of immobile ovaries and/or site-specific tenderness and/or loculated pelvic fluid on TVS have been shown to indicate pelvic pathology at laparoscopy with a positive likelihood ratio of 1.9 and a negative likelihood ratio of 0.2.

Subfertility
USS is used in both the diagnosis and the management of infertility. It can be used to diagnose conditions such as polycystic ovarian disease and hydrosalpinx and to track follicular growth and rupture during normal and stimulated cycles during infertility treatment.
- Oocyte retrieval for assisted conception techniques can be performed under USS guidance.
- Complications such as ovarian hyperstimulation syndrome can also be assessed by USS.
- Hysterosalpingography (HSG) used to be the imaging method of choice to assess the uterine cavity and fallopian tubes.
  - This has now been superseded by hysterosalpingo-contrast-sonography (HyCoSy) where a solution is infused into the uterine cavity whilst performing a TVS.
  - It combines a baseline TVS, assessment of the fallopian tubes and possibly even ovulation if the investigation is correctly timed.

Imaging: masses and urogynaecology

Ovarian masses and gynaecological malignancy

USS is usually the imaging modality of choice to distinguish between different types of pelvic masses. It is easier, quicker, and cheaper than either CT or MRI.

- Experienced sonographers use pattern recognition to make a diagnosis.
- USS has been shown to be as good as or even superior to CT for the discrimination between different types of pelvic mass.
- MRI is superior to CT for discriminating between benign and malignant masses and may be better than USS due to a lower false positive rate.
- Doppler ultrasound and the use of contrast may assist in diagnosis.
- A plain abdominal X-ray may occasionally give further information about a pelvic mass:
  - fibroids may have become calcified
  - dermoid cysts may contain radio-opaque material (teeth or bone).
- A chest X-ray is part of the routine assessment in cases of suspected malignancy (may show pleural effusions or metastases).
- MRI (and sometimes CT) is used in the imaging and staging of gynaeco-logical malignancies.

Urogynaecology

- USS may be used to assess:
  - residual bladder volumes
  - the bladder neck in cases of incontinence.
- Urodynamic flow/pressure studies can be combined with the use of X-ray screening to gain additional information about the anatomy of the bladder and urethra (videocystourethography).
- Intravenous urography may be used to investigate continuous incontinence following childbirth, radiotherapy or gynaecological surgery, which may be due to fistula formation between the ureters or bladder and the genital tract.

Other uses

- USS can be used to visualize intrauterine devices (IUCDs) within the uterus (lost IUDs may be located on plain abdominal X-ray).
- Ultrasound, HSG, and MRI can used to assess congenital abnormalities of the uterus.

⚠ Contrast studies of the renal tract (e.g. intravenous urography) should be considered when congenital malformations of the reproductive tract are diagnosed, as up to 40% are associated with abnormalities of the urinary tract.

Injuries in obstetric and gynaecological practice: overview

Because of their close anatomical relationship, injuries to the genital tract may also involve the urinary tract. Complicated gynaecological procedures increase the risk of urinary tract injury. If an injury occurs, prompt recognition and appropriate management are likely both to prevent long-term sequelae (urinary incontinence, fistulae, and rarely, renal failure) and to reduce litigation related to the injury.

Medico-legal implications

Up to 6% of all medical malpractice claims in gynaecological practice are related to urinary tract injuries. The quantum of claims is probably related to the degree of suffering or perceived suffering by the patient. Thus, urinary tract injuries that lead to litigation are likely to be associated with significant physical and psychological morbidity or loss of income.

Ureteric injury

Incidence

0.5–2.5% of iatrogenic ureteric injuries occur during routine pelvic surgery, mainly gynaecological. Ureteric injury occurs in 0.03% of Caesarean section deliveries compared to 0.001% of vaginal births.

Mechanism of injury

- **Avulsion:** liable to occur when tissues are fragile.
- **Transection** commonly at
  - the pelvic brim (vascular ovarian pedicle is close to the ureter)
  - the broad ligament where the uterine arteries cross (commonly during hysterectomy as the ureters enter the bladder above the lateral vaginal fornix just 2 cm lateral to the cervix)
  - the ureterovesical junction.
- **Ligation** especially during vaginal hysterectomy and repair of procidentia when the ureters also prolapse.
- **Crush** by clamps causing necrosis or stricture.
- **Devascularization** causing ischaemia and necrosis.

Presentation

Only 15–20% of iatrogenic injury presents at the time of surgery.

> **Postoperatively, uretric injury presents with:**
>
> - Fever (sepsis)
> - Flank pain from hydronephrosis
> - Vaginal fistulae
> - Non-specific symptoms of malaise, ileus or the presence of a pelvic mass ('urinoma').
>
> ⚠ Bilateral ureteric injury is very rare, so renal function usually normal.

Diagnosis

- Intravenous urography (IVU).
- Cystoscopy and bilateral retrograde pyelography to identify site of injury, extravasation or ureteric dilatation.
- CT for suspected urinoma.
- USS may also diagnose hydronephrosis or urinoma.

Treatment

⚠ Intraoperative repair has a better long-term prognosis than postoperative repair. Assistance from the urological team should be requested as soon as injury is suspected.

Injuries at or below the pelvic brim:
- **Psoas hitch:** shortens the ureterovesical gap and reduces tension.
- **Boari flap:** creation of a tension-free anastomosis.

Higher-level injuries:
- May require nephrostomy or downward displacement of the kidney with end-to-end ureteric anastomosis with the ipsilateral ureter.
- Ureteroileal anastomosis may be necessary in extensive upper ureteral injury (very rare).
- May need cutaneous ureterostomy or transuretero-ureterostomy.

Risk factors for ureteric injury

- Previous surgery
- Bulky tumours distorting anatomy and/or displacing ureters
- Endometriosis with peritoneal scarring or frozen pelvis
- PID
- Carcinoma of the cervix with parametrial involvement
- Situations that require haste (e.g. Caesarean section)
- Angular or broad ligament tears during Caesarean section.

Prevention is better than cure!

▶ *Identification* of the ureters **prior** to ligation of the uterine artery during hysterectomy should be routine practice.

If difficult surgery anticipated or encountered identification aids include:

- Pre-op ureteric stents (can be 'lighted').
- IV administration 10 ml indigo carmine or methylene blue with 20 mg of furosemide.
  - leakage of dye or contrast is demonstrated with ureteric injury
- Retrograde pyelography under fluoroscopic guidance (identifies ureteric strictures).

Bladder injury

Incidence

Approximately 50% of all bladder injuries are the result of surgical procedures (may occur during hysterectomy and usually involves the anterior
bladder wall). Obstetric bladder injury occurs in 1.4% of Caesarean sections
compared to 0.01% of vaginal deliveries.

Mechanisms of injury

- Mobilization of the bladder to expose the cervix or the lower uterine
  segment during a hysterectomy.
  - previous scarring (Caesarean section, myomectomy, pelvic inflam-
    matory disease, or endometriosis) contribute to an ↑ risk.
- Perforation of the bladder may occur during laparoscopy, hysteroscopy,
  and sling procedures (TVT).
- Ischaemic injury may occur as a result of an inadvertent suture in the
  bladder.
- Prolonged and obstructed labour may compress the bladder leading to
  avascular necrosis and vesicovaginal fistula.
- High forceps deliveries (especially if the bladder is not emptied beforehand).

> ### Risk factors during Caesarean section
>
> - Emergency Caesarean section
> - Low station of the presenting part (especially at full dilatation)
> - Prolonged labour prior to section
> - Pre-term delivery (<32 weeks gestation)
> - Previous Caesarean section
> - Operator skill

Presentation

Bladder injuries commonly present with haematuria and abdominal pain,
but can present with abdominal distension, suprapubic tenderness, and an
inability to void.

Diagnosis

- Cystoscopy is commonly used when bladder injury is suspected.
- Instillation of methylene blue dye into the bladder through a Foley's
  catheter with swabs inserted into the vagina may help identify a vesicovaginal fistula ('three-swab test').

Treatment

- Iatrogenic injuries may be repaired surgically or managed with catheter
  drainage depending on the size and the location of the injury.
- Bladder perforation is repaired in two layers using absorbable sutures.
- A Foley catheter is recommended for 7–10 days with antibiotic cover.

Urethral injury

⚠ Female urethral injuries are rare, and they occur commonly with instrumentation, vaginal surgery and obstetric complications.

Presentation
- Diagnosis can be difficult but they can present with bleeding or an inability to void.
- Fistulae will present with labial swelling or with leaking of urine through the vagina.

Diagnosis
- IVU
- Voiding cystourethrography
- MRI
- Cystoscopy.

Treatment
- For most cases catheterization is sufficient.
- Larger tears are surgically repaired using layered closure.
- Proximal damage to the urethra requires reconstruction surgery including bladder flap–urethral tube reconstruction and vaginal flap urethroplasty.

Communication and record keeping

Good communication, in particular, is as highly valued by patients as any knowledge or technical ability. Repeatedly, the biggest cause of complaints is poor communication (patients will rarely complain about a doctor they like!). The biggest cause of lost medico-legal cases is poor documentation.

Good communication

- Treat your patients as you would like to be treated yourself.
- Always introduce yourself and explain the purpose of any consultation.
- Generally ask 'open' questions ('could you describe the pain you have?') and signpost changes of enquiry.
- Give the patient time to talk (it is her story, not yours, and remember, the patient knows her symptoms better than you do!).
- Listen to the answers (if you don't listen, why ask the question?).
- Summarize your history and invite questions from the patient.
- Always close the consultation with a clear plan of action.
- Acknowledge fear, upset, or if someone looks worried—do not avoid it; the patient nearly always feels better for discussing it.
- Do not be dismissive or appear rushed.
- Doctors who come across as arrogant or patronizing induce anger and resentment in their patients—be wary of this—you will also be complained about or sued if you make a mistake!
- Don't take anger or criticism personally (part of a doctor's job is listening, even when we don't want to hear it).
- Be honest at all times, including when things go wrong.
- Apologize when appropriate. Often this is all a patient wants—things do go wrong, and apologizing is not an admission of guilt or culpability.

Good documentation

- Always record correct date and time of every patient encounter.
- Ensure name, DOB, and identifying number are on every sheet of paper.
- Always write legibly in black ink.
- If entries need to be changed/altered then cross out old entry but leave it visible and sign and date new changes.
- Never alter or remove pages from notes when things may have gone wrong—they have usually been photocopied already!
- Always identify yourself by signature, printed name, and position.
- Identify all people present for any discussions (especially interpreters).
- Keep notes contemporaneously wherever possible (you never remember things quite as they were if there is a time delay).
- Document discussions fully, particularly possible complications; 'complications of laparoscopy explained' will not stand up to scrutiny or challenge after a bowel injury!
- Avoid abbreviations and acronym-itis wherever possible, or explain them (IUD = intrauterine device or intrauterine death!).
- Never make jokes or flippant comments: they are distasteful, notes are a legal document, and patients can access their files—how would you feel if your notes said 'needs a check up from the neck up'?
- For operative procedures or diagnostic imaging, take hard-copy prints or preferably archive images—a diagram may also be useful.

Medico-legal aspects of obstetrics and gynaecology: overview

It is good medical practice for all doctors to have a basic understanding of the law and its relationship with medicine. For the obstetrician and gynaecologist it is essential, because of the many complex medico-legal issues dealt with on a daily basis.

UK law and the court system

The legal system in England and Wales is quite different from that in Scotland, although many of the principles are the same. What is described here is the English system. Medico-legal cases may be heard in different types of court. The court system is hierarchical. The House of Lords is the most senior court in the land followed by the Court of Appeal and the High Court. Laws are made in a variety of different ways.

Common law

This is law which is developed over time through decisions made by judges. These decisions establish legal principles or 'precedent' which can be applied to future cases. Precedent set by a higher court such as the House of Lords, overrules that of a lower court. Medical law regarding clinical negligence is largely derived from common law.

Statute law

These are laws made by parliament. Statute law overrides common law developed by the courts. Many medico-legal issues in obstetrics and gynaecology are governed by statutes, such as the Abortion Act 1967.

Medical negligence

In order to establish that negligence has occurred, it must be shown that on the *balance of probabilities*:
- the doctor or hospital **had** a duty of care
- there was a **breach** of that duty
- the breech of duty **caused harm** to the patient.

What is medical negligence?

- Claims for medical negligence are both more common and more costly in obstetrics and gynaecology than in any other specialty.
- The National Health Service Litigation Authority (NHSLA) has dealt with nearly £2 billion of claims by patients since 1995.
- Usually claims are made against doctors (in practice a claim is made against a hospital trust) in civil law rather than criminal charges.
- Medical negligence is the legal term used when a harm arises because of a breach of duty by an individual clinician or a hospital.
  - An inappropriate treatment or failure to make a correct diagnosis may be found negligent if the patient suffers harm as a result.
  - It may be judged negligent to fail to warn a patient about a risk inherent in an operation, e.g. ureteric injury during hysterectomy.
- The standard used to decide if a doctor breached their duty of care, is whether a responsible body of medical opinion, acting in a logical manner, would have acted differently in the same circumstances.
- It also has to be proved that, on the balance of probabilities, it was the breach of duty that caused the harm.
  - Thus where an abnormal CTG was not acted upon and a baby develops cerebral palsy (CP), negligence will only be established if the CP is shown to be caused by hypoxia during labour and not another cause.

Consent to treatment

⚠ Treating an adult without their consent may lead to claims of negligence or, more rarely, a claim of battery.

In order for consent to be valid the patient must:
- Have the capacity to give consent
- Give consent voluntarily
- Be given appropriate information regarding the procedure.

Capacity

The Mental Capacity Act 2005 has defined capacity in law.

⚠ The pain and distress caused by labour is not enough to determine that a woman lacks capacity to consent.

Assessment of capacity
The person will lack capacity if there is a disturbance in the functioning of the mind or brain so they cannot:
- Understand the information relevant to the decision
- Retain the information
- Use or weigh the information
- Communicate the decision.

Voluntary consent

Consent must be given freely, without undue influence or pressure from others.

Information

To avoid a claim of battery a patient must be aware of the nature and purpose of any procedure to which they consent. For example, when a medical student is to perform a vaginal examination, it must be clear to the patient that the purpose is to enhance the student's training and not for the benefit of the woman. More commonly, lack of information during the consent procedure may give rise to a claim of negligence.

Consent for operations

The law does not specify who can take the consent for an operation but the person obtaining consent should, at the very least, be familiar with the procedure and be able to explain it in detail. Thus in complex cancer or laparoscopic surgery it may be wise for the operating surgeon to obtain the patient's written consent.

The Department of Health has published guidance on what information should be given to patients before an operation. This includes:
- Details of the proposed procedure
- The nature of the condition being treated
- The benefits of treatment
- Alternative treatments
- Serious and frequently occurring risks
- Additional procedures which may be necessary, e.g. blood transfusion.

Consent: other issues

Refusal of treatment

The law allows a competent adult to refuse medical treatment without reason or justification.

Blood products

Religious groups such as Jehovah's Witnesses may refuse all blood products and it is essential that such wishes are very carefully documented. In cases where advanced refusal of blood products is known and the potential for bleeding anticipated (e.g. laparoscopy for ectopic pregnancy) the most senior person available should perform the procedure.

Caesarean section

Several cases have been brought to court challenging a woman's right to refuse a Caesarean section thought by doctors to be in the best interests of her or her fetus.

⚠ The law is clear that the fetus *in utero* has no legal rights up until the moment of birth. Therefore a woman may refuse to consent to Caesarean section even if the consequences for herself or the fetus are death or severe injury.

Consent in children

It is not uncommon for a child under the age of 16 to request contraception or a termination of pregnancy without parental knowledge.

In the case of *Gillick vs West Norfolk and Wisbech AHA (1985)*, the courts ruled that doctors may treat children without parental consent if certain conditions are fulfilled:

- The child understands the advice or treatment being given
- An attempt has been made to persuade the child to inform her parents
- In the case of seeking contraception, the child is likely to have unprotected intercourse whether or not contraception is prescribed
- The physical or mental health of the child is likely to suffer if the treatment is not provided.

Subfertility

The Human Fertilisation and Embryology Authority (HFEA) Act 1990 regulates the area of reproductive medicine covering:

- Infertility treatments using donated genetic material
- Infertility treatments involving stored genetic material
- The creation of embryos outside the body
- Embryo research.

The Act established the HFEA. This body licenses, monitors, and reports on establishments that provide fertility treatments. Individuals undergoing fertility treatments covered by the Act must give written consent to treatment as well as to storage of gametes and embryos. When couples have fertility treatment together, both must consent to the treatment and either may withdraw their consent at any time.

Clinical risk management: identifying and analysing risks

Clinical risk management is a mechanism for improving the quality of patient care. There are several steps in the process.

Identifying risk
What went wrong or what could go wrong?

Local sources for identifying risk
- Incident report forms
- Patient complaints
- Audit results.

National sources for identifying risk
- National patient safety agency (NPSA) alerts
- Reports of national confidential enquiries
- Healthcare commission.

Completing an incident reporting form

Most trusts have a dedicated reporting form to complete. These should be available in all clinical areas. All members of staff of all grades should be encouraged to complete forms when they are aware of risk incidents. A form should be completed for all actual adverse incidents affecting patients as well as near misses.

Many units have a list of specific risk triggers that should prompt completion of a risk form. These might include an unplanned return to theatre, cord pH < 7.10 or an operative blood loss of more than 800 mL.

Incident form information
- Full patient details
- Date, time, and location of incident
- All staff involved (statements may be requested at a later date)
- Brief factual report of the incident.

Serious incidents must be reported immediately to the local lead for clinical risk. All hospitals will have definitions for what constitutes such a serious untoward incident (SUI). When a serious incident has occurred, all staff concerned should prepare contemporaneous statements of their involvement whilst the incident is still fresh in their mind.

⚠ When writing incident reports and statements, only an account of the facts should be documented, **not** an opinion of what went wrong.

Risk analysis

Root cause analysis is a structured investigation that aims to identify the true cause of a problem and the actions necessary to eliminate it.

▶ Adverse incidents rarely occur as a result of individual error alone. Factors contributing to the incident should be identified and an analysis report submitted (see boxes p. 759).

Possible contributory factors to a risk incident

- The patient
- Individual staff
- Communication
- Team working (or not)
- Education and training of staff
- Equipment and resources
- Working conditions.

A risk analysis report will contain:

- Obvious outcomes that occurred
- The chronology of events
- The care management problems identified
- A list of contributing factors
- Recommended actions required
- A timetable for implementation of recommendations.

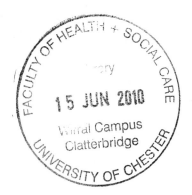

Clinical risk management: risk reduction

Risk reduction
May be achieved by:
- Training
- Introduction of guidelines
- Increasing resources.

Risk elimination
May mean ceasing to provide a particular service.

Acceptance of risk
There is an acceptance that some risk cannot be reduced or eliminated. Hospitals attempt to keep litigation costs to a minimum by joining the Clinical Negligence Scheme for Trusts (CNST—see below).

Dissemination of lessons learned
- **Local level:** sharing information with other units in the hospital
- **National level:** through bodies such as the National Patient Safety Agency (NSPA) or Royal Colleges
- Sharing information should include good practice points.

The clinical negligence scheme for trusts (CNST)

- CNST handles clinical negligence claims against member NHS bodies.
- Membership is voluntary, but currently all NHS and primary care trusts in England belong.
- The costs of the scheme are met by membership contributions:
  - The total projected claims cost are assessed in advance each year and contributions are determined for each trust (influenced by a range of factors including type of trust and specialties it provides).
  - Discounts are available to trusts which achieve the relevant National Health Service Litigation Authority (NHSLA) risk management standards and to those with a good claims history.
- When a claim is made against a member of CNST, the body remains the legal defendant, but the NHSLA is responsible for handling the claim and associated costs.

What risk management is not!

- 'Big brother'
- A vehicle for individual blame or recrimination
- An audit or research tool
- A management policing policy (it is for everyone to learn from)
- Only designed to highlight bad care (good care should also be commended and fed back to staff, even if the outcome is poor or risk has occurred)
- A legal or negligence body.

Index

P

Paget's disease of vulva 714
pain
  abdominal *see* abdominal
    pain
  pelvic *see* pelvic pain
  postnatal 356
pain relief
  cancer patients 684
  in labour 324
palliative care 741
pancreatitis 95
paracetamol 24, 226,
    356, 739
paralysis, maternal
    obstetric 356
parity 3
partogram 265
parvovirus 131, 158
Patau's syndrome
    see trisomy 108
Paulik's grip 8
pelvic examination 448
pelvic floor
  anatomy 644
  muscle training 636, 650
  prolapse 644
pelvic inflammatory
    disease 531
  diagnosis 532
  investigations 532
  treatment 532, 534
pelvic pain 477
  acute 534
  chronic 536
    diagnosis 540
    non-gynaecological
      causes 538
  imaging 745
  treatment 541
pelvis, female 10, 645
  anatomy 453
  assessment of
    adequacy 13
  boundaries 11
  diameters of 12
  inlet/outlet 13
  lymphatic drainage 453
  muscles and ligaments 10
  shapes 11
  see also pelvic
penicillins 365
perimenopause 610
perinatal mortality 406
  classification 407
  key findings 408
  risk factors 408
perinatal mortality
    rate 406
perineal tears 298
  repair 299
  third/fourth-degree 300
  ...ineum 454

postpartum changes 348
pessaries 650, 651
pethidine 324
phaeochromocytoma 244
phenytoin 179
physical examination 6, 7
  abdominal inspection 6
  abdominal palpation 6
physiology of pregnancy 26
  alimentary system 31
  cardio-respiratory 29
  endocrine changes 26
  genital tract and
    breast 30
  haemodynamics 28
  skin 31
  urinary tract 31
phytoestrogens 499
pica 38
pituitary gland 27
placenta
  abnormal site 318
  accreta 316
  at term 20
  circulation 22
  embryological
    development 18, 20
  endocrine functions 24
  fetal surface 20
  manual removal 317
  maternal surface 20
  retained 316
  villi 20
placental abruption 57
placental transfer 25
placenta praevia 55, 56
plasma volume 28
platelets 28
pleural effusion 695
pneumonia 206
  aetiology 207
  management 207
polycystic ovarian
    syndrome 544
  management 546
polyhydramnios 138
posterior urethral valve
    syndrome 120, 121
postmenopause 610
postnatal care 347
  bladder problems 356
  constipation 356
  contraception 358
  deep vein thrombosis 351
  lifestyle 358
  maternal obstetric
    paralysis 356
  mental health
    problems 357
  normal puerperium 348
  pain 356
  puerperal pyrexia *see*
    puerperal pyrexia

pulmonary embolism 351
symphysis pubis
    discomfort 356
  see also breast-feeding
postnatal depression 442
postpartum
  haemorrhage 318
  secondary 350
precocious puberty 466
prednisolone 202, 218, 463,
    518, 613
pre-eclampsia 60
  clinical features 64
  investigations 64
  management 66
  severe 66
pre-existing medical
    disorders 36
pregnancy-related
    death 409
pregnancy test 38
pregnancy of unknown
    location 514
preimplantation genetic
    diagnosis 576
prelabour rupture of
    membranes
  at term 308
    management 310
  premature 100
    management 101
premature menopause 616
premenopause 610
premenstrual
    syndrome 497
  management 498
prenatal diagnosis 106
preparation for
    pregnancy 32
pre-pregnancy health
    check 36
preterm labour 96
  prediction and
    prevention 96, 98
progesterone 26, 499
  injectable 602
progesterone-only
    pill 600
progestogen-based
    hormone replacement
    therapy 618
prolactinoma 250
prolapse 644, 646, 647
  clinical assessment 648
  conservative
    management 650, 651
  surgical management
    652, 654
prolonged pregnancy 102
  management 104
propiverine 643
propylthiouracil 238
  teratogenicity 178